Genius Unbroken

Genius Unbroken

The Life and Legacy of Dr. Charles R. Drew

Craig A. Miller, MD

Foreword by Charlene Drew Jarvis, PhD

Georgetown University Press / Washington, DC

Cataloging-in-Publication Data is on file with the Library of Congress.

ISBN 9781647126117 (hardcover)
ISBN 9781647126124 (ebook)

♾ This paper meets the requirements of ANSI/NISO Z39.48-1992 (Permanence of Paper).

EU GPSR Authorized Representative
LOGOS EUROPE, 9 rue Nicolas Poussin,
17000, LA ROCHELLE, France
E-mail: Contact@logoseurope.eu

26 25 9 8 7 6 5 4 3 2 First printing

Printed in the United States of America

Cover design by Martyn Schmoll
Interior design by Westchester Publishing Services

Contents

Foreword *vii*
Preface *xi*
Acknowledgments *xiii*

Part One

1 A Starlit Southern Night: Washington, DC, 1950 3
2 A Regular Man: Foggy Bottom, Washington, DC, 1904–22 6
3 Growth: Amherst College, 1922–26 23
4 A Chance to Shine: Baltimore, 1926–28 45
5 Let the Rest of the World Go By: Montreal, 1928–35 67

Part Two

6 A Young Man of Ability and Promise: Howard University, 1935–38 113
7 Naturally Great: New York City, 1938–40 131
8 Playing at Bigger Games: Blood for Britain and the Red Cross, 1940–41 168
9 Big Red: Howard University, 1941–45 197
10 This High-Walled Prison: Washington, 1946–50 216
11 Alamance: April 1, 1950 253
12 Epilogue: The Life and Legacy of Dr. Charles Drew 259

Notes *271*
Index *305*
About the Author *311*

Foreword

For many years I collected documents, pictures, articles, and speeches about my father on the third floor of my home in Washington, DC. I shared that information with my siblings, Bebe, Sylvia, the late Charles R. Drew Jr., and with their families and mine. (My brother was a graduate of Howard University, a source of great pride for him and for us.) I also shared this material with my husband, Dr. DeMaurice Moses, a physician with enormous knowledge of, and passion for, the life and contributions of Dr. Drew.

Some of that information was made available to the Moorland-Spingarn Research Center at Howard University, the National Museum of African American History and Culture, the Osler Library of History of Medicine at McGill University, the Charles R. Drew University of Medicine and Science, and with many secondary schools.

Having cataloged this information, my intention was to write a book about my father, but the decades marched on with my work as a neuroscientist at NIH and as an elected official and member of numerous boards and commissions and political appointments.

It was my good fortune after all these years to receive a call from Dr. Craig Miller, a vascular surgeon who had just written a book about the extraordinary work of cardiac surgeon Dr. Michael DeBakey. In short order, Dr. Miller and I agreed that he would write my father's biography, and I would provide access to the material I collected, while both of us continued to do research for the book.

I always thought that making this information about my father's life and pioneering blood research in the laboratory of Dr. John Scudder at Columbia University was important, since my father died at such a young age and his doctoral thesis had never been published.

But in 2023 my husband and I had a fortuitous discussion with a member of the board of the American Medical Association (AMA) at a meeting of the DC Medical Society. That discussion led to an invitation to meet with the board of the AMA.

Recall that the AMA, for many years, refused to allow staff privileges for African American residents in all white hospitals throughout the country, effectively upending their medical careers and leading to a dramatic underrepresentation of Black physicians in this country.

In letters to the AMA written in 1947, my father railed against this exclusionary practice that he knew would derail the production of African American physicians for generations. Not until 2008 did the AMA apologize for these practices.

So, an invitation to meet with the AMA board in 2023 was met with interest and well-submerged anger, but also with the hope of learning about the now published AMA Strategic Plan to finally address equity in training of physicians and in delivery of medical services

One of the people that my husband and I met at that meeting was the impressive CEO of the AMA, Harvard-educated Dr. James Madera. For this meeting, Dr. Madera had read the entire nearly four hundred-page Columbia University doctoral thesis of Dr. Drew, which can be found online at the National Library of Medicine (NLM).

His significant statement to us was that Dr. Drew had not only done extraordinary research in the storage and preservation of blood but he had also actually *founded a discipline*. He didn't just make a discovery, he laid out the rules and methods to be followed by blood bank personnel to always ensure safety in the blood supply. A scientific *discipline* has replicability and continuity. Its variables can be measured and changed systematically.

Unlike my father's dissertation, a doctoral thesis is usually published as a book or as articles in major journals, giving students and researchers alike opportunities to learn, evaluate, and continue the research.

That's why the publication of this book, *Genius Unbroken*, is vital. It not only takes the measure of the man, his upbringing, his drive, his intellect, his expectation of excellence, his students, his wife and family, but it also urges students and researchers to go to his dissertation, look at the data, and continue to increase our knowledge of protecting the blood supply and transfusion techniques. Follow a career in science.

Dr. Drew was a physician, a scientist, and a humanitarian. His voice can be amplified by your knowledge of him.

Dr. Charlene Drew Jarvis

Preface

In the seventy-five years since his untimely death, the story of Dr. Charles Drew has swirled around the rarefied world of American medicine—and the broader landscape of the cultural psyche—like a mercurial vapor. The contributions of the man, a surgeon-scientist of the highest caliber, have often been obscured by his complex, unlikely career trajectory and even more by the circumstances of his tragic death. The result has been that, while the name of Charles Drew has become a familiar one in many segments of the community, the reasons for that notoriety are strangely blurred. It is my hope that the present book will serve to correct this.

Genius Unbroken is the third book I have written on the life of a prominent American physician, following works on the twentieth-century surgical titans Robert M. Zollinger and Michael E. DeBakey. Even before completion of the second of these in 2019 I was approached by colleagues with an interest in medical history regarding what they felt to be a missing piece of the documentary puzzle—a biography of Charles Drew. Like many, I was aware of Drew's name but vague on exactly what he had done, a victim of the historical fog outlined above. Wasn't he an African American pioneer in the development of blood banks? A cursory examination of relevant websites confirmed that much, as well as the surprising fact that, despite the large number of biographical search results that appeared, no actual formal biography of Charles Drew had been written. There were works aimed at children and adolescents, as well as an excellent sociological study on the implications of racism in the events of his death, but no scholarly adult volume about the life of this important man.

At this juncture I reached out to Dr. Charlene Drew Jarvis, a neuroscientist, politician, and recently retired university president who, I had learned, was one of Drew's surviving children. It cannot have been easy growing up with a legend for a father, still more one taken from the family in his prime, but she rose above these tribulations to establish herself as an important figure in her own right. As it happened, Charlene had been contemplating composing a biography of Dr. Drew for some time. Thus began a friendship and close working relationship that has now lasted several years. Charlene opened her heart and home to the picklocks of this biographer, sharing memories, artifacts, and unpublished manuscripts cherished by her family for decades. The result is, we hope, the long-overdue portrait of Dr. Charles Drew, one of the towering figures in American history, whose example even today casts a lengthy shadow over not only his chosen field of medicine but all modern society.

Craig Alan Miller, MD, FSVS, FACS
Dublin, Ohio, August 2024

Acknowledgments

Craig A. Miller, MD, FSVS, FACS
Dublin, Ohio
May 2024

Many individuals and institutions contributed to making this long-overdue biography of Charles Drew a reality.

Al Bertrand, director of Georgetown University Press, provided a steady, guiding hand throughout the work. Per GUP policy, formatting of the text adheres to the standards of *The Chicago Manual of Style*. Mary K. K. Hague-Yearl, PhD, head librarian at the Osler Library of the History of Medicine at McGill University, contributed many important documents regarding Dr. Drew's time in Montreal. Jennifer Ulrich, technical services archivist in Archives and Special Collections at the Augustus C. Long Health Sciences Library of Columbia University Irving Medical Center, was of similar assistance at that institution.

Caroline Overy helped with research regarding John Beattie at the Royal College of Surgeons in London. The staff of the Stuart A. Rose Manuscript, Archives, & Rare Book Library at Emory University assisted in providing material from their W. Montague Cobb collection.

The Moorland-Spingarn Research Center of Howard University in Washington, DC, is the repository of Dr. Drew's papers and is therefore an indispensable resource for any research regarding him.

Dr. E. Christopher Ellison of the Ohio State University, Dr. Patricia Turner of the American College of Surgeons, and Dr. L. D. Britt of the Medical College of Virginia provided important support for this project. I also owe a particular debt of gratitude to Dr. Edward Cornwell for his special insight regarding Drew and the Department of Surgery at Howard University.

I am most deeply grateful to Charlene Drew Jarvis, PhD, and her husband, Dr. DeMaurice Moses, without whom this biography of her illustrious father would not have been possible. In addition to her incomparable knowledge and insight, and her comprehensive collection of family papers and artifacts, Charlene's warmth, candor, and generosity made the entire project a joyous and moving experience.

As always, my wife Mandy and children Mackenzie, Kellen, and Jack provided love and support in a thousand ways, tangible and otherwise, throughout the research and composition of *Genius Unbroken*, and I could not have accomplished this task without them.

Charlene Drew Jarvis, PhD
5/19/24

Serendipity. Craig Miller, MD, came into our lives when I realized that I had amassed so much information as to make the writing of a book about my father a distant dream.

My husband, Dr. DeMaurice Moses, and I had been tremendously impressed by Dr. Miller's biography of the heralded cardiac surgeon Michael DeBakey. A vascular surgeon himself, Dr. Miller's interest in the story of the life of Dr. Charles R. Drew led him to contact me about the opportunity to write about my father. That telephone call led to a collaboration between us that, in short measure, led to this book, *Genius Unbound*.

Craig's reverence for my father as a scientist and a surgeon, his attention to detail, and his verity and alacrity in the actual writing were a gift to me.

I am grateful for the assistance of members of my family in clarifying details that have been included in this work.

My husband drew inspiration from my father's life in his own practice of medicine in Puyallup Washington, in the many years before our marriage in 2013.

My sisters, Bebe Drew Price and Sylvia Drew Ivie, and my brother, the late Charles R. Drew Jr., exhibited love and affection over the years that kept alive the memories of both our father and our amazing mother, M. Lenore Robbins Drew. Nanny, as she was later called by her grandchildren, raised a family of four young children after their father's death with fortitude, intellect, sense of humor, and elegant carriage.

The late Eva Drew Pennington agreed to write the many wonderful memories of her older brother and mentor, Charlie Drew, that have become a vital part of this book in their humor and tremendously insightful understanding of the family in which she and her late sister Elsie, brother Joe, and sister Nora grew up.

Cathleen Drew Botts, daughter of Joseph Drew, is the keeper of the family history in Arlington Virginia, the site of the Drew homestead.

Staff at the National Museum of African American History and Culture assisted in the cataloging of material to be contained at the Museum: Lonnie Bunch III, the founding director of the NMAAHC; Jacquelyn Serwer, PhD; William Pretzer, PhD; V. Andrew Talley; and Elaine Nichols.

The staff at the Moorland-Spingarn Research Center of Founder's Library, Howard University: Joellen El Bashir and Lela Sewell Williams.

Associate provost and professor Angela Campbell at McGill University and Dr. Mary Hague-Yearl and Lily Szczygiel of the McGill Osler Library at McGill University.

A'Lelia Bundles, with whom I first spoke about the possibility of a book publishing effort. Evelyn Favors, PhD, gave me good advice at turning points in this effort.

My son, Ernest (Ernie) Drew Jarvis and his wife have been consistent and loving supporters of my endeavors as they built their own impressive careers. My grandsons, EJ (Ernest Drew Jarvis II) and Jacob Drew Jarvis, the lights of my life, understand that this book is history that they will revere more and more as time goes on; and the late Peter David Jarvis whose memory never fades.

Part One

1

A Starlit Southern Night

Washington, DC, 1950

Around 2 A.M. on Saturday, April 1, 1950, four men wrapped themselves in overcoats against the chill District of Columbia night and piled into the passenger compartment of a late-model Buick Roadmaster. The sky was clear and starlit, and as they wound through the shadowy streets of Washington, a full moon cast brilliant silver beams over the glittering monuments of the nation's capital.

The men were physicians affiliated with the Howard University College of Medicine, one of only two predominantly Black medical schools in the United States. Two of the men, Walter Johnson and John Ford, were interns finishing their first year of training after medical school. The others were professors: Samuel Bullock, who owned and was driving the elegant four-door sedan, and Charles Richard Drew.

Two months shy of his forty-sixth birthday, Dr. Drew was chair of the Department of Surgery at Howard and chief of surgery at its affiliated Freedmen's Hospital. Born just eight years after the Supreme Court enshrined "Separate but Equal" as the law of the land, and only a few miles from the bench where that decision had been handed down, against all odds, Drew had parlayed a soaring intellect and tireless work ethic into degrees from Amherst College, McGill University, and Columbia. Pioneering research on the science of blood preservation and transfusion early in his career had made him perhaps the best-known African American physician in the country. More recently, Drew had turned his relentless energy, scarcely sated by a busy clinical practice, to the twin problems of ensuring the finest care for Blacks while eliminating the specter of bigotry from its delivery.

The two younger men in the car, Johnson and Ford, were living examples of this focus, aspiring African American surgeons molded under Drew's tutelage and soon to commence residency training at one of the few places in the nation that would allow them the privilege: the John A. Andrew Hospital in Tuskegee, Alabama. That southern city, deeply rooted in Black history, was also the doctors' ultimate destination on this trip: a springtime conference and free clinic at the hospital had become Drew's annual pilgrimage.

The two professors had originally intended to fly to their destination, but consideration for their younger counterparts, who could not afford such luxuries as air travel, had caused a change of plan. They would drive to Alabama instead, splitting time at the wheel. Still, at eight hundred miles' distance from Washington, DC, Tuskegee was much too far to reach in one stretch. Today they would go as far as Atlanta, a city where Black men on the road in 1950 could find lodgings, albeit at the YMCA.

Hours passed on the unswerving route of Highway 1 through northern Virginia. Bullock's Roadmaster, filled with the vocal roar of camaraderie, gobbled up miles as the four men discussed topics personal and professional. At around 5 A.M. they passed Richmond, the eastern sky beginning to brighten in predawn twilight. Near the neighboring town of Petersburg, the men spotted a garish neon sign announcing the presence of a roadside café. The lure of coffee and doughnuts was irresistible.

A few minutes later, when the quartet tumbled back into the Buick, Bullock's turn at the wheel was over. He slid into the front row passenger seat and soon joined the younger men in a well-deserved nap.

Drew took over the driving duties. He had spent the whole of the previous day operating, lecturing, and attending to surgery department business. In the evening, he had spoken at a nurses' sorority gathering and attended a student council banquet. It was well past midnight when Drew finished rounding on his patients and, after bidding farewell to his wife, headed to meet

Bullock and the interns—but long days like this were not unusual for the famous surgeon.

Drew shifted the Buick into gear and stepped on the accelerator. Tires spitting gravel, the sedan pulled away from the Petersburg café and merged back onto the interstate. Ahead lay a dim and distant horizon.

2

A Regular Man

Foggy Bottom, Washington, DC, 1904–22

The three acres of Washington, DC, north of the National Mall, between the Potomac River and the White House, have long been known by the romantic name Foggy Bottom. Now home to the Kennedy Center, George Washington University, and a sprawling luxury hotel called Watergate, the district bears little resemblance to the low-lying humid marshland that once covered it, and provided the poetic epithet, in the city's early years.

The demographics of Foggy Bottom have changed over the years quite as much as its physical appearance, and homogeneous affluence now reigns where, a century ago, a bustling and cosmopolitan middle-class neighborhood once stood. In the years following the Civil War, proliferation of small factories in the district fed an influx of immigrants and many newly freed African Americans to the area, looking for livelihood and a place to settle down. The result was an unusually diverse, vibrant, and peaceable community. Black, Italian, Irish, and Jewish families dwelt alongside one another, often but not exclusively in enclaves of voluntary segregation. The streets were paved and lighted, most of the homes were sturdy red brick, and the yards bounded by decorative iron fencing were neatly and attractively kept.[1]

In the spring of 1904, one of the neighborhood's young Black couples, Richard Thomas Drew Jr. and his wife, the former Nora Burrell, was preoccupied with the many preparations that attended the imminent arrival of their first child.

By all accounts the Drews, who had been married early the previous year, led a comfortable life among friends and family in the pleasant neighborhood. At twenty-five years of age, Richard, an affable fellow with light skin, red-tinged hair, and freckles, worked alongside his namesake father as a carpet layer for the city's famous W. B. Moses department store.* In time he would succeed his father as financial secretary for chapter 85 of the American Federation of Labor–affiliated Carpet, Linoleum, and Soft Tile-Layers Union, exceptional positions for African Americans in that day. The need for family income in his youth had forced the teenage Richard to work rather than finish his secondary education at the well-regarded M Street High School, but he was by all accounts intelligent and industrious. He was also highly musical, capable of acquitting himself well on the piano and guitar and fond of singing; one of his favorites was the melancholy Stephen Foster ballad "Old Black Joe." He frequently lent his baritone voice to a local barbershop outfit called the Highwarden Quartet as well as the choir of the famous and fashionable Nineteenth Street Baptist Church, where the family attended the sermons of the noted Reverend Walter H. Brooks, a Foggy Bottom neighbor who had presided at the Drews' wedding. Richard also liked to box for recreation and wore a bushy moustache to hide the scar from one of his less-successful efforts in the ring.

Twenty-three-year-old Nora, eldest of nine siblings, had more formal education than her husband, having graduated from the famous Miner Normal School for Colored Girls as well as nearby Howard University—a remarkable achievement. She was trained as a teacher and vainly sought work in this competitive field after her graduation in 1901. After she was married, though, Nora's home was her full-time career, and she never took other employment.[2]

---

*Richard's parents were Richard Thomas Drew Sr., who was born in Charlottesville, Virginia, around 1853, and Martha Taylor, who hailed from Winchester. Richard Sr.'s parents were Thomas Drew and Elizabeth Morris, who appear in the 1850 United States census as free mulatto individuals. Nora's parents were Joseph Burrell and Emma Mann. By family tradition, Nora, who was much older than her eight siblings, was fathered by Day O. Crane, formerly a white officer in the Union army, and adopted by Joseph Burrell when he married Emma. Emma's parents were Robert Mann and a white woman named Margaret Freeman.

From the time of their wedding the couple lived with Richard's family—his parents and two siblings, Martha and Charles—at 821 Twenty-First Street NW. When Nora became pregnant, though, she wished to be close to her own mother, Emma, who was a midwife, for support. Accordingly, the expectant pair packed up the essentials and temporarily moved several blocks to the Burrell house, a massive three-story, sixteen-room structure at 1806 E Street.[3] This was where they welcomed their firstborn, a son, on June 3. Although Nora's mother was present, the family physician, Dr. Charles Marshall, delivered the baby (in time he would deliver all five of Nora and Richard's children). The new arrival was named Charles Richard, but from his earliest days everyone called the boy "Charlie."[4]

In his early days Charlie Drew had a bellowing cry that he exercised with such frequency and vigor that his mother lived in fear that the neighbors would think she was beating him.[5]

Soon after the happy event, the little family returned, perhaps to the relief of the Burrells, to Richard's parents' house for a brief time before all the Drews moved down the street to 1149 Twenty-First Street NW. They were living here when a second child, a daughter named Elsie, arrived on August 16, 1906. After Richard's mother Martha passed away in 1908, the families separated and Richard, Nora, and the two children returned to the big Burrell residence at 1806 E Street, where they welcomed two more additions to the family: a son, Joseph, on July 20, 1909, and daughter, Nora, on May 10, 1913.

In these early years one of Charlie's closest friends and playmates was the youngest of the Burrell siblings, a daughter who shared her mother's name Emma. As it happened this Emma, who was so diminutive she was nicknamed "Midget"—soon shortened to "Midge"—was the same age as Charlie. Whenever the two reached any sort of disagreement in their play time Midge would place her hands on her hips in a stern fashion and wag a scolding finger at Charlie, reminding him that he had to obey her wishes—after all, she was his aunt.[6]

When he reached school age, Charlie attended one of the two segregated Black grammar schools in the neighborhood, the highly regarded Thaddeus Stevens Elementary, also on Twenty-First Street, between K and L Streets. Although the classroom instruction at the school was exemplary, at this age, and for some time to come, the young man's interests lay nearly exclusively in athletics. This was natural, since Charlie seemingly excelled in every sporting endeavor he attempted. Before long he would dominate the usual

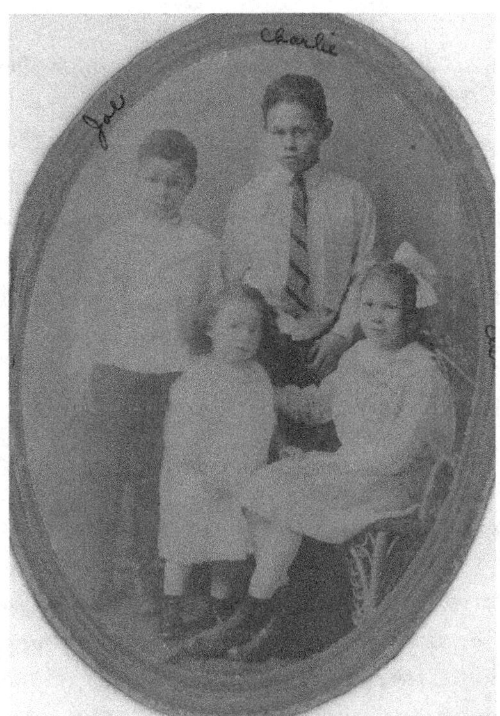

Figure 2.1 The Drew children circa 1911. Clockwise from top: Charlie, Elsie, Nora, and Joe. Personal collection, Charlene Drew Jarvis.

schoolyard standards like baseball and football, but his earliest exploits came in the water.

Richard Drew was an excellent swimmer who thought nothing of diving into the Potomac River for a few relaxing strokes on a summer day. When they were old enough, he took his boys along and taught them to swim in the muddy waters. Around the time Charlie turned eight years old, the Twelfth Street YMCA opened—and with it the first swimming pool in the city available to Black children. Here Charlie met another lad of similar age and temperament, William Montague "Monty" Cobb, who would remain a friend for life. The boys enjoyed playful races in the small pool at the "Y," but the directors there had more ambitious goals and set up competitions at another new segregated facility with a bigger pool near the Washington Monument. Charlie was the consistent winner here and, as the pastime gained popularity, at yet another new pool that opened on Howard Playground across the street from the Lucretia Mott Elementary School at Fourth and W streets NW.[7]

While Charlie's athletic exploits were celebrated at home, Richard and Nora never showed favoritism, nor did they waver in emphasizing to all their children the value of education—both for its own sake and, to be sure, as a path to success in life. In about 1915, the Drews finally moved into their own place at 1826 E Street, just down from the big Burrell house. Shakespeare and other classics adorned the bookshelves, alongside novels and texts on art and music. All the family read regularly and were avid patrons of the public library; one of the children's worst punishments was to have their library card confiscated. Richard frequently shepherded the children on tours of the many historical monuments of Washington, DC, as well, including the Lincoln Memorial, which was in the process of being built. Hand in hand with this enlightened encouragement in intellectual pursuits, the young parents taught their children the importance of serving the community and taking an active role in the local congregation: Richard eventually became music director and Nora a member of the Board of Trustees at the Nineteenth Street Baptist Church. Socially conscious sermons from Reverend Brooks helped to bolster the sense of community service that pervaded the Drew household, and scripture was never very far from the forefront.

As Drew's sister Nora recalled, weekends were particularly special: "I remember Sunday mornings my father always read the Bible, and we all knelt and prayed before breakfast. And there were always hot rolls. The rolls were made the night before and stayed up in the warmer all night. And then my mother got up early in the morning and made the rolls—pretty different from today."[8] Eva, the youngest sister, added: "We, the children, wished he would hurry and finish before Mama's hot rolls got cold. They were delicious when hot and hard as bricks when cold. Mama was not a gourmet cook."[9]

When the children needed new clothes, Richard would take them to Hahn's shoe store on Pennsylvania Avenue, to Kann's on Seventh Street, or to Park and Bridges, which specialized in boys' clothing.[10]

Although he took the high-minded tenets of his parents to heart, young Charlie was not above engaging in a little mild mischief, particularly when accompanied by his willing younger brother, Joseph. When they were still very young, the brothers sometimes took the nickel they were supposed to give to the Nineteenth Street Baptist Church Sunday School and instead spent it on a bag of chocolates at Lottie's candy store on Ninth Street. Later, their questionable antics created greater fireworks.

In those days, streetcars were a prime source of transportation, and Charlie was fascinated by the mechanisms that powered the lumbering behemoths. He noticed along nearby Virginia Avenue that the electrical cables lining the car tracks were punctuated every fifty yards or so by iron-lidded junction boxes, set flush with the street. One day, Charlie and his brother Joe pried the lid off one of these boxes and dropped a tin can down into the circuitry, just to see what would happen. They were astonished and thrilled when, accompanied by a smoky sizzle, the can melted—either from the current or friction with the streetcar wheels. They decided to submit another object to the experiment and located an iron rod nearby. When the boys dropped this into the box, though, it did not melt. Instead, the box burst into flame and exploded with a deafening report. If that was not sufficient to scare them, the fire then shot off along the electrical cable down the street and ignited the next box, then the next. Terrified, the boys fled. Back at home, Charlie's mother was momentarily panic-stricken at the sound of the detonations, thinking the city was being bombed. It was only when her boys dashed through the door and, without speaking, shut themselves in their room that she realized the true source of all the ruckus.[11]

Later, Charlie began to apply his seemingly boundless energy in a more entrepreneurial direction. Wishing to augment the family's income, as well as have a few dollars to spend on himself, at age twelve he started his own newspaper stand at the corner of Eighteenth and E Streets. As this little enterprise grew successful, Charlie expanded operations and soon employed ten of his classmates, as well as Joe, peddling the capital's dailies—the *Washington Times*, *Washington Herald*, and the *Evening Star*—at street corners across Foggy Bottom. At its zenith, the small brigade of young salesmen under Charlie Drew was peddling two thousand newspapers a day.[12] In these years and beyond, he and his brother also made a little extra money assisting their father at his job, pitching in at local construction sites, and lifeguarding after school and during the summer.

The two-story house at 1826 E Street was typical of those in the neighborhood: compact but well appointed. In front, a wrought iron fence separated the small yard from the sidewalk. Across the street from the house was Rawlins Park, whose grass fields and magnolia trees the Drew children could not help but consider their own.[13] One day in this park a very young Charlie and his mother encountered President William Howard Taft. Eyeing the rotund chief executive, who tipped the scales at more than 300 pounds, the boy observed, "You're so BIG!" Nora was aghast, but the president merely replied, "So I am."[14]

The green front door of 1826 opened into a small hallway and front parlor whose centerpiece was an upright piano, around which the family, or occasionally Richard's Highwarden Quartet, would gather in the evenings to sing and play. A doorway in the back of the parlor opened into the dining room, where the family ate and, after dinner, the children did their homework. In the rear of the first floor was the kitchen with a coal-and-wood stove, and, through the back door, a porch and larger yard with shade trees and more play space. The bedrooms were on the second floor, one each for the brothers, the sisters, and the parents. The upstairs hallway was illuminated at night by the gentle amber of a gaslight, shaded by a tulip-shaped globe. At the end of this hallway were the Ivory soap–scented bathroom and a sunroom, where Nora tended to her children whenever one fell sick, believing that "the sun would take care of any germs we might have."[15]

The Drews and their neighbors in Foggy Bottom had a special bond, born of shared experiences, backgrounds, and values. As Charlie's sister, Nora, later recalled:

> The fathers were busy people. I didn't know very many mothers who worked. The fathers were those who supported the families. And the emphasis was upon family life. The stress was upon the children's religious lives and their educations. . . . I think that we as a family were raised not only by our parents, our grandparents, our aunts and uncles, but we were also raised by the community, the school, the church, and the neighbors. We were a part of that community.[16]

The pleasant and privileged experience of the Drew family in early twentieth century Washington, DC, was by no means typical for African Americans of the time. Extreme poverty and few opportunities were the norm for most Blacks in the United States in this era, as race relations ebbed to some of the lowest points since Reconstruction. The nation's capital, however, harbored a far greater concentration of Black families of means than was typical in other parts of the nation, primarily due to the presence of unusually large numbers of long-established free Blacks (some families dating their residence here to

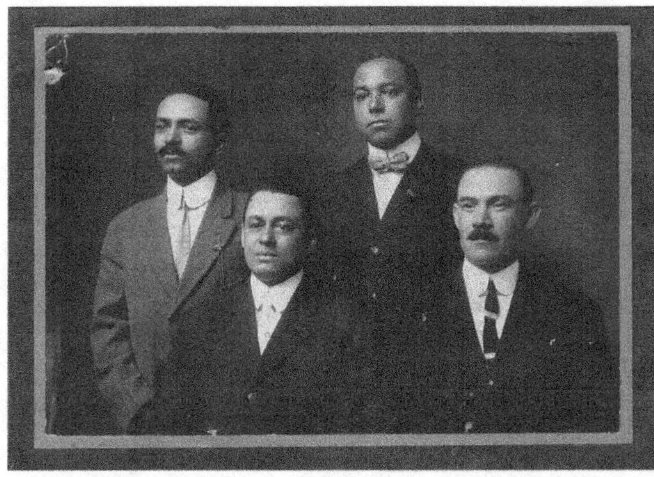

Figure 2.2 The Highwarden Quartet, Richard Drew's vocal ensemble. Richard is at bottom right. Personal collection, Charlene Drew Jarvis.

the eighteenth century) as well as the availability of relatively lucrative employment (most of the African American men in the neighborhood worked as chauffeurs, waiters, janitors, or porters in the District's many hotels). The stability and economic advantage that came with all this was reflected in the lifestyles and culture of the close community. A step in the wrong place might earn a thrown brick, but regarding the amenities of life, the white middle-class families of Foggy Bottom had no great advantages over their African American neighbors. As Charlie's brother Joseph would say, many years later, "We were aware of discrimination, yet we lived in our own little world. There could be some prejudice, but it never touched us. The whites weren't any better off, and they were not as well off educationally."[17]

One of the outstanding reasons for Joseph Drew's remarkable assertion of the superiority of African American educational opportunities in his youth was Charlie's next scholastic destination after Stevens Elementary: Paul Laurence Dunbar High School, located a few miles away in Truxton Circle. If the scholastic reputation of Stevens was justifiably esteemed, that of Dunbar High was revered.

Founded in 1870 as the Preparatory High School for Colored Youth, this was the nation's first public high school for Black students. Between 1870 and 1916 it was known as the M Street High School (attended by Richard Drew), but two years before Charlie's matriculation the institution was renamed for the great Black poet. At this time Dunbar High was, by any standards, one of the finest academic facilities of its kind anywhere in the United States.[18]

Since the school's inception, the prosperous and influential among the District's African American community had made a special effort to ensure that this was the case, providing ample support of every kind. The physical facilities included thirty-five classrooms, a 1,500-seat auditorium, a pipe organ, five pianos, a large swimming pool, a 4,350-volume library, an armory, a rifle range, and even a greenhouse.[19] In any effort to develop a first-rate educational institution a clear priority, naturally, is the faculty, and Dunbar's—not incidentally, paid at the same rate as the district's white teachers—was extraordinary. Advanced-degree graduates from some of the nation's finest universities taught the classes and assembled the curriculum, which was rigorous and uncompromising in the true classical tradition (every student, for example, was required to study Latin). Because of this commitment to excellence, Dunbar attracted outstanding African American students not only from every corner of Washington but from surrounding cities and even distant states.

Given his general lukewarm attitude toward scholastic matters, Charlie's academic performance in this rarefied setting was, perhaps predictably, not impressive—although he passed all the challenging classes without difficulty. On the other hand, the athletic promise he had displayed in elementary school came to full fruition.

Growing into a solid six-foot, 180-pound frame, Charlie emerged as an exceptional four-sport star at Dunbar. He was a standout end on the school's championship football team, captain of the baseball team, and excelled in track-and-field, especially at the high jump. Drew also captained the league-champion Dunbar basketball squad, where he fell under the masterful tutelage of Coach Edwin Bancroft "E. B." Henderson, one of the pioneers of the relatively new sport.*

---

* A member of the Naismith National Basketball Hall of Fame, Henderson was a pivotal figure in encouraging the participation of African American players in the sport.

In the spring of his senior year, the *Sunday Star* summarized Charlie's high school athletic career:

> Charles Drew is considered one of the greatest high school athletes in this country. He has been a consistent performer in all branches of sport—football, baseball, basketball, and track—for four years. He is an end and will start for some eastern or western college for the next four years, thus bringing honor to Dunbar and to the race in general. In baseball he is a good batter and can play almost any position, his forte being catching. In basketball his play had featured nearly every game Dunbar has played. A fine shot, excellent guard and center, he should have no difficulty making his alma mater team no matter where he goes. In track Drew has broken all records for the running high jump by leaping 5 feet 10 inches at the recent Hampton meet, thereby setting a mark that has never been reached by any high school athlete in the District of Columbia and which, it is believed, would win him a place right now in most college meets. He can put the shot over 30 feet

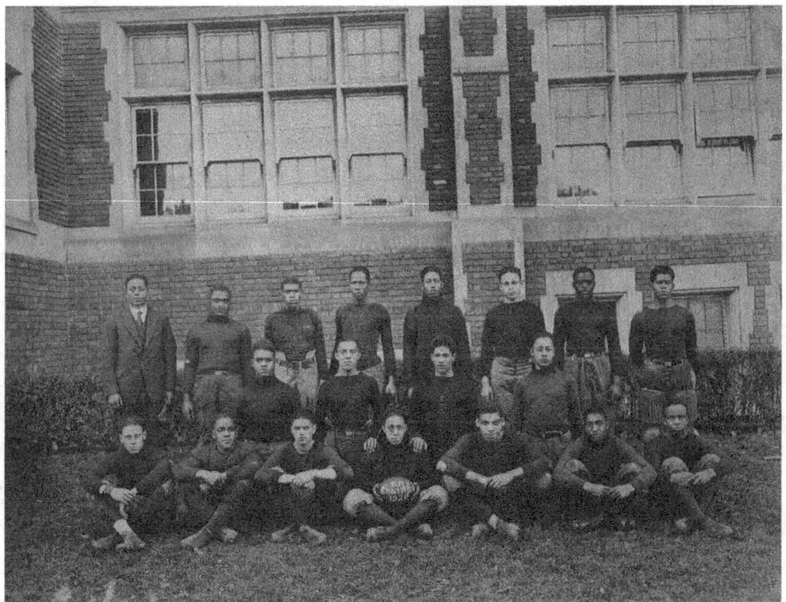

Figure 2.3 The Dunbar High School football team, 1920 season. Drew is top row, third from right. Personal collection, Charlene Drew Jarvis.

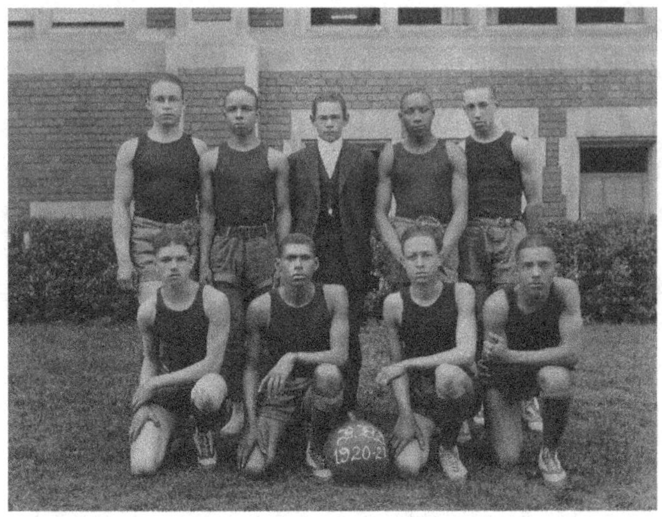

Figure 2.4 The Dunbar High School basketball team, 1920-21 season. Drew is top row, extreme left. Personal collection, Charlene Drew Jarvis.

> and can broad jump over 20 feet. The track coach predicts that in time Drew will rank among the premier athletes of the country.[20]

Drew earned Dunbar's James E. Walker medal from the faculty for all-around athletic performance in both his junior and senior years. As his brother Joseph later remembered, "(Charlie) was always very ambitious and restless. . . . He had a tremendous will to win, to get ahead. It devastated him if he didn't win."[21]

Despite this drive, young Charlie was very well liked by his peers, selected by them in his senior yearbook, *Saturae*, as not only "most athletic boy" and "most popular" but as the "student who has done the most for the school."[22] His sister Nora recalled many years later, "Charlie was a happy person, popular, outgoing . . . with definite charm. Girls loved Charlie."[23] During his time at Dunbar, Charlie was elected president of the Athletic Association (the first junior ever awarded this honor) and the Rex Club (a large group of boys dedicated to "uplifting through example"). In addition, he was voted president of the junior class as well as captain of Company E in the school's Cadet Corps. The annual Cadet Review was held at Griffith Stadium, home of Major League

Baseball's Washington Senators on the campus of Howard University and was one of the outstanding events on the community's social calendar.

His siblings tended to look on Charlie with a mixture of affection and awe. The youngest sister, Eva, recalled, "Charlie was very handsome . . . Girls really loved him. But Charlie was the reliable one . . . He worked hard and was very conscientious. He was totally organized down to the last tee. . . . I adored him and was a little bit afraid of him. He had very strict ideas about the way he wanted me to grow up and dress."[24]

Nora agreed with this assessment: "He commanded respect by his presence. He stood very straight—a big, powerful man. If I was reading a magazine he'd say, 'Aren't you going to school in September?' I don't think Charlie knew it, but he was always something of a legend, as the first child."[25]

The figure of authority who led by example as well as the spoken word also knew when it was time to use a gentle hand. As Nora observed, "He was the one who when one of us would cry would come by and say, 'That's all right.'"[26]

Charlie, in turn, revered his father Richard: "He thought Pop was the quintessence of all that was wonderful," remembered Nora.[27] In addition to the general qualities of personal responsibility, hard work, and faith, the young man tried to emulate his father's other talents, especially in music. Whenever the family gathered in the parlor for a musical interlude, he would pitch in, albeit without as much success. "He played the saxophone badly, the piano loudly," Nora recalled. "He whistled alto and soprano parts at the same time, and he sang—we called them 'Charlie's shouts.'"[28] Later, in college, he picked tunes on a ukelele.

Despite limited ability to play it himself, Charlie loved music passionately and made it a point to attend live performances whenever possible. In this more innocent era, public band concerts were regularly held at the baseball fields (called the White Lot) then present south of the White House. This was within easy walking distance of the Drew home, and Charlie and the rest of the family were frequent attendees. Wanting the best vantage point possible, he would sometimes arrive early and climb a tree near the bandstand, patiently waiting on a low-lying limb for the concert to begin. On one occasion he was either too early or the musicians were late because the young man drifted off to sleep while waiting in his comfortable perch. When the band started their concert with a blast of fortissimo brass, he was jarred awake and promptly tumbled onto the bandstand below.[29]

As close as Charlie was to his father, his bond with his mother was even greater: a deeply devoted relationship that would last the whole of his life. Mrs. Drew provided her eldest son with many lessons and practical instructions in his youth. Among these was the skill to sew, which would be useful in caring for his clothing in the economically challenging times to come and would eventually pay even greater dividends in his professional life.

Likely through his mother's influence, by his teen years, Charlie had developed a sweeping, exceptionally graceful longhand script. In one essay for an English class, he displayed this penmanship while describing his vital role on the Dunbar gridiron squad:

> September 29, 1920
>
> Some of the Duties of an End on a Football team.
>
> The end has to be fast enough to beat the ball on the kickoff down the field and he has to stay on the sideline to run the play toward the center of the field or stop it if it come his way. His duty when scrimmaging when on the defensive is to go behind the opponent's line with the snap of the ball and break up the play before it is in fast motion. The end if possible has to be a fast and sure tackler. His work while on the offensive is to block or upset his opponent so that the man carrying the ball can run free. The end also is the receiver of the forward pass and this requires a keen and cool head. On the whole an end is a very essential part of the team and one bad play on his part may lose a game.[30]

Even as the young man's formative years took shape, though, significant changes rocked the Drew household. Several months before Charlie submitted his elegantly penned essay on football to the Dunbar English faculty, Elsie, Charlie's eldest sister at thirteen years of age, had fallen gravely ill. Petite and pretty, Elsie had always been somewhat frail, especially in contrast to her robust siblings. In the spring of 1920 she came down with symptoms of tuberculosis, possibly acquired from Grandmother Drew, who was known to harbor the disease.[31] When the little girl's dreaded diagnosis was complicated by a case of influenza, coming at the tail end of the great pandemic crisis that followed World War I, the outcome was sadly inevitable. Elsie died on May 22, 1920. Naturally, the shadow of this tragic event hovered over the family like a pall for months, if not longer. Richard, who adored all his children but particularly doted on his girls, was devastated. In later years Drew, who also held a job during the pandemic as a special delivery postman taking the mail to temporary emergency hospitals established in buildings around Washington, would mention his eldest sister's untimely death as one of the events that influenced his decision to pursue a career in medicine.[32]

The desire to live in the healthier climate of the countryside was one of the motivating factors in the Drews' decision, several months later, to move from Foggy Bottom across the Potomac River to then-rural Arlington, Virginia.[33]

Their new home, located in a sparsely populated Black neighborhood called Butler-Holmes, was a two-story white-frame structure dating from 1912, complete with tin roof, French doors, glass knobs, and a charming wraparound porch. Richard and Nora bought the property, which had no formal address but lay on lots 24, 25, and 26, for $2,100—a $500 down payment and the rest on a bond at 6 percent interest, which amounted to $25 a month.[34] Although there were only two bedrooms—which meant that Charlie and Joe had to sleep on a pullout couch—the new property included one-third of an acre of yard space and several plum, sweet cherry, and apple trees. Most of the neighbors had chickens and other farmyard animals, as the Drews soon did. Mail was delivered to a nearby box by Rural Free Delivery. At the time of purchase, the house did not have an indoor bathroom, nor did it have electricity or gas, and the city girl Nora Burell Drew sometimes lamented the decision to move away from the conveniences of Foggy Bottom. Those amenities would come, though, within a few years (along with a new bedroom addition for the boys).[35]

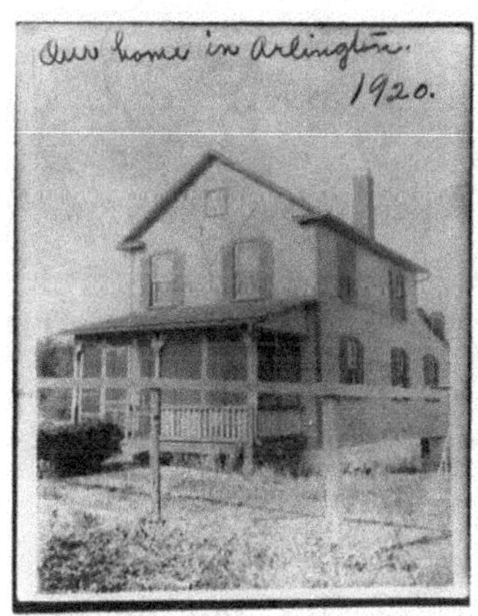

Figure 2.5 The Drew home in Arlington, Virginia, circa 1920. Personal collection, Charlene Drew Jarvis.

The pain of losing Elsie was somewhat assuaged by the arrival of the final family child, a daughter they named Eva Virginia Drew, who was born at the new home in December 1921. Although Charlie initially found her to be something of an embarrassment—some school friends jokingly asserted that Eva was not, in fact, Charlie's sister but his daughter—in time these two siblings of such disparate ages would grow close. When it was Eva's turn to be a teenager, she could look to her mature, successful, and self-assured older brother as a role model and, after their father Richard passed, paternal figure.[36]

Despite living across the Potomac, the Drews continued to be a part of the Foggy Bottom community—attending school and church in their old neighborhood and socializing with the same close friends. Charlie caught a streetcar that took him, for three cents, across the Aqueduct Bridge to and from Dunbar. About a year after the family moved to Arlington, his father—who now primarily worked for a former colleague named Ericsson, who had started his own carpet-laying business—bought an automobile, which eased the commute even further.[37]

On May 5, 1922, Charlie capped off his illustrious career as a high school athlete in the District of Columbia by helping Dunbar vanquish its rivals in the annual championship track-and-field meet of Washington's Black high schools. Dunbar tallied more than twice as many points as the nearest competitor, and Drew was high scorer, winning the shot put, high jump, and broad jump. This victory, combined with championships in football and basketball, gave Dunbar the coveted Major Walter Loving Trophy as all-sports winners of the unofficial league.[38]

The stellar reputation of Dunbar opened many a door to higher education that would have otherwise been irrevocably shut to its students. In this era, and for many years, Dunbar graduates could apply to some of the nation's best colleges and universities with confidence that their likelihood of acceptance was high; some favorites included Harvard, Yale, and Oberlin. This was another reason for the affinity with which the well-heeled local African American community showered the school with funds and attention. In turn, Dunbar alumni went on to great distinction at these institutions and beyond.[39]

One of the schools that had developed a pipeline of sorts from Dunbar in the preceding years was Amherst College, a little institution with a big academic reputation in faraway inland Massachusetts.[40] In the spring of 1922, Drew received a letter from Amherst offering him the opportunity to continue the Dunbar-Amherst axis in person, along with a tempting financial incentive:

May 20, 1922
Mr. Charles Drew
Arlington, Va.

Dear Mr. Drew:

I am glad to inform you that you are awarded a scholarship in Amherst College for the academic year 1922–23. In accordance with our regular rules of procedure, this aid will not be given to you unless your admission to college is free from conditions. If you have fully met all the entrance requirements, you will be granted a credit of $100.00 on your first tuition bill. The amount of your credit for the second half of the year will be determined on the basis of your grade in the studies of the first term.

May I send you my congratulations on your securing this award and my best wishes for your success in the college course?

Sincerely yours,

Alexander Meiklejohn
President[41]

Tuition for the 1922–23 academic course at Amherst was two hundred dollars, payable in two installments, "one of one hundred and fifteen dollars at the opening of the college in September, and one of eighty-five dollars on or before February first."[42] Thus, the offered scholarship would nearly cover the cost of attendance—at least for the first semester. The combination of Amherst's reputation and its generosity made any choice about collegiate destination easy for Charlie and his parents: he would be traveling north in the fall.

Charlie worked through the summer with his father, at construction sites, and as a lifeguard at the pool, earning as much money as possible for the family and his own coming needs (he had ceded his newspaper business to his brother Joe on entering Dunbar). As the shadows grew longer in late September, Charlie gathered a few things, said goodbye to his tearful, proud parents and siblings, and boarded a train bound for New England and a vast, unknown future. The strapping young man may have harbored some trepidation as he put all that was familiar behind him, but he was rarely one to lack confidence or show doubt. Alongside the photograph of a cadet-uniformed Drew in the 1922

Dunbar High School yearbook, below the many accolades and honors from his educators and peers (and his stated intention to become an electrical engineer) was a quote, succinct and sincere: "You can do anything you think you can."[43]

Charlie also clipped a prayerful poem to carry in his wallet for inspiration in the years to come:

Lord let me live like a Regular Man,
With Regular friends and true,
Let me play the game on a regular plan
And play that way all through
Let me win or lose with a regular smile
And never be known to whine
For that is a regular fellow's style
And I want to make it mine;

Oh give me a regular chance in life;
The same as the rest I pray
And give me a Regular girl for a wife
To help me along the way
Let me know the lot of humanity
Its regular woes and joys
And raise a regular family
Of regular girls and boys

Let me live to a regular good old age
With Regular snow-white hair
Having done my labor and earned my wage
And played my game for fair
And at last when the mourners come to scan
My face on its peaceful bier
They'll say Well he was a Regular Man
And drop a Regular tear![44]

3

Growth

Amherst College, 1922–26

A few weeks before his undergraduate classes began, Charlie Drew received a small book in the mail from the Christian Association of Amherst College. Bound in figured black leather with a stylized "AU" and the Amherst seal embossed on the cover, this little volume's appearance was a good match for its title, *The Class of 1926 Freshman Bible*.[1]

Contained within the pages of the handbook were all the tidbits of information that the upperclassmen and faculty considered to be useful for the incoming men.* There were sections on the administration of the college, lyrics to the school songs (no fewer than nine of them, including the Alma Mater, "To the Fairest College"), maps, points of interest, and many other items—not least a brief history of the institution.

Here the freshman learned that Amherst College was named for the otherwise nondescript rural town where it arose (which, in turn, was named for a British general of colonial vintage—Lord Jeffrey Amherst). The school was founded in 1821, a century and a year before Charlie Drew first set foot on campus, having evolved from a less ambitious local academic endeavor called the Amherst Academy, augmented by premature presentiments of nearby Williams College's foundering. Although it endured the teething pains common to any

* Women were not admitted to Amherst until 1975.

new institution, Amherst College saw great growth as the years passed, employing a classics-heavy curriculum deeply rooted in the Calvinist worldview of old Massachusetts. By the third decade of the twentieth century, the college sprawled over one hundred acres (including playing fields) and was a major cultural, political, and financial force in the west-central part of the Bay State.[2]

The faculty had also embraced a cultural pivot toward the educational philosophy of newer liberal arts colleges.

Classes in theology and Bible literature, though still present, were gradually giving way to the pure and social sciences. As President Meiklejohn described the atmosphere at Amherst in his day—which was also Drew's, "The College is called liberal . . . because the instruction is dominated by no special interest, is limited to no single human task, but is intended to take human activity as a whole, to understand human endeavors not in their isolation but in their relations to one another and to the total experience which we call the life of our people."[3]

As an African American, Drew's presence in his class was unusual but not unique. Few Blacks attended institutions of higher learning in the United States at this time, north or south, but Amherst had been admitting men of color (albeit in small numbers) almost since its founding.[4] When Drew arrived, he could count about a dozen other African American men among his schoolmates, including fellow Dunbar graduates William Montague Cobb (his friend since the days of the Twelfth Street YMCA), W. Mercer Cook, and William Henry Hastie, who were all in the class ahead of him. Drew was assigned a room in the dormitory at old South College Hall, one of the original campus buildings. This unadorned red brick structure, which housed about 150 students, was erected in the colonial style of Harvard and other New England educational institutions. It sported a cornerstone laid by the famous educator and lexicographer Noah Webster, a local resident, in August 1820.[5]

The official enrollment day for the incoming class of 1926, the largest admitted to the school to that point, was September 19. Most of the new freshmen had been on campus for at least a few days already, preparing for fraternity rush. These new men learned firsthand about all the traditions of the school that they had read about in their freshman Bibles, including the figurative dues they were required to pay as neophytes.

Chapel was held every weekday morning at 8:15, and attendance was mandatory. Freshmen were permitted to enter the Johnson Chapel building through

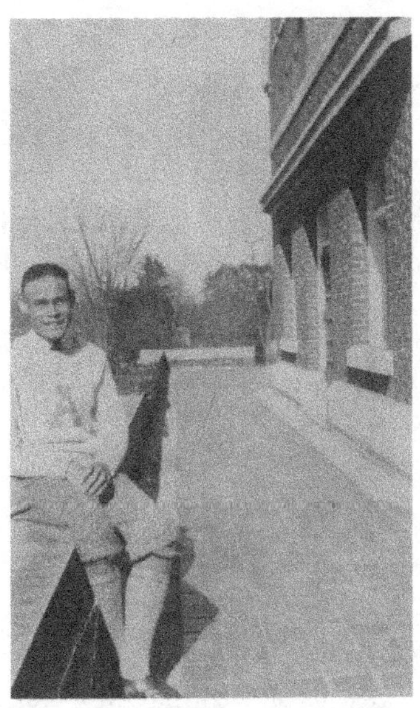

Figure 3.1 Charles Drew on the campus of Amherst College. Personal collection, Charlene Drew Jarvis.

the side door only, and, after the services, they had to stand at attention while the faculty and upperclassmen left the building; they could not so much as move until that process was complete. No smoking was permitted by freshmen on the streets of campus or the town, and, for some reason, they could not carry canes, either. Most humiliating, though, was the requirement that the newcomers wear pea-green Eaton caps "with a black button not less than one and one-half inches in diameter," although in severely cold weather they might substitute a regulation Freshman Toque, which was no kind of improvement. As their Bibles succinctly reminded them, "Above all things, remember that you are a Freshman."[6]

As they absorbed these degradations, the Class of '26 also engaged in more pleasant pursuits, such as the long-standing traditional interclass competitions Chapel Rush and Flag Rush, in both of which they prevailed over their predecessors from the Class of 1925. They also saluted the unofficial school mascot, "Sabrina," a four-foot tall, three-hundred-pound bronze statue of a nymph that had been donated to Amherst back in 1857. The new men first glimpsed Sabrina, who had a collegiate mascot's lengthy history of prank abductions and rescues, when she was trotted out for a class photo in front of the columns and cupola of old College Hall on September 22.[7] Classes had formally begun the previous morning.[8]

Charlie's high school work at Dunbar had earned him a total of sixteen "Entrance Credits" at Amherst (fifteen were required for admission, although they could be made up before the Junior year). He had four in mathematics, three each in English and Latin, two each in history and Spanish, one each in chemistry and physics.[9]

Amherst operated on the semester system and enforced a rather rigid set of course requirements for its incoming students; opportunities for electives were few. Over the course of the 1922–23 academic year, Charlie would attend the year-long classes Chemistry 1, Physical Education, Public Reading, and Spanish 2. In addition, he had the semester-length classes English A and B, as well as Mathematics 5 and 1.[10]

Amherst's ongoing focus on the classics required that students with less than four full years of Latin education in high school either take two years of Latin or three of Ancient Greek to qualify for a degree. Charlie evidently decided that the path of least resistance involved continued study of the language with which he already had some familiarity, so he opted for the two-year Latin pathway. He enrolled in what was called Latin A, a reading of Vergil's *Aeneid* taught by Professor William Tingle Rowland four times a week. The class met in one of the recitation rooms at Johnson Chapel, vintage 1827, which was located adjacent to Charlie's South College dormitory. Here, in the main hall, the flag of the Amherst Ambulance Corps from World War I hung soberingly, complete with Croix de Guerre and fourragère. Since they had to wait in this building at morning chapel, standing, for the several minutes it took the faculty and upperclassmen to disperse, the freshmen had plenty of time to appreciate the relics from the recent Great War.[11]

Chemistry 1 was an elective course in general chemistry, with a weekly lab (and $10 annual lab fee) taught by an up-and-coming young associate professor and Amherst alum, George Scatchard. English A and B were required semester-length courses. English A was called An Introduction to Literature, while English B covered Literature of the Old Testament and was taught by Professor Albert Parker Fitch among the oak panels and stained-glass windows of the college's ornate Morgan Library. Mathematics 5 covered the topics of descriptive geometry and mechanical drawing, while Mathematics 1 involved study of elementary functions of algebra and trigonometry, especially as applied to geometry and physics. These half-year classes were of obvious value for Charlie's avowed interest in electrical engineering. Professor Stewart Garrison instructed the students in the oratorical art of public reading. Spanish 2 was made up of selected material from sixteenth and seventeenth century Spanish literature, the *Siglo del Oro* of Cervantes and contemporaries. This was taught in Barrett Hall, a long-time gymnastics building that was now home to Amherst's modern language departments.[12]

This was a formidable set of classes by any measure and a daunting introduction to the world of higher learning for eighteen-year-old Charlie Drew. In addition to this challenging coursework, Charlie had several opportunities to display his exceptional athletic prowess while contributing to his class's efforts against the sophomores in an ongoing series of intramural underclass sporting events through the fall and winter. The results in these were mixed for the '26ers, but Charlie generally performed well and was one of the stars of the series. He particularly excelled on the freshman football team, which walloped the sophomores 26–6. Word of Drew's arrival at Amherst made it back to one of his hometown newspapers: "News has been received at Dunbar that Charles Drew of the class of 1922, one of the best all-around athletes and scholars ever graduated from Dunbar, in a recent physical test given to all freshmen at Amherst College was found to be the best developed man in the class. Drew has also been made a member of the freshman football squad."[13]

In the spring of 1923 the level of competition took a noticeable upturn when Charlie went out for Coach Richard Nelligan's varsity track team. Drew made the squad—he was the only freshman to do so and, as it turned out, the only one in his class to earn a varsity letter in any of the major sports. Although the "Lord Jeffs," as all the Amherst teams were informally known (they were also called the "Sabrinas" or the "Purple and White," for the school colors) struggled to a winless season, Charlie gave a yeoman effort at the New England Intercollegiate Athletic Association (NEIAA) meet at Harvard Stadium in Cambridge late in May, where he tied for fourth place in the running high jump with an effort of 5 feet 8 and one-half inches, helping Amherst to a fifth-place team finish.[14]

Charlie made even larger waves by winning the Samuel L. Cobb Pentathlon Trophy. This award, named for a captain of the team from the previous decade, was given to the champion of an intrasquad competition involving a series of events: 100-yard dash, shot put, 220-yard hurdles, broad jump, and a mile run, all of which had to be completed within a two-hour period. Drew defeated three of his teammates, including his Dunbar friend William Hastie, in winning the trophy.[15]

When the academic dust settled at the close of Charlie's freshman year, it was clear that whatever scholastic light might be shining beneath his quiet demeanor had yet to be revealed fully. Still, he passed all courses, recording C's in English, math, public reading, and Spanish, and D's in chemistry and Latin. The brightest spot, likely to no one's surprise, was physical education, where he earned a B.[16]

Although Drew passed the two semester-length English courses, since these only met twice a week, he was awarded just four credit hours in this subject, as opposed to six for Spanish and eight for Latin. These were the only courses in English that Charlie took at Amherst, and his limited credit hours in the subject would come back to haunt him a few years down the line.[17]

Charlie returned to the family home in Arlington for the thirteen-week summer break, where he could look forward to spending time with his parents and siblings and earn some money working odd jobs as well as lifeguarding. She was too young in the summer of 1923, but in years to come little Eva waited at the front window for him, running down the road when she spotted his approach, intent on being the first in the family to welcome home the eldest brother she so adored. He would swing her onto his shoulders, and together they would rush past the hedgerow that adorned the front path to meet the others at the door.[18]

When he returned to Massachusetts to begin his second year at Amherst in September 1923, Charlie was assigned a room at the North College Hall dormitory, a structure nearly identical to his freshman dormitory, South College Hall, and only slightly less ancient. As he perused the course catalog, Drew would have learned that sophomores had a bit more leeway than first-year students in terms of elective class choices. He decided to study German 1 (an introductory class), Latin 1 (which, somewhat confusingly, was not an entry-level class but required working knowledge of Latin grammar and covered readings from the likes of Cicero and Tacitus), Oratorio (vocal chorus performance and instruction), Philosophy 1 (an overview of logic, ethics, and something called social psychology), and the required physical education. His high school goal of a career in engineering apparently intact, Charlie also selected challenging courses in Mathematics 2 (calculus and analytical geometry, taught by Professor George Daniel Olds) and Physics 1 (electricity and magnetism, thermodynamics, and the relatively new electron theory of matter).[19]

That fall he also went out for football and made Coach DeOrmand "Tuss" McLaughry's varsity team. As was the case at colleges and universities across the country in the early twentieth century, at Amherst football was king. Every season was highly anticipated, the seats at the school's Pratt Field were typically filled to the last, and more ink was spilled in newspapers and yearbooks to describe and glorify gridiron heroics than for any other collegiate activity. The Amherst football season always culminated with a fierce contest against the school's nearby archrival, Williams College. Together with Wesleyan University in Middletown, Connecticut, Amherst and Williams comprised an unofficial mini conference of bragging rights self-styled the Little Three (in reference to the Big Three Ivy League colleges, Harvard, Princeton, and Yale). Although there were no coeds to impress, football stars nonetheless held considerable cache on the quads of Amherst and the streets of its namesake town.

On paper, the 1923 Amherst football team had considerable weaknesses, but Coach McLaughry, who had played both collegiate and professional football himself, was a determined, skilled instructor. The previous season had been his first as head coach at Amherst and, despite an unimpressive 2–6 final record, knowledgeable observers had detected a disciplined, skillful coaching style that boded well. The roster for McLaughry's second "Lord Jeffs" squad may not have been ideal for his vision, but there were certainly some bright spots.

Unquestionably the most luminous of these was Charlie Drew, who shone as a budding star on both sides of the ball. Since the freshman football team sometimes scrimmaged the varsity, McLaughry may have witnessed Drew's talents firsthand the previous year. He cannot have failed to hear word of mouth about the young man's ability and must have eagerly anticipated his eligibility for the varsity team. Many years later, McLaughry recalled:

> As a football player, Drew was great. He could have played regular on any team in the country, both in his era, and any time since. I am qualified to say this because I coached in the East-West Shrine Game four years . . . and when I was not coaching, saw these games as a spectator.[20] Each year the players included the very best of the previous season. Charlie was a halfback of tremendous speed and quick reactions, a great second effort, a splendid passer. He could hit a bull's eye with the old ball at any distance up to fifty yards. Furthermore, he was a tiger on defense. When he tackled, the runner went down as though he were shot. His playing weight was 190–195 and his height was six feet plus. His physique and walking carriage were superb.[21]

On October 6, 1923, at Baker Field in Upper Manhattan, Amherst played favored Columbia University to a scoreless tie. Drew caught the eye of the sportswriter for the local African American newspaper, *The New York Age*: "In Saturday's game, Amherst was represented by a colored boy, Charles Drew of Washington, who plays left end. Drew is a former Dunbar High School star and played a brilliant game. He was unusually fast in getting down under punts, a deadly tackler, and good on catching forward passes."[22]

The most exciting and dramatic example of Drew's talent came in the contest against Wesleyan, held at Pratt Field on the unseasonably mild afternoon of November 3. Stymied much of the game, and trailing 10–6 as the clock wound down, the Amherst team was facing certain defeat at the hands of its Little Three rival. In desperation, with twelve seconds remaining in the game, Coach McLaughry pulled the strong-armed Charlie from his end position to field the snap for the final play. As Wesleyan defenders closed in on him, Drew launched a forty-yard strike to the end zone, where the usual quarterback, John McBride, made a spectacular catch over the outstretched arms of his opponents for a touchdown.* The electrifying score meant a 12–10 victory and sent the astounded Purple and White faithful into a jubilant, raucous celebration.[23]

Although the "Lord Jeffs" limped home to a 3-3-2 record after a loss to hated Williams, the seeds of success had been sown and would, before long, bear fruit.

In December of that year, after the football season had come to an end, Charlie became a member of the Alpha Psi chapter of the fraternity Omega Psi Phi. This organization had been founded in 1911 at Howard University and was the second-oldest African American fraternity in the country. The Amherst chapter, which had no "house," had only come into being the previous year and had not garnered official recognition from the school.

In the spring of 1924 Charlie prepared for a return to the track-and-field team. By now his athletic excellence was known all over the Amherst campus. As aware of this as anyone, the school's baseball coach decided to make a play for the talented young man's services. Charlie, of course, had been a multifaceted

---

*This memorable play eventually took on legendary status. An article about Drew that appeared in the *Amherst Alumni News* upon his death noted, "Each college generation treasures its recollection of some particular pinnacle of athletic achievement. The men of Drew's time will never admit that any other high moment could approach his forty-yard touchdown pass to John McBride, which, in the last minute of play, defeated Wesleyan in 1923."

baseball standout at Dunbar High School and seemed a natural to excel on the collegiate diamond as well. When Coach Nelligan got wind of this tampering with his star athlete, he hastened to intervene. W. Montague Cobb later recalled that "the track and the baseball coach fell out with each other" over Drew's springtime athletic pursuits.[24]

After he made the decision to stick with track-and-field, Charlie competed in several events, including shot put, high and low hurdles, long jump, and broad jump. One writer called him "a one-man track team, being a consistent winner in every track meet which Amherst entered."[25] The season was brief, comprising only three dual meets in May, two of which Amherst won. Drew was high scorer for the Purple and White; he also won the Cobb Pentathlon Trophy for the second consecutive year. He literally took the prize home this time—rather than merely having his name inscribed on it—because, according to donor Samuel Cobb's instructions, anyone winning the competition twice in his four years at Amherst was to keep the actual trophy.[26]

As had been the case at Dunbar and his freshman year at Amherst, Drew's performance in the classroom did not match his exploits on the playing fields. He scored C's in German, Latin, and philosophy and D's in the difficult physics and mathematics courses. Physical Education remained a bright spot with a B, and Charlie did even better in Oratorio, earning an A.[27]

When he returned to the classroom for his junior year in September 1924, Charlie's choice of elective classes indicated a shift in focus away from mathematics and physical science, perhaps reflecting a diminishing interest in engineering. His classes were Biology 1 (a general course), Chemistry 2 (inorganic chemistry), French 1, German 2 (a survey of literature, including works by Schiller and Goethe), Philosophy 4 (which was titled "Psychology" and purported to address "theories of behavior"), and Physical Education.[28]

Of course, autumn also meant football season. The 1924 "Lord Jeffs" started promisingly as they earned a 3–2 record by mid-season, one of the losses being by just two points to a scrappy squad from Bowdoin College in Maine. In a preview for that game, a sportswriter from the Portland, Maine, newspaper called his readers' attention to the threats Amherst posed to the home team:

> Then there is Charlie Drew, the fleet-footed Negro, who was Amherst's one (man) track team last Spring (sic). Drew may not be the most shifty runner in the world,

> but once he takes the pass from center he must be watched and watched with an eagle eye. It was Drew who hurled the long forward pass that spelled defeat for Wesleyan in the closing seconds of play on Pratt Field, Amherst, last year. It was Drew who hurled the passes that bothered Williams' fine eleven.[29]

The Purple and White rebounded from the Bowdoin loss to post an impressive 33–13 win the next week over their Little Three rival Wesleyan. The once again promising season was threatened with a serious setback, though, on the afternoon of Saturday, October 25. Late in a lopsided, 48–0 victory over Hamilton College, Charlie, who had scored two touchdowns in the game, suffered a significant injury to his right ankle on a hard tackle. After the game, Coach McLaughry drove Charlie twelve miles to Northampton, the nearest town where X-rays could be done.[30] No fracture was reported, but the pain and swelling were dire enough to indicate either a severe sprain or ligament tear. In any event, it seemed clear that Drew would not be able to play football for some time.

Local sports pages ran headlines in subsequent days such as "AMHERST CRIPPLED BY DREW'S INJURY," so it was not much of a surprise when the team, "demoralized by the absence of Drew," lost in depressing fashion on the following Saturday to the Aggies from the crosstown school, Massachusetts Agricultural College (now known as the University of Massachusetts, Amherst).[31] Charlie also sat out the next game, but the magnitude of the season's closing contest against rival Williams, a victory over which would mean a Little Three title for Amherst, was enough to make him take the field. "The morale and actual strength of the team has been increased by the return of Charley Drew," reported a local paper, but, unfortunately, the matchup was not a good one for the "Sabrinas," who fell 27–6.[32] Despite being hobbled by his painful ankle, Drew was able to generate more heroics as he scored the team's lone touchdown when he "made a brilliant catch behind the goal line after evading three defenders."[33]

Despite the 1924 Amherst football team's mediocre final record, observers found cause for optimism. Most of the best players would be returning for the 1925 season, along with the proven coaching staff. As was recounted in the Amherst yearbook *Olio*, "the season can by no means be regarded a failure . . . a new fighting spirit was aroused, not only on the gridiron but also in the student body." Charlie won the Thomas W. Ashley Memorial Trophy in 1924 as the Most Valuable Player on the team.[34] "Drew's exceptional passing and receiving, powerful running, and hard tackling were responsible for many of the team's touchdowns this year."[35]

As the most valuable player on the squad in his junior season, by Amherst tradition Charlie should have been made captain for his final year. However, at the close of the 1924 season a white player named Moore was selected for the honor. Although he was disappointed and angry, as were the other African American players and students, Drew heeded the advice of the team's fatherly old Black trainer, Doc Newport, and defused what could have been a serious disruption to the promising team by stepping aside graciously.[36]

With the football season over, Charlie could focus on his schoolwork and healing up. Alarmingly, though, the pain and swelling in his right ankle failed to improve. Soon it became clear that his injury was more severe than had been thought. After the first of the year, dire reports began to appear:

> The Amherst College athletic forces have suffered one of their most serious losses when it was learned today that Charlie Drew, the wonderful football and track star, will be out of participating in any sport for the rest of his college course. This loss is due to the injury Drew suffered way back in the middle of the football season last fall in a game against Hamilton. At first it was thought that merely a tendon was broken but treatments at this time have confirmed the fact that it was a bone, which makes his right ankle useless for running.
>
> It will be remembered by the followers of the Amherst backfield wizard that he could not use his leg in his accustomed speed in the later games this season. What speed and work he could do must have been mainly done on pure sand because the ankle now gives him difficulty in even walking fast.
>
> He is considered one of the best backfield men around these parts and if he had played on a team of a bigger university would have won a national reputation.
>
> In addition to his football ability Drew has been the outstanding track star. He was good for many points in the dual meets and was the only Amherst man to place in the national intercollegiate races.[37]

As Drew's symptoms worsened over the winter, concern arose that he had developed an infection in the injured ankle. In this era before the advent of antibiotics such a complication could be extremely serious—even fatal. Only the previous summer, the entire nation had followed with worried fascination the case of sixteen-year-old Calvin Coolidge Jr., the son of the president, who had developed an infected blister after playing tennis on the White House lawn. Sadly, the infection—caused by staphylococcus bacteria—spread to his bloodstream, and the young man died of septicemia.[38]

President Coolidge was an Amherst alumnus—his other son, John, was in the class of 1928—and the death of Calvin Jr. had a profound impact on the little college community. The fact that the school's most accomplished and renowned athlete had developed a similar malady to that which felled young Calvin was on the mind of many. Not least among these was Coach McLaughry, who doubled as coach of field events in the spring and whose high opinion of Drew extended beyond the playing fields. In March, as track season began, he took Charlie to see a renowned orthopedic surgeon in Boston, bringing along the X-rays from Northampton. The doctor made the diagnosis of a "periosteal tear with complications," to the considerable relief of all involved.[39] He also taped Drew's ankle up and, in what must have seemed a moment from a dream to the athlete and his coach, cleared him to rejoin the track team. McLaughry and Drew took their leave of the Boston specialist and hastened off to join their comrades, who were preparing for a dual meet against Brown in Providence, Rhode Island, that same day. Charlie's surprise appearance was met with "great rejoicing" by his teammates.[40]

Unfortunately, the joy was short-lived. Despite Drew's heroics in winning four events while struggling with his taped, ailing ankle—shot put, broad jump, and both hurdles—this contest was the occasion not only for a close defeat but also a sad incident of bigotry remembered later by W. Montague Cobb:

> There were four colored boys on that team. . . . After the meet we found ourselves last to leave the dressing room. As we emerged the rest of the team was standing unusually quietly over by the convoy of limousines by which we usually travelled. The head coach (Nelligan), the coach of field events (McLaughry) and the student manager were in a huddle, but still we did not catch on. Then the manager came over and said he was very sorry but that during the meet the Narragansett Hotel had heard there were colored boys on the Amherst team and had sent word that they would not serve them with the team although they would serve "Doc"

Newport, the colored trainer. The manager continued that he had called every other hotel in Providence and none could serve so large a group on such short notice. Would we mind, therefore, taking dinner in the Brown University commons?

We were caught flatfooted, fatigued from the rigors of the meet and momentarily silenced by the fact that the team had deserted us by being willing to go ahead and eat at the Narragansett anyway, which they did. The four of us went to the Brown commons, but it was a silent, spare meal. The convoy picked us up and we each rode in different cars, but the night ride back to Amherst was painfully silent in those four cars. That was such a bad one that it was seldom mentioned afterward even among ourselves.[41]

As with football, the captaincy for the subsequent year was voted on at the end of the season. After the controversy over leadership of the football team, Charlie was unanimously elected to head the Amherst track team in the spring of 1926, his senior year. For the third straight time, Drew triumphed in the Cobb Trophy pentathlon.[42]

As part of his philosophy class, with its emphasis on psychology, that spring Charlie wrote a paper called "The Psychology of Music, Especially Its Effect on Man," which he delivered to the professor in late May. For this assignment he displayed a flowery, ornate writing style: "Now that I am in the midst of this pleasing, though none too easy subject, fair would I extricate myself from this entangling mesh . . . I shall not attempt to give a complete study of this phase, but shall be content, nay overjoyed if I am successful in portraying a few of the fundamental elements."[43]

The professor found this baroque composition amusing but ultimately counterproductive, awarding a C+: "These expressions were good English style 75 years ago, or so, but would better be left to the poets now. . . . It's hard to grade your essay. You have put a good deal of sincere poetry into it, and have made a good effort to deal with important aspects of the subject. All that deserves a much better grade. But, in connection with the course, poetry can hardly take the place of science."[44]

Charlie completed his final exams with the rest of his class in June. He must have been well pleased with the B's he earned in both Biology and Chemistry 2, which may have evened the scale for the D he got in French. Philosophy and

German were both C's, and Physical Education, the usual bright spot, this time an actual A.[45]

It may have been at this penultimate homecoming from Amherst that Charlie announced to his young sister Eva, who, as usual, met him at the street in front of the Drew home in Arlington, that she had grown too big and he could no longer carry her to the doorway. When she began to cry, he reassured her that the two of them would, from then on, walk hand in hand together to the door. Her greeting was, he told her, his way of knowing that he was really home. As Eva later remembered, "It made me feel really special."[46]

Over the years to come, Drew observed that three events shaped his decision to become a physician. One of these was the sad death of his sister Elsie. On his medical school application in 1928, Drew wrote, "My first real urgent desire to study medicine came when my sister died with an attack of influenza in the great epidemic here in 1920. No one seemed to be able to stop it and people died by the hundreds every week. I have studied the sciences diligently since that time."[47] Another seminal moment involved the care he received while recuperating from the ankle injury he sustained on the football field against Hamilton College in the Autumn of 1924: "[I] got banged up in football and wanted to know how the body works."[48]

The third came in his senior year at Amherst.

That year commenced on September 24, 1925, at which time Charlie's course selections hinted that his academic interests were veering in a new direction: he took both Biology 4 (comparative anatomy and embryology of vertebrates) and Biology 8 (a self-designed class that had to be specially approved by a professor). These were buttressed by the challenging curriculum of Chemistry 4 (organic chemistry). French 2 and German 3 rounded out Drew's formidable senior year schedule.[49]

Both of the biology classes Charlie had selected were taught by Otto Glaser, a forty-five-year-old full professor (soon to become department chair) who originally hailed from Germany. Compact and energetic, with inquisitive, careworn eyes, Glaser had an instructor's charisma that caught Charlie's attention in a way that most of his other teachers up to this time had not. Inspired by his new mentor, Drew applied himself in the classroom with a nacsent energy, a zeal that, from this time forward, he never relinquished.[50]

As opposed to the classroom, inspiration was never a thing Charlie lacked on the playing field. Excitement reached a new level, though, in the fall of his senior year.

With seasoned veterans on the lines and star athletes at the skill positions, Coach McLaughry's 1925 Amherst football team was one of the most anticipated in the school's history.

True to the hoopla, on a mild September 26 afternoon at Pratt Field, the Purple and White opened their season with a resounding victory over the University of Rochester, 26–6. Buoyed by this success, the team went into its next contest, on the road against a highly regarded Princeton Tigers squad, with cautious optimism. Although acquitting themselves admirably—the second team held Princeton scoreless in the first half and Drew, in particular, had an outstanding performance—the Amherst men eventually fell by a score of

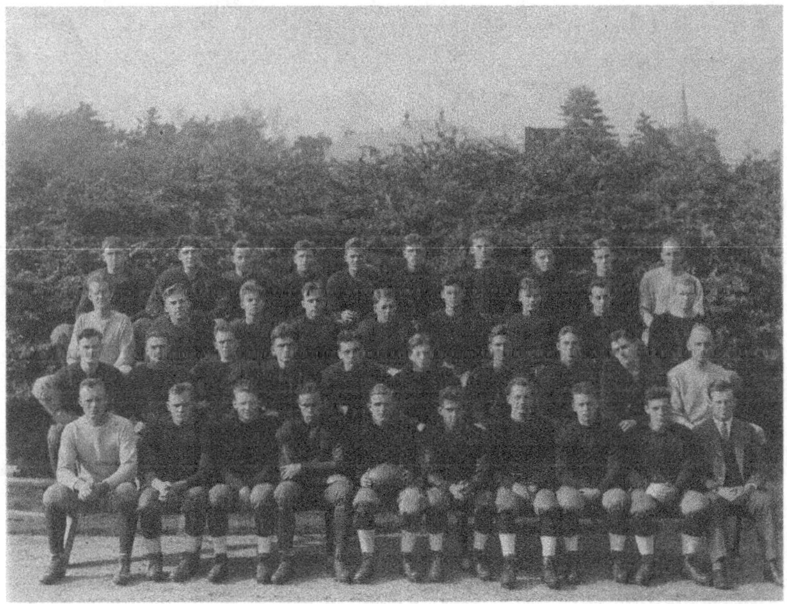

Figure 3.2 The 1925 Amherst football team. Drew is bottom row, fourth from left. Coach DeOrmand "Tuss" McLaughry is bottom row, far left. Personal collection, Charlene Drew Jarvis.

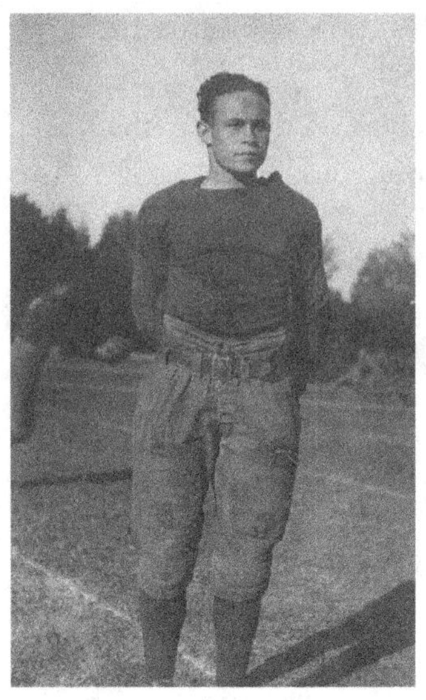

Figure 3.3 Drew as a star player for the Amherst football team. Personal collection, Charlene Drew Jarvis.

20–0 in a contest that was closer than the score indicated. Unfortunately, Princeton's field was the scene of more racial animosity.

W. Montague Cobb later recalled that "Princeton had been famous for breaking up any colored player."[51] Intending to forestall anything of this nature, McLaughry had contacted the Princeton coach in advance and was told that there would be no incidents on the field. Although this was true, nothing could stop the Princeton fans from shouting ugly epithets at Drew and the other Black players and equally hearty cheers whenever one of them absorbed a heavy hit.[52]

As disappointing as the atmosphere and outcome of the Princeton game were, it was the last defeat the Amherst team would taste that year. McLaughry's men swept their next five games, including a 73–6 demolition of their Little Three rival Wesleyan. This set the stage for the year's finale: a winner-take-all match against their arch-nemesis, the team from Williams College. Many students and fans joined the team in the trip to Weston Field in Williamstown, swelling the stands with over six thousand raucous voices that even a cold, rainy November afternoon could not silence. After a mud-drenched slog, the teams battling hammer and tongs, the visitors saw their wishes fulfilled and joined hands to celebrate a 13–7 win, the first by Amherst in the series since 1920. Jubilant song reached into the gray Massachusetts sky:

Come fellows, now, and join the chorus,
Together, every Amherst man;
With white and purple waving o'er us,
Victorious since our course began;
Behind our team we stand united,

Behind old Williams' goal-line, too;
And well her sons may get excited,
Today's her Waterloo![53]

These victories made the Purple and White, who surrendered just twelve points in the entire season after the Princeton loss, champions of the Little Three. As the sportswriter for the *Olio* put it, "It is safe to say that no Amherst football team in history has had greater honors come to it than those which piled upon the 1925 eleven."[54]

Several members of the team, including the star halfback Charles Drew, were named to all-league, all-New England, and even All-America teams.

Many years later, Coach McLaughry would write about Drew in an article for the widely circulated *Saturday Evening Post* titled, "The Best Player I Ever Coached."

> In all of Amherst College's long history, no campus generation treasures a more glorious football memory than the graduates of 1923–26. Easily their most memorable thrill while I coached there was given them by a tall, well-built Negro halfback from Washington, DC named Charlie Drew. And he did it as a sophomore.
>
> Near the close of the 1923 season, Amherst was trailing helplessly behind Wesleyan. On the last play of the game, Drew tried a desperate pass. With tacklers hanging all over him, he got off a tremendous forty-yard throw to John McBride. It was good for a touchdown and a precious 12–10 victory. Better still, it built up such team faith in Drew that he was able to lead Amherst to its largest scores in Little Three history at its peak in 1925, two seasons later. That year, Amherst lost only to Princeton and, even in losing, Drew gained more than 160 yards and was the outstanding man on the field.
>
> One hint of Drew's phenomenal speed, for the benefit of those who never saw him in action, is the fact that when this six-foot-one, 195-pounder turned to track, he won the junior national A.A.U. hurdles championship.
>
> In football, he was lightning-fast on the getaway and dynamite on inside plays, plowing on with a "second effort" that brought him yardage long after he should have been stopped. He threw the old pumpkin-shaped ball farther and with more

accuracy than anyone else I ever saw, and was also an excellent receiver. He was equally effective on defense, a true tackler and pass stopper.[55]

Despite the playing field accolades, there remained for Charlie and his African American classmates boundaries that could not be crossed, entrée that remained denied. Perhaps the most august of the student groups at Amherst was called Scarab. As Cobb later remembered: "There was a student group called 'Scarab' composed of ten or a dozen seniors who were recognized as the most outstanding men on campus from the standpoint of all-around achievement. Scarab tapped its own successors each year from the Junior Class. Charlie was a logical choice, but again he was passed over."[56]

As with the sports captaincies, this slight of Drew created ripples among members of the student body. In this instance, his exclusion from Scarab "produced a split within the group itself, some demanding vainly that he be inducted *post facto*."[57]

While these struggles peppered Drew's extracurricular world, the mundane necessities of the classroom went on.

In the spring semester Charlie was once again under the auspices of the charismatic Otto Glaser, who led the young man through the special Biology 8 research class. Influenced by Glaser's own research, which focused on embryology and other aspects of animal development, Drew composed his senior thesis from this class on the subject of "Growth." The finished product was sixty-four pages long, handwritten in his characteristic sweeping script. Although the compositional style remained ornate, it was not as frankly poetic as the music paper. Drew began his magnum opus with a weighty quote,* "As Thompson has so well put it, 'The world of things living, like the world of things inanimate, grows of itself, and pursues its ceaseless course of evolution.'"[58]

Years later Drew would remark that this work, assembled under Glaser's tutelage, was not only the first salvo in a career that would produce many research papers, but one of the best things he ever wrote. It earned an excellent grade. Most importantly, Glaser, through his influence in exciting a

*The quote is from the monumental work, *On Growth and Form* (Cambridge University Press, 1917), by the Scottish mathematical biologist D'Arcy Wentworth Thompson.

passion for the life sciences, had provided the final lynchpin that set Charles Drew on the path to becoming a physician.

That spring also saw what seemed to be Drew's final season of intercollegiate—even competitive—athletics. Of course, he was now captain of the track team and expected to lead, not only by example. Unfortunately, injuries to other athletes would have a detrimental effect on the team's success.

On Saturday, May 8, Coach Nelligan's squad traveled to Williamstown to take on their rivals from Williams College. Anticipation for this meet was, as usual, high, and the local papers met the demand for information: "Capt. Charley Drew, college record holder in the high hurdles, stands as sure winner in this event over the Williams field, and on a good track has a chance of at least equaling his former mark. Drew also looms as a sure first place winner in the high jump."[59]

The pressure of expectations did not affect Drew as he lived up to the lofty predictions of the journalists, but Williams emerged victorious in the dual meet,

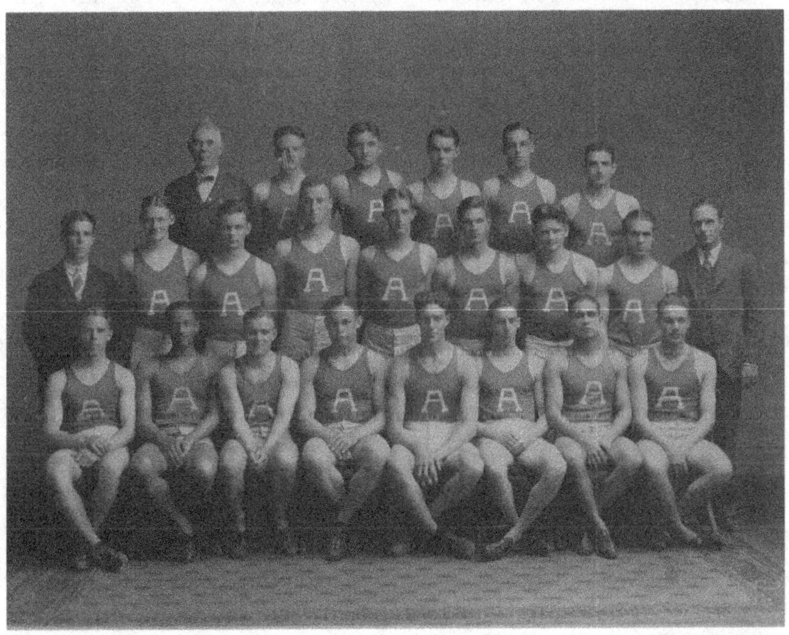

Figure 3.4 The 1925 Amherst track team. Drew is bottom row, fourth from left. Coach R.F. Nelligan is top row, far left. William H. Hastie is bottom row, second from left; W. Montague Cobb is bottom row, second from right. Personal collection, Charlene Drew Jarvis.

a disappointing outcome that would be uncomfortably common that season for the Lord Jeffs. Amherst eventually finished with a losing record, although Charlie performed to his usual standards, showing as the team's high scorer at every contest and winning events at both dual meets and the annual NEIAA grand gathering in Boston. He also won the intrasquad pentathlon for the fourth consecutive year. On the Harvard track at Cambridge, in his final competition while a college student, Drew dominated what had become his favorite (and best) event, the 120-yard-high hurdles, setting the Amherst school record.[60]

Final exams came a few weeks later. Although Drew's grade in French 2, another D, demonstrated that this was not a language he was likely to continue to embrace after college, he performed very well in Glaser's biology classes, earning a B for Biology 4 and an outstanding score of A for Biology 8 with his "Growth" paper. Organic Chemistry, notoriously a "weed-out" class for premedical majors with its complex symbols and carbon-based reactions, proved a struggle for Drew, who scored a D in this, too. For the third straight year he earned a C in German.[61]

Although his performance in the classroom was not stellar, he had passed every course and earned his degree of bachelor of arts. The graduation ceremonies were scheduled for the third week in June.

As the arrangements for commencement began to take shape, Charlie's classmates of 1926 composed a sort of *chanson de geste* for their esteemed friend and colleague by way of a profile for the *Olio* yearbook:

> Yes, this is Charlie Drew about whom you have heard so much, the terror of football opponents, the young ladies' delight, and the frank straight-forward lad in whom all mothers put their trust. Charlie's good nature is known wherever he is known, and that is over a rather extensive area vouch the Post Office clerks. Like a knight of old is our hero. His straight arm is the trusty lance that has battered the helm of many a foe. His ukelele is the melodious harp whose sweet lays accompanied by his own caroling conquer the stoniest heart. And Lizzie is the fleet steed which carries its knightly master in search of nightly adventure.[62]

Drew's parents made the long drive up from Virginia—one of their rare trips outside the Washington, DC, area—to see Charlie graduate. They brought along a carsick young Eva, too. It was a busy commencement weekend.[63]

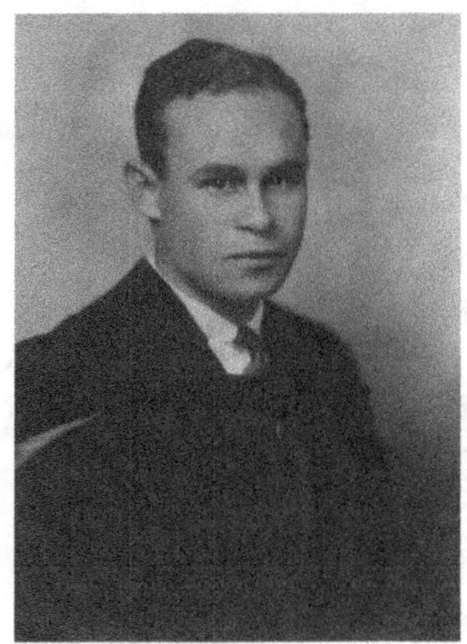

Figure 3.5 Amherst graduation portrait, spring 1926. Personal collection, Charlene Drew Jarvis.

On Friday, June 18, the graduating "26ers" had Class Day, an Amherst tradition. In the morning, they planted ivy at the College Church and listened to the class oration at College Hall. That afternoon there was a reception at the home of President George Olds (Drew's Mathematics 2 professor from his sophomore year, who had taken over when President Meiklejohn resigned in 1923) followed by a concert, senior service, and dancing, which stretched into the early morning hours.[64]

At the Alumni luncheon on Saturday, it was announced that the poet Robert Frost would be joining the Amherst faculty. Three cheers were given for John Jeffrey Archer Amherst, Viscount Holmesdale, a direct descendant of the town and college's original "Lord Jeff," who was on hand for the festivities. Finally George Pratt, an Amherst alumnus and member of the philanthropic family for whom the football field and gymnasium were named, announced that Charlie had been awarded the Howard Hill Mossman Trophy as the member of the Senior Class who brought "the greatest honor in athletics to his Alma Mater—the word honor to be interpreted as relating to achievement and sportsmanship."[65] By adding this large and impressive cup to his mantle Drew had made a clean sweep of the named athletic trophies at Amherst College.

The actual 105th Amherst College Commencement came at 10:30 A.M. on Monday, June 21, 1926, the first day of summer. After a prayer and rendition of "Memory Song to Amherst," followed by three valedictory speeches by top members of the class, the bachelor's and master's degrees were conferred. Ceremonies closed with a benediction and the singing of "The Soul of Old Amherst."

A song let us sing of the soul of old Amherst,
That soul deep and true, the Alumni well know;
'Tis not to be heard in loudness and clamor,

'Tis not to be seen in confusions of show;
The soul of old Amherst is loyal and tender,
For loved Alma Mater to guard her high fame
Her welfare to prize and staunch to defend her,
By honor and truth in the class and the game.[66]

Months before the words of the venerable Amherst hymn were echoing off the red brick walls of College Hall, Charles Drew, moved by the threefold inspirations of his sister Elsie's death, his experience with the medical system in treatment of his football injuries, and the brilliant, charismatic life scientist Otto Glaser, had resolved to pursue a career in medicine. He had also learned that doing so would present him with new challenges and daunting pitfalls, some of which—for the first time in his life—he could not conquer by surpassing talent or simple hard work.

4

A Chance to Shine

Baltimore, 1926–28

There was no money for medical school.

Despite the scholarship Drew had generously received from what was now his alma mater, he had always been on a shoestring budget while at Amherst. His parents had sent what support they could, but money was tight at the house in Arlington, too—even apart from the efforts to secure a top-flight education for their eldest son. In fact, Drew had been forced to take out student loans with the college, significant amounts that would take many years to pay off. The wherewithal for graduate professional school simply did not exist. There were other, more insidious barriers, too, but these were not yet factors.

Drew was aware of the lack of funds long before he donned the mortar board on the green at Amherst on June 21, 1926. Since he would not be dissuaded from the career path he had chosen, his solution had been to secure employment in the meantime and save what funds he could, hoping to apply for medical school in a year or, more likely, two. In fact, he had already found a position before leaving Amherst. A week before graduation Drew received a letter, along with a proposed contract, from the president of Morgan College, a Black school in Baltimore at which he had interviewed. He was offered a job as director of the physical education programs and would be expected to do some teaching in the classroom as well:

June 14, 1926
Mr. Charles Drew
Amherst College
Amherst, Mass.

My dear Mr. Drew:

Confirming our various conversations and your acceptance of position in Morgan College by wire, I am now placing in formal manner our agreement as per contract enclosed.

Kindly send me as soon as possible a good sharp cut photograph of yourself together with a brief sketch of your life, especially as related to athletics, in order that we may use the same in some publicity which we plan for the summer.

We are congratulating ourselves and the public in having you with us for the coming year and feel sure that if you will throw yourself heartily and enthusiastically into the work you will not only make a great reputation for yourself but will lay the foundation for a most successful career.

Of course, as noted in our conversation here, you will meet conditions vitally different from anything which you have experienced in your college life at Amherst. We must stress economy in our program and attempt much with small equipment and space. But you can adjust yourself and can go forward to success. In the social, literary and religious life of the campus we shall need your cooperation and it is here that your real self will be developed.

With best wishes,

J.O. Spencer
Morgan College

By action of the Board of Trustees of Morgan College you are hereby appointed Physical Director for young men in Morgan College and Academy from September 15, 1926 to June 15, 1927. You will receive a salary of two hundred ($200) per month, paid at the end of each calendar month. In addition to salary you will be given use of (a) room with heavy furniture, heat and light free. Board will be had in the school dining hall at cost of $16 per calendar month. Extra cost of board during training table will be met by the College.

> Your duties will be as follows: Act as director of physical training for the young men in general and coach the teams in all sports in vogue at the College. You will teach two classes in science in the Academy. . . .
>
> You will be a member in full standing of the faculty . . . You will be expected to lend your support to the out of class activities of the school such as social, literary and religious programs, as largely as may be possible.[1]

Two hundred dollars a month (about $3,500 in present day value) was nothing to sneeze at—for example, his parents' mortgage payment, as noted earlier, was $25 a month. Such an income would be enough to set aside some cash for medical school, while also helping his family and, of course, making his own way. As the summer of 1926 wound down, therefore, Drew accepted the offer and prepared to settle into the role outlined for him in President John Oakley Spencer's letter and contract.

The roots of Morgan College could be traced to the founding of the Centenary Biblical Institute of the Methodist Episcopal Church in the years immediately following the Civil War. The original mission of the institution was to train young African American men for the Methodist ministry, but in the ensuing decades this focus broadened to include the education of teachers, even women. In 1890 the school was renamed Morgan College (after a philanthropic trustee) and the scope of courses enlarged to a comprehensive curriculum. The institution moved to the site Drew would know (which it still occupies) in 1917, an upgrade funded by the ongoing benevolence of the aged robber baron, Andrew Carnegie. Long after Drew's tenure the private college became state funded, at which time it acquired the name it has gone by since: Morgan State College.[2]

Before beginning a new—if temporary—life at Morgan, though, Drew had what appeared to be one last exclamation mark to add to his illustrious career as an amateur athlete. Although no longer associated with Amherst, he was eligible to compete at the national Amateur Athletic Union track meet as the finest track and field athletes in the country (including past and future Olympians) gathered in Philadelphia on July 3. Drew was part of an outfit affiliated with the Century Athletic Club of New York, an organization put together only the previous year to sponsor amateur African American athletes. Concentrating on just one event, Drew rocketed to victory in his favored

120-yard-high hurdles, nosing out a talented athlete named Harrison Flippin at the tape.[3] This triumph would give him the title "AAU champion" forever afterward.

The two classes Drew was assigned to teach at Morgan coincided well with his putative interest in medicine and some of his greater success in the classroom at Amherst—biology and chemistry. He held the rank of assistant professor and, like many new possessors of that academic rank, approached his nascent responsibilities with a combination of enthusiasm and angst. No such conflict applied to his efforts in the athletic realm, though—here he profited from having been tutored by two eventual legends in the coaching profession: E. B. Henderson and Tuss McLaughry. In the autumn of 1926, it certainly appeared that he would need the strength of their example.

The Morgan College Bears football team had, to put it mildly, a lackluster history. The outfit had tallied just one winning season so far in the century (in fairness, the school only started formally playing football in 1913). There were some years in which the Bears scored no points at all—*for the entire season*. Defeats by scores such as 69–0 and 85–0 were common, and in 1919 they were even beaten by Dunbar High School (during young Charlie's freshman year). Drew's predecessor, Coach Jim F. Law, had begun to make some inroads toward fielding a competent team, but there was no question that the new coach would have his work cut out for him.[4]

Only weeks past his twenty-second birthday, Drew was barely older than most of the seniors at Morgan. Surveying the students who came out for the squad, he could identify talented athletes among them: left end and sometime receiver Talmadge "Marse" Hill (playing his coach's old position), quarterback "Pinky" Clark, Captain Dick Thomas, and others were all capable men, if provided the proper instruction.[5] Unquestionably Drew himself was the finest player on the practice field, which must have provided him equal measures of amusement and frustration as the season unfolded.

The Morgan schedule for 1926 was brief by modern standards—just seven games. Since white schools would not play them, assembling a slate of opponents required determination and some creativity. The season opened on October 2nd with a home game against the Newark Athletic Club of Delaware. Drew's men scored a decisive win, 27–0. Although the opponent was not particularly formidable, this dominant score must have raised some eyebrows among the fans and onlookers. The following week saw an even more lopsided victory, 39–0 over the Bordentown Manual Training team from New Jersey. If Drew's men were feeling their oats, the next week's road trip to Charleston and a date with the West Virgina Collegiate Institute squad brought them back down to earth to the tune of a shutout defeat, 19–0. Over the next two weeks a home-and-home two-game series ensued with the Ward Athletic Club of Annapolis, Maryland—another improvisation required by the scarcity of potential opponents. Drew's boys took the first game on their home field, 27–0, but the score of the sequel is lost to history.[6]

The season wrapped up on Morgan's home field with November games versus Storer College and the Lions of Lincoln University, a rival. In the school newspaper, the *Morganite*, several of the players previewed this clash, among them Captain Thomas, who noted that "the Coach has struggled hard on the problem of 'The Superiority of Execution,' which will be the greatest factor against Lincoln." Talmadge Hill went further, pledging in colorful language that "I shall do all in my power to smear all end runs, stop all slashing backs, and rip up all interference before it forms. In brief, I shall give my best and then some in a supreme effort to reduce the mighty roar of the Lions to the low bleating of a lamb."[7]

Unfortunately, the fiery bluster went for naught as the Bears lost to the Lincoln Lions in a hard-fought struggle, 9–6.

In the same issue of the *Morganite* that previewed the Lincoln game, Drew was accorded four columns for a lengthy essay in which he dwelt, with observations often applicable even to the present day, on the meaning of college football to the community at large as well as its impact on the students, faculty, and alumni of an institution. The baroque compositional style he developed at Amherst had not been fully exorcised by this time, although the imagery employed was undeniably engaging, and even cinematic:

> The autumn sun again beams down, striving with radiant countenance to beguile the bleak north wind with its chattering jaws into lands far removed for a few more days. All over the country surging throngs are making weekly pilgrimages toward some appallingly monstrous stadium or less elaborate edifice or merely place to see the greatest of college games, football.
>
> From great distances the grads come, some but recently departed from the glorious life of college, others bent with the weight of years, their white hairs

adding a touch of sobriety and dignity to the occasion, but their hearts like the hearts of the young ones are full of expectation, their minds turned to thoughts of days gone by. For a short moment their youth is survived by this flood of fond reminiscences and youthful enthusiasm.

At their journey's end there is to greet them the exuberant, victory-seeking band of undergraduates, with their white bedecked, exhorting their followers to get behind "that team," show some pep and help "those boys" win "the old game."

A sudden hush—then a great spontaneous shout and the main cause for this great and motley gathering puts in its appearance.

Twenty-two young men, nearly perfect physical specimens of the human race, red blooded and wide awake.

The show is on. Staid old matrons lose their austere dignity and applaud and cheer with an abandonment that surprises themselves; arrogant captains of industry and learned professors elbowed by a jostling, happy crowd bind themselves unconsciously in a close brotherhood of emotions with the man of the ditch peeping through the gate and the street urchin perched in the tree outside. There is a spirit of united purpose on each side of the field and most of the crowd is cheerful and happy. This fact alone should in some small manner justify college athletics. It has been said that a poem is worthwhile if it contains one needed message or one beautiful thought. If this be so, and if, as some philosophers think, happiness is the ultimate goal of all human endeavor, then, anything that stands to increase the amount of happiness in the world, fosters a spirit of cooperation, or united purpose, and a bond of common brotherhood must have some virtue, some intrinsic worth. This college athletics in a small way does. It is for a continuous state of affairs such as this that the great souls in the world strive.

This, I realized, is not the usual or orthodox method of discussing athletics. What we are accustomed to hear is the uproar from the battle between the financial fanatics who are looking for big profits, large scale production, and the best buy in so-called amateur athletics and the super intellectual morons who think that the colleges are going to the dogs because their teams draw such crowds when a lecture on some prehistoric fossil remain, or something of the sort, draws only a meager handful.

But let us confine ourselves at present to the college athlete himself; his attitude toward his school and work, and the benefits he made derive from athletics.[8]

Drew went on to discuss, from his unique perspective, the role of athletics in the present and future lives of the student-athlete, revealing what the years on the playing fields of Dunbar and Amherst had wrought in his own psyche:

> A college athlete should be made to meet all the curricula requirements of his school just as rigidly as his less versatile fellow student. He should be in the truest sense of the word an amateur athlete, playing the game for the love of playing and for the honor of his alma mater. A man playing under such conditions with the sportsmanlike spirit of the true amateur is far more likely to keep unsullied the name and traditions of the institution he represents and keep the game on a high plane than one who plays because he is paid to do so and has no scholastic or sentimental obligations to meet which are worth mentioning.
>
> College athletics are to me a means, not an end in itself, for considering it as an end or ultimate goal in itself, even when a boy is the idol of the school and the hero of myriad hosts of rabid fans, he shall have profiteth himself very little if he goes no farther nor makes what he has acquired in his battles of play serve him in battles of life when his college days are over.
>
> Those who take part in athletics have a wonderful chance for physical development at a time when it will do them most good. Their growing period is about over or had advanced far enough not to weaken or stunt them when forced to train hard for long periods of time. Their training as a rule is done under the instruction of efficient men, they themselves being well schooled in theory and practice. No idiot ever has his name flashed across newspapers as a great college athlete. It takes brains to win most anything and all college teams strive to win. The man who has not the head can't stand the grade, though he may have the courage of a lion and the strength of a bull. This physical development and training is great. Anything that makes a fellow think and think fast and accurately is surely of some value, but these to my mind pale in comparison to the test that competitive college athletics give a man's character, his very soul.
>
> Here, early in life, in play he becomes accustomed to meeting all kinds of odds, and overcoming them, if he is made of the right stuff. Here he has to subordinate self for the good of the whole team. Here he learns to keep plugging away, to give more than he has, when his body is worn out and every move is pain. In the throes of impending defeat, in agony of a losing battle he learns to fight and fight till the end, with nothing to drive him but his own indomitable will that says, fight

> on, and the knowledge that others have fought the same battles and won. Such a test tries a man's mettle, and if he survives the battle and comes out "bloody but unbowed" a new world of confidence will be born for that man and this confidence will give him faith enough in himself to face the problems in the battle of life with the firm belief that he has the stuff to see it through. If he has got all the benefits from his college athletics that they had to offer, and has passed their stringent tests, he should be able to leave college with a sound, ready brain, a well developed body and a faith in himself acquired through previous struggles to meet life as he finds it and dare to live it.
>
> On the other hand the man who is physically and mentally fit to play at games, yet fails to make good when put under fire, knows himself for the coward and laggard that he is. Some hope lies in this knowledge. Maybe the yellow streak can be purged in time by real red blood. I do not say that the fellow who does not engage in this killing competitive life lacks any of the finer qualities of manhood or possibilities of heroic action in the case of emergencies; what I do say is that we cannot guarantee these untested goods. We can put our stamp on a man whom we have seen go through the fire and come out more glorious for his having gone through, strong and clean and true like bright new steel. The tragedy of athletics, like that of most other things in college, is that so many are just exposed to it, sip but lightly and delve no further, thereby failing to get much that is to be had for the taking.[9]

Drew's *Morganite* essay captured the attention of African American news editors, and the second part was syndicated into Black papers across the country.*

The autumn of 1926 had proven to be a tumultuous one for the beleaguered Morgan College Bears, but when the dust settled at Thanksgiving, Drew's "Eleven" had notched what had been, up to this point, a rarity for the team: a winning season. Although the players and their fans could not have known it, the tide had turned for the team from Baltimore's African American college. Expectations of defeat on the gridiron would soon be a thing of the past.

---

* One of the most important of the Black American papers was the local *Baltimore Afro-American*, which was established in 1892 and is still in publication. During this era the Associated Negro Press, a global news service based in Chicago, provided stories and other items to more than 150 Black publications.

No sooner did the football season end than basketball commenced. Although Drew had not played the sport (except intramurally) while at Amherst, he had the advantage of having learned at Dunbar at the figurative feet of E. B. Henderson, a consummate instructor with deep understanding of the game. Several members of the gridiron squad, known commodities to Drew, went out for the basketball team, too—"Marse" Hill and "Pinky" Jones among them.

One of the first contests of the season was against Drew's hometown school, Howard University, in Washington. Two thousand fans filled the stands of Howard's newly opened gymnasium on the evening of Saturday, January 8, 1927, hoping to see the home team vanquish the Baltimore visitors. Morgan's standout center, "Lanky" Jones, hit the first basket. After that, a newspaper reporter wrote, "the game was hard and fast." Howard struggled against the tough, disciplined defense Drew put on the court. The score was tied at the half, but Morgan pulled away after the intermission and finished on top, 24–19. The reporter noted, "It was hard to pick the star man on Morgan's team as they played in a unit with clever passing in working the ball to the basket."[10]

Coach Henderson would have been proud.*

The Morgan College basketball team under Drew went on to a spectacularly successful, undefeated 1927 season. One African American newspaper, the *Pittsburgh Courier*, which named "mythical" national champions among the Black college athletic programs, called the Bears "the class of big college teams" and awarded them the unofficial national title.[11]

Things quieted down some for Drew in the spring. Although he had physical education classes to supervise and, of course, lectures to give in biology and chemistry, Morgan College had no baseball or track teams. Lack of the latter was a particular disappointment for Drew since he had much to offer as a coach. He hoped to lay the foundations for these sports, although he realized that his time at the school was limited due to his own plans.

Drew filled what little leisure time that arose with constructive entertainments. According to his long-time friend and colleague, W. Montague Cobb, Drew began a flirtation with the saxophone during his time in Baltimore, "practicing

---

*Henderson was still working in physical education in the Washington, DC, schools at this time and may well have been in attendance.

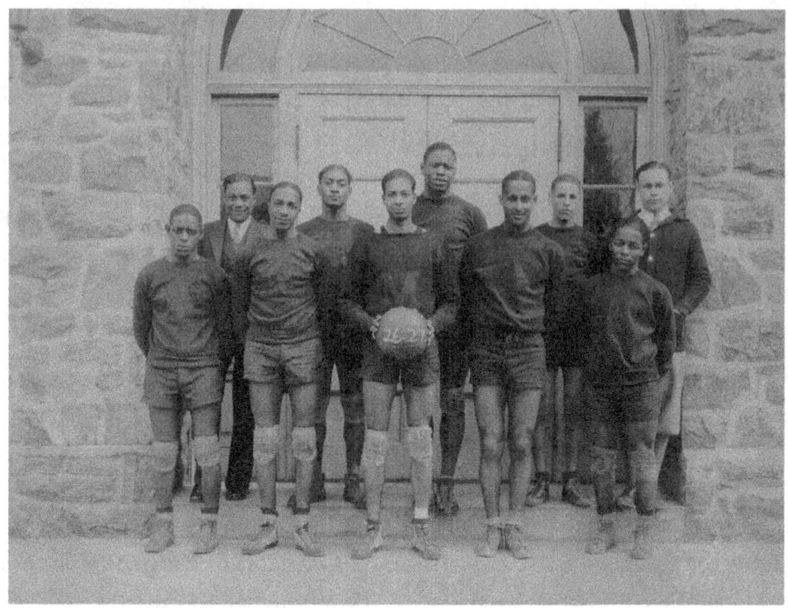

Figure 4.1 Drew as coach of the 1926-7 Morgan College basketball team. Personal collection, Charlene Drew Jarvis.

on a battered second-hand instrument from which he claimed he produced musical tones."[12] It was also during this period that he cowrote the hymn "Omega Dear" for his college fraternity, Omega Psi Phi. W. Mercer Cook, his friend from Dunbar High School and Amherst, wrote the music and first lyrical stanza while Drew penned the last two measures.[13] This piece soon became the official hymn of Omega Psi Phi across the nation:

Omega Dear, we are thy own
Thou Art our Life, our Love, our Home,
We'll Sing Thy praises far and nigh
We love Omega Psi Phi.
To all thy precepts make us true;
Live Nobly as all real men do;
Let manhood be our eternal shrine;
With faith in God and Heart and Mind.
Through days of joy or years of pain;

To Serve thee e'er will be our aim;
And when we say our last goodbye;
We'll love Omega Psi Phi.[14]

During his time at Amherst, Drew had struck up a friendship with a young lady from nearby Springfield, Massachusetts, named Lelia Waller. Intelligent and athletic, at age seventeen "Lee" was finishing high school when Drew graduated from college. She was the daughter of the Reverend Garnett Russell Waller, who was pastor of Springfield's Third Baptist Church.

Reverend Waller had a national profile, having grown the Trinity Baptist Church—ironically in Baltimore, where Lelia was born—into a major force in the community. Along with W. E. B. DuBois and other luminaries, he also was one of the "original twenty-nine" members of the Niagara Movement, a foundational organization in the Civil Rights efforts of the twentieth century. The National Association for the Advancement of Colored People (NAACP) was one of the first direct fruits of the Niagara group, and Reverend Waller was made national vice president in 1912.

How Drew and Lelia Waller crossed paths is not known, but surviving correspondence from the young lady composed in 1927 indicates that their friendship was a close one, at least from her perspective:

Darling darling—

I want so to see you—and tell you how much I care
"bushels" seems too childish
"loads" and "heaps" are trite
"with all my heart" is too prosaic
Nothing seems quite right
Perhaps if you would open wide
Your arms and hold me close
And kiss me
You'd know, don't you suppose?

What do you think about girls smoking? Almost everyone wants to know what you think. And I have meant to ask you before. All the girls I go with in school smoke. . . . I do once in a while, mainly to show off, as I don't enjoy it. My family would die if they knew, but what they don't know of things like that, won't hurt them. They object on moral grounds. Personally, I don't think that enters into that at all. Physical grounds are the main things. I know pretty well my own limits by now, so I'm not likely to harm myself by smoking.

It would be foolish for either of us to say that we would love each other until death do us part for, as you say, we don't know that now - perhaps we may never know it, but there are two things that I can do - one, to pray that we will . . . two, to never forget that I have loved - I do love you. Crushes I have had before, many of them - but never before have I loved anyone dear. Please send my best regards to your mother and dad.

Lee

Dear Charley

It's raining out and it's cool and damp. . . . The skies are gray. . . . But what do I care! I'm about the happiest person for miles and miles around and nothing but blue skies do I see.

I got your sweet long letter this morning. It's been a mighty long time since I've seen that big strong scroll and every time I do see it my heart just pounds and leaps and bounds (is that why you don't let me see it more often?) Thanks awfully for the snaps the one of you is sweet. You look just as if you were going to step straight out off the step and say hello Lee.[15]

Whether due to her youth, his burgeoning ambition, or other reasons, the relationship between Charles Drew and Lelia Waller was not destined to blossom, and they went their separate ways.[16]

School holidays during the summer and Christmas seasons were an opportunity for Charles to return to Washington to visit his friends and family, although other responsibilities were never far removed. In December of 1927, for example, while home for Christmas, he accepted an invitation to speak before a crowd of two hundred at a special fathers and sons banquet in the familiar setting of the Twelfth Street YMCA.[17]

During the more extended warm-weather breaks Drew made the most of his time at home, helping out with improvements to the house and yard and earning some extra money as a lifeguard at the little segregated swimming pools around their old Foggy Bottom neighborhood.

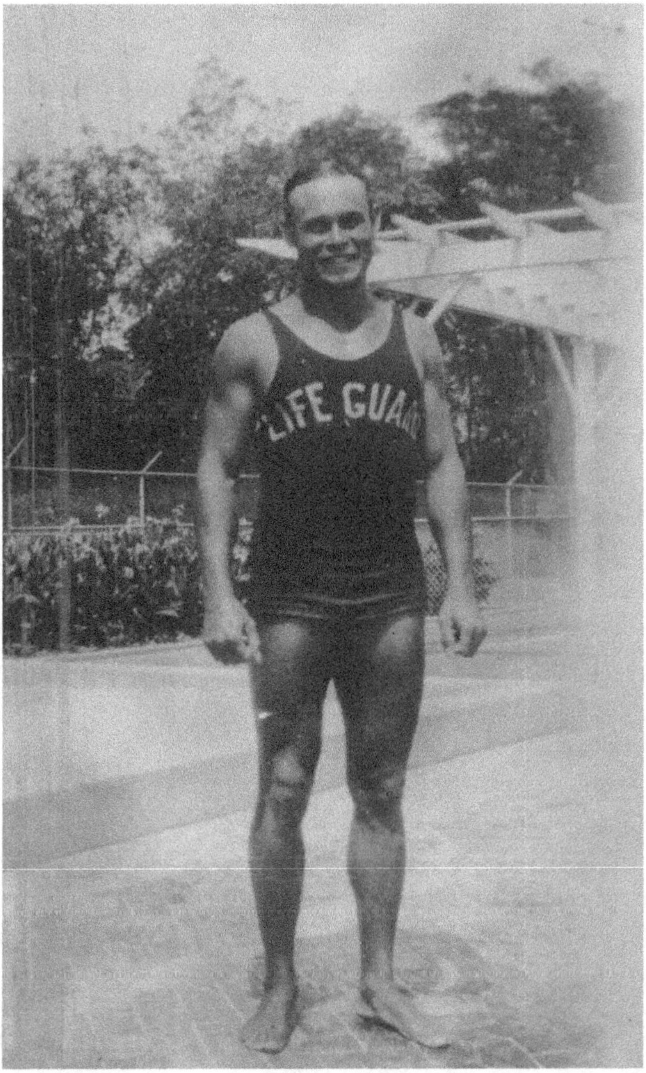

Figure 4.2 Drew as a lifeguard on summer break. Personal collection, Charlene Drew Jarvis.

When Charlie returned to the Morgan College campus in Baltimore for the 1927 fall session, there was excitement in the air regarding the Bears football team, akin to that seen on the Amherst campus two years before, and for similar reasons. The nucleus of what had gelled as a formidable squad by the end of the previous year returned for Coach Drew's second season, and onlookers were eager to see how they would fare.

Things started with a bang on October 8 as the home-field Bears drubbed Pennsylvania's Cheyney Training School by the sort of score they had once endured on the losing end, 57–0. "Pinky Clark" and other stars thrilled the crowd as they "passed and ran at will around and through the Pennsylvanians' defense."[18] By the second quarter Drew substituted his whole second string, which demonstrated scarcely any drop-off from the starters in completing Cheyney's demolition.

A trip to New Jersey the following week resulted in another blowout victory for Morgan, 40–7 over the Bordentown School. On October 22 Drew's team faced Annapolis Athletic Club and came away with one more lopsided win, 32–3. All eyes were then focused on the next date on the schedule, October 28, and a rematch with the only team that decisively handled Drew's men the previous year, the West Virginia Collegiate Institute. On an unseasonably warm Baltimore autumn afternoon, with temperatures reaching the 70s, 1,500 spectators watched the Morgan squad battle evenly for four grueling quarters with its nemesis from the west. The game ended in a scoreless tie.[19] The following week the Bears traveled to Harper's Ferry to take on the Storer College Golden Tornado. Although trailing the whole game, the Morgan team was able to eke out another tie, this time 13–13, behind a late long run by Clark.[20] On November 19 the still-unbeaten Bears traveled south to battle Howard University in Washington, DC. Unfortunately, this homecoming for Coach Drew was an unhappy affair, at least on the gridiron, as Morgan suffered its first defeat in the year's final contest, 26–6.

In the spring of 1928, in adherence to his original plan coming out of Amherst, Drew turned his attention toward applying for medical school. His commitment to this objective was so strong that the young faculty member took the somewhat treacherous step of resigning his position at Morgan College before securing a spot in a medical school.

The *Baltimore Afro-American* revealed the news in headline form on a June sports page:

DREW RESIGNS
Morgan Coach Gives Up Job To Study Medicine
Former Amherst Track and Field Star Quits This Month

Looking back on his two years in Baltimore, the outgoing coach summarized his achievements and encouraged the gathering fans to continue their newfound support of Morgan's athletic endeavors:

I came direct from Amhurst as a student to Morgan as a teacher and coach; very naturally, there were a great number of things that I might have known which I was entirely ignorant of, yet all of my unlearned efforts were met with and sustained by patience and kindness on the part of the administration, my colleagues, the students, and the people of the city as a whole. For this, I am thankful. So far as I know, I have made nothing but friends; it's always with a feeling of regret, a little mixed with sorrow that we leave friends.

Morgan had good material when I came, some of her athletes now are as brilliant as any that I have known. My part was to give this brilliance a chance to shine where it would count most, that is in big collegiate competition. This to some extent has been accomplished. Next fall the football season opens in Petersburg on October 6. On October 20. The team plays Charleston. On the 27th the national champs, Bluefield, will make their appearance in Baltimore, followed in quick succession by Storer, Lincoln, and Howard. These are good names, and the people will have no excuse for not turning out with the alibi of previous times that the games were not worthwhile.

Few losses of men

Morgan's team for next year remains practically intact, led by Captain Dick Thomas, and with a nucleus of two seniors, 11 juniors and 14 sophomores, it should make itself felt throughout the season.

Basketball

The basketball team loses two men in Hill and Sheffey. Men have been trained to fill their places, and the team should go forth to its fourth collegiate title. The schedule includes as home games, Bluefield, West Virginia, Institute, Virginia Seminary, Morehouse, Wilberforce, Howard, and Lincoln.

Much expansion

Under Coach Drew's direction, athletics of Morgan have attracted nationwide attention, and due to his program of expansion, Morgan has made somewhat of a start in baseball and track. Due to the shortage of athletic funds, spring athletic activities were brought to a premature close this year, but with the realization of the crusade drive, adequate funds should be available for a furtherance of a greater athletic program at the school.

Championships

Morgan's football team came up practical obscurity to a prominent place in the collegiate horizon and proved no set up. The basketball team won national honors by carrying off three collegiate crowns. Limited funds forced Coach Drew to curtail his pet activity, track, but much interest was stimulated by him in that bridge of sport during his two-year sojourn.

He has not yet decided just what school he will attend next year.[21]

Although correct in its succinct particulars, the last sentence of the article failed to capture the spirit of the actual story. There is a venerable saying in medical education circles that, as far as the prospective trainee is concerned, "it is not where you want to go, it is who wants you." Drew's first choice for medical school was Howard University in Washington, DC.

The attractions of Howard were obvious: it was in his hometown, and he could be close to his tightly knit family, perhaps even stay at the Arlington house. Not only would this cut down on expenses but it would also allow him to help with chores, odd jobs, and so forth. After all, his father, Richard, the undisputed man of the house, was getting up in years (he would turn fifty in August).

On top of this was another practical advantage: Howard was one of only two medical schools in the United States committed to educating Black physicians (the other was Meharry Medical College in Nashville, Tennessee). The match seemed tailor-made: local boy returns from major successes at colleges

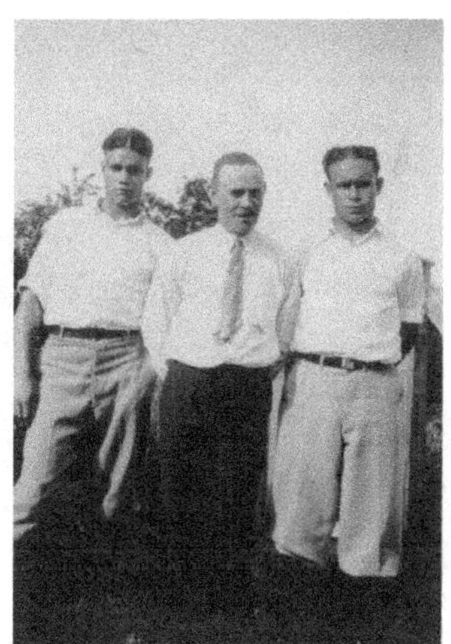

Figure 4.3 The Drew men, late 1920s: Charlie with his brother Joe and father Richard. Personal collection, Charlene Drew Jarvis.

far afield to become a doctor at the hometown school, one that will admit him without reservations as an African American.

Thus, it came as a devastating shock to everyone when Charles was denied admission to the Howard University School of Medicine.

It was at this juncture that Drew's lack of English credits from college came back to haunt him. Howard's rejection of his medical school application was not based on his college grades, his highly successful two-year stint as a coach and instructor at Morgan College, or any question about his character, but was based, ostensibly, on policy alone. There was a requirement, evidently unbending, for candidates to have completed at least eight hours of undergraduate English. Although Drew's Amherst freshman English class was a year-long one, it only met twice a week and so yielded just four credit hours on the college's scale. There was never any question about the quality of the instruction; as Joseph Drew observed with likely accuracy in that era, "One year of English at Amherst was probably worth two at Howard."[22] But nothing of that sort mattered: he did not have the hours and that was that. Brother Joe also remembered the anger that Charles expressed at this rebuff, pledging that one day he would "come back here and run the damned place."[23]

Before that could happen, Drew needed to find another medical school. Being forced to cast his net wider, one fish he hoped to catch swam in the familiar waters of Cambridge, Massachusetts, where many of Drew's collegiate track highlights had taken place. Harvard Medical School was known to accept the occasional Black student, why not Charles Drew? He evidently contacted the school sometime before June 1928, but whether Drew actually applied is unclear. The existing communication from Harvard is, however, unequivocal.

Harvard University Medical School
Boston 17, Massachusetts
June 4, 1928
Mr. Charles R. Drew, Director
Morgan College
Hillen Road and Arlington Avenue
Baltimore, Maryland.

My dear Mr. Drew,

I am sorry to say your earlier letter cannot be found and I am sending you a catalogue under separate cover, and am enclosing an application blank. However, the class has already been chosen and there is quite a long waiting list, so there is probably very little chance that you could be considered.

Yours very truly,

Louisa C. Richardson
Secretary[24]

This terse letter made it clear that, at best, Drew might have a chance at joining the Harvard class entering in 1929, but there was certainly no guarantee that he would be accepted. The specter of delaying his medical education yet another year under such circumstances, while he might save a bit more money to defray the inevitable costs, was too high a price. In any case, his resignation from Morgan College rendered this an untenable alternative; he had closed that door himself.

In the meantime, having rejected Drew as a medical student, Howard University reached out to him from its athletic department. A cryptic letter from Edwin Porter Davis, a professor of languages who doubled as the school's athletic director, read thus:

Board of Athletic Control
Howard University
Washington, DC
July 30, 1928
Mr. Charles Drew

Box 326
Rosslyn, Va.

Dear Mr. Drew:

Please call to see me in Room 314, Main Building, Howard University, on Wednesday or Thursday, August 1 or 2, between 11:00 A.M. and 1:00 P.M. on a matter that may be of interest to you. If it is not possible for you to call in person, please telephone Columbia 8100 for an engagement.

Yours truly,

E.P. Davis
Chairman[25]

What business Davis and the Howard University Board of Athletic Control had with Drew is not mentioned, but family members confirmed in later years that he was being considered by his hometown institution for a faculty coaching position (evidently, with regard to their opinion of him as an athletic instructor, the sound defeat Drew's Morgan basketball team had placed on the Howard "five" outweighed the reverse outcome in football). The irony of his lack of English hours being an obstacle to joining Howard as a student but not as a faculty member was not lost on Drew, but in any case, he was no more inclined to continue as a sports coach in Washington, DC, than he was in Baltimore. He had resolved to go to medical school, and now was the time. But would he be accepted, and where? As he returned to the family home in Arlington that June, the anxiety felt by Drew must have been acute.

Sometime during the summer, he received an envelope with a return address in Canada.

The events that led to Charles Drew's matriculation at the McGill Faculty of Medicine in Montreal comprise some of the enduring mysteries of his life. The impetus for his application is as unclear as the circumstances of the school's acceptance of it. Biographical materials dating from Drew's lifetime up to the present day have suggested or even flatly stated that a less stringent racial admission policy existed for the Canadian school than for those in the United States and that knowledge of this drove the young man's interest. As an example, in her excellent book, *One Blood: The Death and Resurrection of Charles*

Drew, the late author and social scientist Spencie Love states that Drew applied to McGill because the school "had a decent record of enrolling black students and treating them fairly."[26] Love provides no citation for this assertion, but if it were true, it would obviously explain Drew's rationale in applying to the far-off university in Quebec.

However, existing documents reveal that very few Black medical students were admitted to the McGill classes of the 1920s and 1930s, and these were mostly from other British Commonwealth sites in the Caribbean (British West Indies) such as Jamaica, Barbados, and Trinidad. Moreover, the number of Blacks was not significantly greater than that of Harvard, Yale, or other similar US institutions that accepted one or two African American medical students each year. Only a few years before, in 1916, the Black Caribbean medical students at McGill had staged a formal protest against what they perceived as a racial quota system at the University. Although they were able to marshal the support of their own national governments in their efforts, these students made no headway with the school, probably because no *official* quota system was in place.[27] But that does not mean there were no limitations.

An important letter on the topic of racial quotas at McGill from around this time, addressed to University Counsel from the associate dean of the faculty of medicine J. C. Simpson, can be found in the University Archives. Although primarily a discussion of admission policies regarding Jews, the letter also broaches the subject of Black candidates:

> 14th January, 1938
> L.W. Douglas, Esq., B.A., LL.D.,
> Principal, McGill University
>
> Dear Mr. Douglas,
>
> I have received your memorandum of the 13th enclosing a letter from Mr. Walter Menaker, dated the 10th instant, which I am returning herewith.
>
> Mr. Menaker's contention that no American Jews are admitted to our Faculty of Medicine is not supported by the facts, since there are at present three (I believe there are four, but am not quite sure of the race in one case) American Jews registered with us. As each year we receive some hundreds of applications from

> Jews resident in the United States, the acceptance of only four in the last five years might, of course, seem like a policy of exclusion.
>
> We have never established a quota for Americans. Naturally, our first duty is toward Canadians, and we do give them some preference. We have always welcomed as many Americans as we have had places for. In the present freshman class, we accepted 38 out of a total of 104, that is, about 37%.
>
> Some years ago, after consulting many Jewish students and graduates and several prominent Jewish citizens of Montreal, we decided that we would keep about eight places a year for Jewish students. In view of the population ratio, and of the difficulty that Jews have in securing hospital internships, our Jewish friends thought that this was a generous quota. We have never fallen below this number; usually we have ten.
>
> I would like to point out that this decision was a purely administrative one, and was never brought to the attention of either the Faculty or Senate. . . .
>
> . . . For your information, I might add that the only other apparent discrimination against Americans is in respect to the negro. Because of hospital restrictions, particularly in obstetrics and gynaecology, we can take very few negroes. Feeling that our first duty is toward those of British extraction, we generally refuse the American negro, though, here again, we occasionally make exceptions.[28]

Simpson went on to cite the example of Drew, whom he had personally taught and even financially supported. At the time of the letter Drew was favorably advancing in his career.

All this serves to deepen the mystery of Drew's application to McGill. The influence of his graduation from the prestigious Amherst, irrespective of his grades, and his remarkable athletic record were key in his acceptance; enough to supersede the race-related administrative obstacles in place at McGill. Years later, John C. Mackenzie, then superintendent of Montreal General Hospital, noted in a recommendation letter for Drew that his race "was very fully discussed at the time of his appointment which was based on his outstanding undergraduate achievements both academic and in the field of sport."[29]

Drew, however, can hardly have anticipated this from his office in Baltimore or his home in Arlington in the summer of 1928. Perhaps the most likely explanation is that he applied to several medical schools, rejections (or even acceptances) from which became insignificant when he was offered a position in Montreal (of note, McGill's Faculty of Medicine did not have specific English admission requirements).

Whatever the circumstances were that led to Drew's matriculation at McGill, in the late summer of 1928 he was once again on a train headed north—this time, beyond the borders of his country—ready to begin the next chapter in what was already an extraordinary life.

5

Let the Rest of the World Go By

Montreal, 1928–35

In September of 1928 Drew arrived at the McGill University campus in Quebec, twenty-six sprawling acres in the shadow of Mont Royal that were a home to over three thousand students.

The school had been founded in 1821, the same year as Amherst College, with money and land left for the purpose by a wealthy local merchant of Scottish birth named James McGill. Legal wranglings delayed the opening of the institution until 1829, the same year the physicians of Montreal General Hospital "engrafted" their unchartered Montreal Medical Institute with the fledgling university to create the McGill Faculty of Medicine, the first faculty of Quebec's new university.[1]

Throughout the nineteenth century the medical school grew and modernized at a conservative pace, pushing into the increasingly scientific consideration of human health and disease that characterized medicine worldwide. Along the way, McGill produced many medical graduates of high achievement and renown. Unequivocally, the greatest of these was Sir William Osler.

A native of Ontario (then known as Canada West), Osler graduated with the McGill medical degree of MDCM (an abbreviation of the Latin, *Medicinae Doctorem et Chirurgiae Magistrum*, meaning "Doctor of Medicine and Master of Surgery") in 1872, then trained for two years with the great Rudolph

Virchow in Germany before returning to his alma mater as professor. He later joined the faculty of the University of Philadelphia before becoming the first physician-in-chief of the new Johns Hopkins Hospital in Baltimore in 1889. After his indispensable role in raising that institution to world-renowned greatness, Osler closed his career as Regius Professor of Medicine at the University of Oxford.

Osler inaugurated a host of innovations in medical education. He is credited with being the first to move such teaching from the lecture hall to the bedside, initiating didactic rounds on the ward and outpatient units, a methodology so ubiquitous today that it is difficult to conceive that it had a discrete origin. As he put it, "To study the phenomenon of disease without books is to sail an uncharted sea, while to study books without patients is not to go to sea at all."[2] Osler has also been credited with introducing the residency system in North America, a distinction that likely earned him few admirers from the ranks of medical trainees but proved of immense value over the years.

Osler was also one of the greatest diagnosticians of all time. Working in an era long predating sophisticated imaging modalities, he relied on an "incomparably thorough physical examination" and diligent history-taking to guide him to conclusions with a level of accuracy that often struck contemporaries as preternatural.

Among his many other interests and talents, Osler was a bibliophile as well as an important leader and advocate of medical libraries. If the reflected glory of Osler's achievements were not enough, McGill benefited incalculably from its greatest graduate's decision to bequeath his own personal library, consisting not only of up-to-date publications but historic medical books and artifacts of inestimable value, to the University upon his death in 1919. As Drew arrived in Montreal, McGill was basking in the honor and pride of the still-new Osler Library collection.

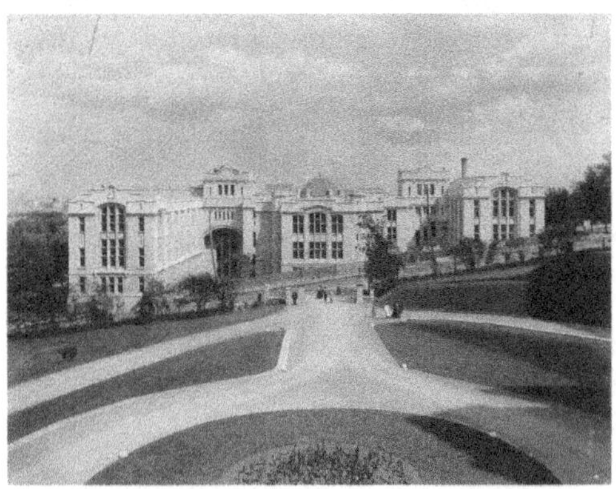

Figure 5.1 Strathcona Hall. Courtesy of McGill University Archives.

The Faculty of Medicine physical plant, comprising three large buildings of relatively recent vintage, was located on the edge of the main McGill campus. This proximity to the bulk of the university was convenient for administrative purposes but also fostered cooperation with the affiliated pure science departments such as biology and chemistry. The medical school structures were called the Medical Building, the Biological Building, and the Pathological Institute. All were in the northeast section of campus, adjacent to the Percival Molson Memorial athletic stadium. In the years to come Drew would become a familiar figure in all these places.

The main Medical Building, a magnificent, ornate edifice of Montreal limestone with an interior arrayed in oak and stained glass, was the oldest of the three, having opened in 1911 at the southwest corner of the broad thoroughfares University Street and Pine Avenue. Sometimes called the Strathcona Building after the landed benefactor whose generosity led to its construction, this colossus housed the administrative offices of the medical school as well as the departments of histology, hygiene, pharmacy, and anatomy (complete with a fifty-table dissecting room). This was also the site of a world-class medical museum, along with the medical library, where the great Osler collection was held.

Three hundred feet south, past the university greenhouse, was the Biological Building, only seven years old. This imposing, blocky structure housed the departments of botany, zoology, biochemistry, physiology, and pharmacology. A sculpted frog stood whimsically atop the McGill crest at the main entrance, apparently to confirm the identity of the nondescript structure to any confused students. A two-story Laboratory for Experimental Surgery was adjacent, connected to the Biological Building.

The most recent addition to the medical school campus was the Pathological Institute, completed in 1924 at the northwest corner of University and Pine. Nearly two hundred and fifty feet of facade greeted the street-side visitor, and the limestone edifice contained seemingly endless labs and offices, as well as the departments of pathology, bacteriology, and medical jurisprudence.

A tunnel beneath University Street, offering protection from both traffic and the often-harsh Quebec weather, connected this Pathological Institute with one of the main teaching hospitals of the university, the Royal Victoria Hospital.[3]

The course of instruction at the McGill University Faculty of Medicine was five years in length, with three ten-week terms each year—fall, winter, and spring (summers were, for the medical students, thirteen weeks of *les vacances*).

Most of the work of the first two years comprised subjects grouped together as the "First Division." This was similar to curricula of medical schools in the United States in that there was a focus on what were called (then as now) the "basic sciences": anatomy, physiology, biochemistry, bacteriology, and histology (the study of tissues). The final examinations for these subjects had to be successfully completed before the third year (seventh term) began. This was ostensibly when the medical student moved on to the Second Division, comprising pharmacology, pathology, and, in a departure from most American institutions, medical jurisprudence. These courses covered six terms or, if the student were on the standard schedule—some variations were permitted—up to the spring stanza of the third year.[4] It was required that the Second Division exams be passed before commencing the tenth term. The Third Division represented the long-awaited introduction to actual hospital ward work; it included seven terms in internal medicine and six in surgery, encompassing these fields in general as well as some of their branching subspecialties. To qualify for the final examinations in medicine, surgery, and obstetrics, the would-be graduating students were also required to complete courses and examinations in ophthalmology, otolaryngology, abnormal psychology and psychiatry, infectious diseases, anesthesia, and post-mortem examinations.

Grades were awarded in five categories. Honors level worked earned an A, "good" a B, and "fair" a C. The grade of D was reserved for a "doubtful" performance and, of course, F constituted "failure."

The total fee for the first year was $317 Canadian. This included $250 tuition, payable in two installments, one in September and one in February, $17 for a student union and athletic fee, $10 for a deposit euphemistically called "Caution Money," and $32 for a microscope. The microscope was actually $105, but this cost was divided into annual installments over the five years:

> Each student is required to provide himself, on beginning his studies, with a first-class microscope for laboratory and private study throughout his course. . . . Such an instrument will last a lifetime and is an essential part of the equipment of a practitioner in medicine.[5]

When it came to the cost of attendance at the McGill Faculty of Medicine, the university fees were, of course, only part of the story. Books were a separate—and considerable—expense, not to mention room and board. Generally, the full cost of a year was about $1,000, subject to the tastes and wherewithal of the student as well as the vagaries of the unexpected.

At this time there were no university residence halls for McGill medical students, although about sixty rooms were available at Strathcona Hall (a different structure from the medical building of the same name) courtesy of the Student Christian Association, which was headquartered there. Representatives from this organization regularly met new students who were strangers to the city on arrival and, if no room was available at Strathcona Hall, helped them find lodging elsewhere. Given the proximity of the school to the major metropolitan center of Montreal, plenty of private boarding houses or rooms were typically available for rent, the usual rate at this time being in the vicinity of $60 per month for room and board. Inexpensive board was also available at the McGill Union, which had a large dining room offering prepared meals and an *a la carte* lunch counter.[6]

After a brief but intense search, Drew was able to locate a room at 3580 Durocher Street, on the northern edge of the McGill campus. He wrote a letter to his father shortly after moving into the new address:

> Dear Pa,
>
> Just got settled at the above address. I'm living with a private family (ye goode ol Irish stock, by Jesus). The room is quite decent, front on the third floor next to the bathroom and she swears its warm in the winter, let's hope so for its cold as blazes here already.
>
> Frankly speaking, the going's going to be a bit hard. The school is in the most aristocratic part of the city and there is simply nothing cheap to be had anywhere. I walked for two whole days trying to find a room for less than $20 a month, most of them are $25 and $30. I pay $20. Board can be had for as little as $35 a month, but you see what that adds up to at a minimum $50 to $60 a month. Doesn't look so good does it? But that's not for us to worry about yet. I've got enough to make this year and maybe by that time I will have learned to turn a few tricks here. I always luck out.[7]

Time and circumstance would eventually throttle the confident optimism of the letter's final sentence.

Charles Drew's initiation into medical school and the First Division began with classes on Wednesday, September 19, 1928.

For generations, formal medical education has commenced for the new student in a sort of *rite de passage* with gross anatomy—the study of the structures of the human body that can be examined with the naked eye (as opposed to microscopic anatomy, for example). Drew's case at McGill was no exception.

The anatomy course covered all three terms of the first year and was divided between lecture sessions of three hours per week and laboratory dissections of fifteen hours (one less in the spring). The professor was an Englishman named Samuel Ernest Whitnall, and the texts were the venerable atlas *Grey's Anatomy* and Professor Whitnall's own dissection guide, *Study of Anatomy* (Whitnall was well known for his contributions to the study of the ocular orbit, where two structures named for him, the Whitnall Tubercle and Whitnall Ligament, can be found. He was also a humorist who published satirical medical student guides under the *nom de plume* Dr. Tingle). Whitnall was assisted by another Englishman, an associate professor named John Beattie, who was to play an important role in Drew's life years later.

Running in tandem with anatomy for the first two terms was histology, which also included the subject of embryology. This class, taught by Professor J. C. Simpson (who later composed the letter about Jewish and Black quotas cited above), met three hours per week, with an accompanying lab occupying seven additional hours.[8]

Drew related his feelings about the beginning of medical school and his classmates in the same letter to his father that described his new apartment:

> I started classes this morning. My class is 125 strong and most of them look like students, very, very few of the typical college looking fellows and they all seem as though they are here on business and the professors look that way, too—still, they haven't anything on me, if I ever meant business I mean it now.[9]

Although he professed dedication to his studies, Drew was not yet prepared to give up on the avocation that brought him the most satisfaction—not to mention renown. Barely two weeks into his medical school classes, he had the first opportunity to showcase his athletic talents in a Canadian venue at the annual Freshman-Sophomore intramural track-and-field meet held in the Molson Stadium at McGill on October 5. Freshmen medical students qualified the same as undergraduates, and at a fully mature twenty-four years of age Drew had no problem dominating the field.

A week later he demonstrated his prowess again in leading the Faculty of Medicine team to victory in the annual interfaculty track meet:

> Drew swept through to brilliant victories in both track and field, winning the high and broad jumps, the shot-put and the high hurdles. Drew, on his performance yesterday, should be a big point winner for McGill in the intercollegiate meet here next Friday, for in all four events none of the performances in the Varsity interfaculty meet measured up to Drew's sensational showing yesterday.[10]

Unlike in the United States, Canadian universities did not restrict intercollegiate athletic competition to undergraduates, which afforded Drew the opportunity to shine even more brightly in his new environs than he had at Amherst. He represented his new school in a victorious meet on October 19 against the University of Toronto (referred to as the "Varsity" in the article above) and Queen's University:

> Individual honors for the meet fell to Charlie Drew, former Amherst College track and football star, who did the expected by capturing the aggregate by a good margin.
>
> Drew swept through to take two first places and two seconds for a total of 16 points and shattered the only intercollegiate record to go by the boards during the afternoon. In the first event of the day, Drew started McGill off on the right foot by winning the 120 yards high hurdles in the record-smashing time of 14 4–5 seconds, two-fifths of a second better than the old mark set by Sid Pierce in 1923. Pierce, incidentally, sat in the stands and watched Drew smash the record without being extended, finishing yards ahead of the second-place man.[11]

Drew also triumphed in the shot put while finishing second in both the high and broad jump competitions as McGill won the Tait-Mackenzie Trophy as Canadian Intercollegiate track champions.

The local offshoot of American football, sometimes confusingly referred to as "rugby" despite obvious and significant differences from the old English game, was well-ensconced in the Canadian collegiate setting by this time, in fact dating as far back as the 1870s at McGill. Fan enthusiasm for the contests mirrored that at colleges in the United States, as well. Naturally, Drew's presence as a bona fide American college football star had fueled speculation in the autumn of 1928 that he might bring his considerable talents to the modified pitch for his new school, even before his scintillating track success. After Drew's show-stopping performances in the hurdles, shotput, and jumping events, rumors about the dominant young athlete took flight and even made it onto the sports pages of the *Montreal Gazette*:

DREW, McGILL TRACK ACE, MAY TURN OUT FOR SENIOR RUGBY

Star of Last Friday's Meet Was Picked on Second All-American Team in 1926

McGill rugbyists and rugby enthusiasts are not going to let Saturday's defeat crush their hopes for that title that has evaded them for nine long years. Although it was blue Monday at the stadium and all the footballers were enjoying their usual post-game holiday, the campus was buzzing with football gossip. . . .

The chief reason for the optimistic outlook was the news that Charlie Drew, star of last Friday's intercollegiate track meet, was seriously considering turning out for football. Drew's imposing record was the talk of the day. Besides being national junior hurdles champion of the States in 1925, Drew starred at football at Amherst College and in his final year was captain of the varsity team. Drew was picked that year for the second All American team and was rated as one of the best fullbacks in the east despite the fact that injuries kept him out of over half the games. . . .

If Drew decides to turn out with the red seniors, he will have two weeks' practice in which to accustom himself to the Canadian style of game before McGill goes into the next intercollegiate struggle, and he will also have the opportunity of playing in an exhibition contest to find his bearings under the strange code of rules. . . .

United States college football stars in the past have failed to cut very much of a figure under the Canadian code, and the history of the game is filled with

> stories of many that have failed and of few that have succeeded. Drew has this in his favor, that he is as fast as any man that has trod Canadian cinder paths, and he is a born athlete, both in physical build and mental makeup. These last adjuncts should stand him in good stead if he decided to turn out for the MGill senior team.[12]

Despite this fanfare, Drew eventually decided not to don the red McGill jersey for the school's varsity team, probably determining that the time commitment and risk of serious injury were too great. He did, however, contribute to the Faculty of Medicine's intramural rugby squad that fall, leading them to a league championship over McGill's agricultural college on November 14. In the process Drew gave his classmates a glimpse of the speed and strength that had graced the gridirons of autumn New England a few short years before:

> Medicine captured the Wood Cup, emblematic of the interfaculty rugby championship, when they swamped MacDonald College under a 22–3 score in the final played yesterday afternoon at Ste. Anne de Bellevue. . . . Drew three times raced thirty yards down the field, to put his team in scoring positions, taking the ball across the goal line himself for the second Medicine touchdown.[13]

That winter, to help make ends meet, Drew began to referee basketball games in the Montreal Basketball League. Later he would also officiate football games. These extracurricular efforts typically yielded five to ten dollars a week in extra money.

Thrilling and rewarding as athletics were for Drew, he fully grasped that the true business at hand was scholastic. As his freshman year in medical school began to gather momentum, the young expatriate, whose lifelong love of poetry rivaled his passion for music, took the unusual step of describing a typical day for his mother in the form of a verse:

> *This is the hour between supper and night, I allot to myself each day*
> *To forget the stiffs and books and things, a time for my mind to play,*
> *It's only a short while, but gee! how it helps to get one's self straight, you know,*
> *To look o'er the past, to peer just ahead, to muse at one's fate don't you know,*

Then you never can tell when you set your mind free, where it'll end
If it's just let alone—it may wander a while, maybe stray far away, but usually come back with a friend
Though you can't talk with the friend, nor feel the warm clasp of the hand,
Across the miles that lie between go thoughts that you both understand.
This hour is for peace, for rest and quiet—my dream hour of the day
In contrast extreme to the rush I'm in preparing for exams next May.
At 8 A.M. I sleepily arise with anatomy heating my head,
I stretch and yawn—then jump in my clothes—scattered around my bed
To clean my teeth and wash my face and work on this hair of mine,
Then a rush to grab a bite to eat and make that morn's class by nine.
From nine till one I cut and dig into some unfortunate fellow,
Who didn't die for this I know—but—by George this guy is mellow.
By that I mean he is ripe you know, in fact very mature to smell him,
But the poor cuss is doing the best he can, I'm grateful, but I can't tell him.
When the clock strikes one with my nostrils full, I go to fill my belly,
Now that doesn't sound nice, and it's not so nice, his fat's like scrambled jelly.
It runs and oozes over everything, its hard to keep anything neat,
But after standing four hours straight, what a man needs is meat.
It's a rush to dinner and a bigger rush back—Histology lab at two,
When you're given a slide you just and see (sic) and are told "You know what to do."
For the next two or three hours with my back in a cramp, I peer in a microscope,
And draw as I peer—things I ought to see—things that are there I hope.
From there to the track to take a workout, to keep in shape my big aim
But the track coach thinks with a little hard work, I'll add some fame to my name
Then a shower and rub until the skin glows—feeling pretty good again,
The grand old feeling I've known before but I'm getting too old for the game
Then I hike on down to the feed bag once more,—then home to my house of rest
My day is all good for I'm learning so much—but out of it this is the best.
It's the sweet hour—when I dream—make plans—sing—or just sit
And wonder how my little plans, full of hope, into the great plan will fit.
Today I have spent this dream hour with you, Mother mine, as many, many before
For me you are still the best sweetheart of all—the one whom I most adore.
You're smiling now—that sweet bright smile—that warms my heart clear through
Sounds like a school kid writing his girl, but I know that you know it's true.[14]

After McGill closed for Christmas break on December 19, Drew took the train on the long trip home to see his family. It was a time to catch up on all that had transpired among the family members, with Charlie—the favored son on an exhilarating academic adventure in a foreign land—inevitably in the spotlight. The Drews cherished these times together, and the festive and profound nature of the holiday only served to draw them closer in celebration.

Many years later Eva, the youngest child, recalled some of the efforts Charles and his brother made to capture the essence of the season for their family:

> No one on earth loved Christmas any more than my brothers. They would decorate the house with colorful lights, select the trees, decorate inside with pine and cedar branches. The house even smelled like Christmas. All in back of our house where Arlington Boulevard and Lyon Park are there were woods. Pine trees, cedar trees, hickory nut trees—all kinds of trees and ferns and mosses grew there. Each year the boys would take Papa's trusty hatchet or axe and make their pilgrimage to the woods to find the perfect tree. They felt each tree was prettier, greener, more fragrant than last year's.[15]

When histology ended after the winter session, its place on the first-year students' schedule was taken by an introductory course in physiology, six hours of lectures a week in the frog-adorned Biological Building from a renowned Scottish physician and scientist named Professor John Tait and his teaching staff.[16]

In the meantime, the full-year gross anatomy class continued. As the lectures and dissections unfolded at Strathcona, Drew became familiar with the course's assistant professor, John Beattie.

Like many of the faculty at McGill, Beattie hailed from Great Britain. He had graduated from Queen's College, Belfast, with the degree of MB, ChB, in 1923 and later received the MD and DSc from the same institution. From 1924 to 1927 Beattie worked with Professor Sir Grafton Elliot Smith, the world's leading expert on evolution of the brain, at University College, London. In 1927 he was appointed assistant professor of anatomy at McGill and would be promoted to associate professor in 1930.[17]

Judging from the papers Beattie published during his career—*Hypothalamic Mechanisms*, *The Neurology of Micturition*, *The Importance of Anomalies of the*

Superior Vena Cava in Man—his scientific interests within the realm of anatomy were many and varied. In a period to come, though, he would focus his attention on the field of blood physiology and fluid balance in health and disease—and a decade after their interaction as pupil and instructor, Drew and Beattie (who returned to England in 1934 to become conservator of the Hunterian Museum and director of research at the Royal College of Surgeons in London) would cross paths as scientific peers in important roles as leaders of their nation's efforts to procure blood for victims of the German Blitz.[18]

After successfully completing his final exams in May of 1929, Charlie Drew returned for the summer to the familiar environs of Washington, DC, and the family home in Arlington. The gigantic new segregated Francis Municipal Swimming Pool had opened at Twenty-Fifth and N streets near Rock Creek the previous summer, and Drew's old friend Monty Cobb, who was a student at Howard University Medical School, was the superintendent. Charlie had worked at this facility briefly before heading to McGill the previous autumn, and now, in the summer of '29, he found steady employment there as a manager, lifeguard, and swim coach—sharing some duties with his brother, Joseph. He made $160 a month and would continue this pleasant summer occupation for the next several years.[19] Cobb and the Drew brothers began to develop what would become a highly competitive Francis swim team this summer, dispatching a visiting squad from Baltimore, 60–10. Although neither Charles nor Joseph Drew swam in the races, they teamed up with Cobb to win the Water Polo event.[20]

When he returned to Montreal for his sophomore year in the Faculty of Medicine, Drew again took up residence in his room at 3580 Durocher Street, north of campus. This year he faced the remainder of the First Division subjects: the final two terms of the physiology course, the two-term series in biochemistry, and the single-term class in bacteriology. He would also have his first Second Division class, an introduction to pharmacology course.

The final two physiology courses, in the fall and winter terms, comprised three lecture sessions under Professor Tait with six hours of laboratory work per week. The autumn course focused on study of the nervous system, while the winter series concentrated on mammalian particulars. The two-term biochemistry course was four lecture hours per week from Professor J. B. Collip and his assistants, augmented by a daunting twelve hours of lab time. The first half of the course was an overview of the chemistry of "the products of the activities of living matter," while the second centered on digestion and nutrition. Readings came from Cameron's *A Textbook of Biochemistry*. Both physiology and biochemistry were conducted in the squarish Biological Building, which, charming door-frog aside, must have seemed a particularly tiresome quadrilateral by the end of winter term.[21]

Extracurricular activities afforded a welcome change of pace, not to mention surroundings. Picking up where he had left off the previous track season, Drew led the medicine club to a resounding win in the interfaculty meet at Molson Stadium on the warm and sun-drenched afternoon of Friday, October 11, 1929. He must have been stunned, however, to finish second in his signature 120-yard-high hurdles event (a man named Howie Baker from the Faculty of Commerce set a meet record in defeating Drew by inches). Wins in the high and broad jumps, combined with a second-place finish in the shot put, gave Drew 16 of his team's winning 51-point total.[22]

The following week in Toronto, the McGill track team lost the intercollegiate meet to the host squad despite a heroic effort by their star performer, who rebounded from his hiccup in the interfaculty meet to win the high hurdles as well as the long and broad jumps.[23]

Drew also returned to his sporadic employment as a referee for the Montreal amateur basketball leagues, earning a few extra dollars here and there. Money had always been an issue, of course; soon it would be on everyone's mind.

At the end of that portentous month of October 1929, in the financial capital of his home country some four hundred miles away, the stock market crash on the 29th—Wall Street's "Black Tuesday"—heralded the onset of the worldwide Great Depression, an economic calamity that would affect prince and pauper alike for the next decade. Among those who felt the deleterious financial impact were an already-struggling medical student in a nearby foreign country and his family back home.

Now in his early fifties, Richard Drew was slowing down some (Drew and his brother, now full-grown men themselves, had taken to calling him "Pop" or "Pa" instead of the former "Papa"). Most of the work he still did was with his old colleague Ericsson's outfit, laying carpet in private homes in Northern Virginia as well as the occasional theater or other public space in the District.

His income had been drifting down even before the advent of hard times; now that money was scarce for everyone, people were decidedly less interested in luxuries like new carpeting. Eva and Nora still lived at home. To top it off, Charlie's brother Joseph, who graduated from Dunbar High School in 1927, was now a student at Howard University, adding another tuition to the family's burden. Consequent to all this, the amount of financial support Charlie received in faraway Quebec trickled down to almost nothing. He felt it acutely.

McGill closed for Christmas break after lectures on December 21. It is not known if Drew took the train home to Arlington, but with funds so scarce, he probably remained in Canada over the holiday week, saving the train fare. He was certainly in Montreal on December 31, even though resumption of classes was still a week away. Given the importance the family placed on being together at the holiday season, it must have been extremely difficult for Drew to stay at school.

Indeed, New Year's Eve of 1929 was among the darkest times of Drew's life. Bereft of funds and friends—at least for the evening—he walked the cold, dark streets of cloudy Montreal numb and alone for hours with no destination. Finally, footsore and chilled to the bone, he retired after midnight to his room on Durocher Street and, while revelers celebrated all around the city, sat down in lonely silence to compose a melancholy letter, addressed (at its close) to the new year of 1930. As the words spilled onto the pages and the clock circled hour after hour, Drew revealed in startling candor the depths of depression that threatened to overwhelm him at this difficult juncture in his life. He clearly missed his close and supportive family, but there was more than homesickness at work. Wherever he turned, Drew could not escape the specter of poverty, and the pernicious tentacles that stretched from its bitter reality to choke nearly every endeavor he contemplated:

> 12:30 A.M. Jan. 1, 1930
>
> What a hell of a new year! As the year entered was paying the cashier at the Northeastern Lunch. Ten cents for tea and toast. I was cold from walking all over the city—looking for what? I don't know. Excitement maybe, trouble—most anything out of the ordinary just like the hordes I passed—some laughing young couples—they looked the happiest, other more elderly couples—out seeking a

return of the youth from which they had drawn away with the passage of days—days which had turned their temples grey and slowed their steps. Gay young fellows in bands and small groups, yelling, playing, making believe they're having a good time, men and boys drunk and puking all over the sidewalks—noise, taxicabs, streetcars, lights whistles—all a jumble, all moving crowds in front of the Theaters, a few quietly entering the churches,—a sign in one church "Where do us go from here" by Rev. Dr. somebody. I wonder? Wished the boy at the counter in the lunch room a happy new year, but expressed regret at being at that particular place just then. He returned my greeting with the rejoinder that it wasn't such a bad place. The Northeastern never jipped me; then he thought my bill was 15 cents. I corrected him—a few words—I paid a dime. That's how my new year started—with words over a nickel. All signs tend to point out that this whole year and few more right behind it will be spent in this way.

Today I have not been hungry, I was well dressed, I am not sick and have had no great sorrow yet I have felt poorly today as I have never felt it before. I have a dollar. Thought I wanted to join the merry making in some form or another so bad that my very heart ached. I couldn't go far on a dollar, not even alone, and solitude is the only thing I enjoy alone. But tonight I didn't want solitude, I wanted companions, gay companions, girls and fellows, music, laughter, food and soft words, maybe a stolen kiss in the middle of a dance when soft arms are around my neck, when my breath itself is drawn then the aroma of brown curly hair or any kind of hair that's soft to the touch and sweet smelling, when flickering lights of delicate hues play in the depths of brown eyes that have that merry twinkle in them that you believe is for you alone, or black eyes that intrigue, draw you into their depths but tell you nothing, holding you in the ecstasy of expectancy, or blue eyes, clear, appealing, like the angels must have, oh any kind of eyes that are kind, or mischievous or luring that look into your own and pause to linger awhile. My arms tonight should hold close to me some warm, vibrant body whose touch would thrill me and make me forget that a thousand miles lies between me and those dearest to me. No, but this cannot be so. I have a dollar—I am afraid to spend it—tomorrow I must eat and the day after, and many days after that. How? Who knows. For days now I haven't been sure whether I'd eat or not. Tomorrow I know I will because I've been invited to dinner but the next day? Yet I find no bitterness in me—just a touch of sadness, a sort of infinite yearning.[24]

In the pit of this despair, though, Drew recognized that there were others in worse circumstances throughout this foreign capital and around the world and found room for both understanding and charity for these forgotten souls. For his own part, pride and the need for independence prevented Drew from asking for financial assistance from friends or family. He would rather suffer than ask for help:

> But a smile always breaks thru. When beggars stop me I enjoy it, perhaps I feel the attachment of a brother, I smile I don't know why, perhaps because man is so vain and their assumption that I have money is such flattery that I can't resist the temptation to feel inflated. When prostitutes stop me I believe that the look or answer is kind, for they, like me, have nothing. I sympathize with them, perhaps even envy them that they have something to sell while I have nothing. Once from my virtuous pedestal of ignorance I hated prostitutes, had no place in my idealistic world for such persons, considered them lower than beasts, earths vilest and most despicable lot. I still fear prostitutes, fear them for the harm they might do my body that I have cherished and taken such good care of, but my scorn has turned to pity in most of their cases. Their crudeness, their dirt I still loath, but their souls I no longer damn. They have missed so much of life that is worthwhile, they have seen so much that isn't, they need so much. Their dreams, imaginations, hopes have either been taken from them or crushed, why not sell what they have left that is desirable to save the rest. Need is such a tough mistress. Today I got a card stating that there was a box for me in the post office. I didn't know what was in it. I didn't know what the duty would be. The day before Gladys had sent me a pair of bedroom slippers that cost $3.13 to get thru. It broke me, ruined my chances of having any fun tonight. I didn't have any money to get the package from my own family—yet I must get it or it would go back and they would know that something was wrong. Where to get it? That is the question. I never ask favors. It is one of the things I am proud of. Rightly or wrongly proud I do not know. This I know—that this pride sustains me when otherwise I would sink, not only in the eyes of others but in my own. To Mrs. Dowson I am Mr. Drew, one of McGill's best athletes and students, kindly, friendly, of happy disposition but not intimate. That must remain, I cannot borrow from her. My friends are home with their parents and families. I took my tuxedo and suitcase to the pawnshop to get money to save myself from embarrassment if there should be duty on the goods. Luckily there was none, so I got my tux and bag

back. In the end I had gained nothing, had just a little less money and my outlook just as dark, but if necessary I can sell both of them. If I should sell all I own and then find myself hungry I have no doubt but that I would steal. Here after my judgment of crime, my code of ethics shall be more tolerant than ever before, because now I know in slight measure what it means to be downhearted, worried, lonesome, even hungry. Yet my condition is as that of a prince when compared to many that I have passed tonight. For them even hope has been shut out, faith long ago blotted out, ideals perhaps never born or if born so ill-nourished they never had a chance to grow, under developed in body and mind and spirit a hard cold indifferent world shoves them to the wall and they haven't the strength to fight back. Like animals they are treated, yet when they protect themselves and retaliate in the only way animals can, they are put in jail or made outcasts. Do I condone lawlessness, or filth? No, decidedly not, but I have come close enough to the causes of some of it to become a little taken back, in suffering a little I have learned much, have learned to understand. Truly a great prophet or wise man was he who said, "Get wisdom, but above all things get understanding." How little we understand, how little we try to. It is not meanness, heartlessness, sometimes not even thoughtlessness, just a lack of experience which could make certain ideas comprehensible. My class mates today could not understand why I wouldn't go to the dance with them tonight. When I told some of them frankly that I was broke, they simply thought that I had over spent my allowance or my check hadn't come in or something to that effect. They don't understand that while $10 to some of them will mean—well just ten dollars and maybe a note to Dad that to me it means a whole weeks living, or from my father it would mean an actual sacrifice for the rest of my family. Even an offer was made to pay my way. The fellow couldn't understand why as a friend I wouldn't accept it, especially when I had both admitted that I was broke and would like to go. If I accept gifts without the potentiality of repaying them I give up a part of my independence, I become indebted. My independence must maintain, as long as I am not obligated to any one in any way even poverty does not make me humble, as a man, I am the equal of any man I meet, I have to lean toward no man in either fear or gratitude, no one can make my decisions for me. When I allow myself to become obligated, I put myself in a position in which my judgments may become prejudiced by these obligations. Natural obligations, or fate if we choose to call it that, circumscribes us enough, voluntary limitations of this already cramped freedom are certainly contraindicated.[25]

As the night wound on, Drew's mind drifted to other, related thoughts—questioning his choice to follow a career in medicine rather than the offered job in athletics at Howard University and lamenting the long road he saw stretching ahead of him:

> I have wondered far in the three hours I have been writing, many things I have thought are not put down, many things written are not clearly so, for in my mind I am not clear. So many thoughts rush in, I am almost swamped. Why do I go on like I am? Living harder than I ever did. I don't know. I only know I must. It would be so much easier to do many other things. I gave up the chance to be a real leader in the field of physical training and athletics for my whole race. In it was honor enough to gratify most men, money enough to live on, social position if I desired, and close proximity to everything that I had known as dear and close to me. Yet here I am, a stranger amongst strangers in a strange land, broke busted, almost disgusted, doing my family no good, myself little that is now demonstrable. Yet I know I must go on somehow—I must finish what I have started—though no sure reward waits for me when I again go out to begin once more at the bottom and work up. This series of steps up to now are but stepping stones to reach the bottom round of the ladder which should lead me after many days of thinking to that common place of all who pass this way. This is not a beautiful future, yet this is my life and my life it shall be. I like to take the responsibility for the finished products of this life by thinking as someone has said that "Life is the final expression of the universal Will" It is the inner meaning of evolution. That "this Will be done" in me I suppose is the final end of my daily aspirations and struggles. To something like this I must attribute the urge which forces me on, for I can find in my conscious experience any inspiration capable of such dynamic power. My family love me and I gloat in this love but they cannot inspire me to such efforts. They encourage by every word and deed, they are proud of me and for me, their prayer I know go with me, but I feel that some other power drives me and would continue to do so even if I should fulfill the fondest dreams of my parents.[26]

With the predawn glow already filtering through his window, Drew turned finally to what was, perhaps, the greatest source of his depression:

> Love of women or some woman has inspired some men. I cannot claim this motive. I have known many women, many have held a big share of my heart, no one ever has had complete possession. For this I don't know whether to be glad or sorry. My mind I believe has always played too big a part. It has repeatedly inhibited my heart when there was danger of attachments which might interfere with already existing plans. I have felt this inhibitory warning and have shied from love, Perhaps I am a fool to do so, but who can judge. The present throws this daily into my face, only the future can answer it for me. Many women have told me they love me, many of them, I believe I could love with all my heart if I dared. Together we would be happy. But damn it I can't take care of a wife and medicine too and as yet I haven't worked out any plan, besides I'm having one hell of a time with medicine alone. Money, that two-fold curse and boon to man. Ah what's the use. Can't figure it out but I know it's not as it should be . . . all the desirable girls are either married, planning to get married or in attempting to be decent and wait around for a proper proposal are so repressing and sublimating themselves or maybe something worse that by the time I'm able to take care of one of them there won't be anything but brain left and that darn soft in its ways. The hearts probably will be the seat of exact philosophic ratiocination instead of anything as gloriously foolish as love, while passion of any kind will have been suppressed in the name of virtue so long that it has given up trying. . . .
>
> I'm getting sleepy now, so babe 1930 looks like the going is going to be hard for you so far as I'm concerned. Your birth was under an ominous sky, your early moments most inauspicious, you don't look a bit healthy but I'm going to try like the devil to make something out of you. Maybe your prognosis isn't as fatalistic as the present diagnosis indicates, but don't expect anything sudden or big to happen. Got to handle you awful carefully, I won't have to make many slips to make you count for naught so if you have any good luck with you spread it on thick or I might lose you. I'll check up with you in twelve months. In closing I must say again—this is a hell of a New Years day.[27]

Not long after penning this extraordinary document, a kind of Montreal Testament, Drew realized that, personal pride notwithstanding, he must reach out for help. There was no other way to remain true to his dream. He contacted his former football coach from Amherst, D. O. "Tuss" McLaughry, who had moved on to sparkling success as the head coach at Brown University in Providence, Rhode Island. At this time, in addition to his freelance refereeing, Drew had taken on a job waiting tables in order to bring in more desperately needed money.[28] Unfortunately, as he related to McLaughry, his old ankle injury had temporarily flared up, making it difficult for him to continue this rather physically demanding job. As he had confessed in the testament, all his funds were drawn into his tuition, room, and books. Food was last on the list, and now he had no money for it, an admission to his mentor that must have come with enormous pain for a man of Drew's manifest pride.

McLaughry told Drew to hang on and went to work at once:

> I immediately wrote to some of his class mates and told them of Charlie's predicament and his need of a loan. Within a few days, I received enough money to pay for his board for an extended period. Years later, after he had completed his broad medical education, and was beginning to earn money, he paid back every cent of the loan. He never knew the names of the friends who helped him. All I ever told Drew was that they were class mates who considered it a privilege to be able to come to his aid.[29]

Buoyed by the assistance of his old friends, Drew managed to make ends meet through the last few months of his second year at McGill.

Despite these overwhelming distractions, he also somehow managed to remain focused on the daunting academic tasks at hand. In the spring term Drew learned about microorganisms from Professor F. C. Harrison in bacteriology and devoted his attention to pharmacology professor R. L. Stehle as he made "a serious attempt to familiarize the student with the chemistry of the drugs studied in so far as it is known."[30] Pharmacology was a Second Division course; Drew's passing the examinations of all the First Division classes meant he could continue in his progress in the curriculum with formal advancement into his seventh term, and most of the other Second Division subjects, the following autumn.

Back home in Washington for the summer months, Drew continued his employment at the Francis Pool. In some ways returning to the facility was as much like coming home as going to the Arlington house. As Eva recalled: "The staff was like family. Several of the fellows were classmates—all had attended Dunbar.

They were all protective of the women who worked there and were especially caring for the children who swam there. It was also a social thing. Going to Francis was special, like going to a party. Charlie liked to dive—somewhat unusual for such a big man."[31]

Early on, the swimming and diving instruction had evolved into organized teams and meets—including both intramural events that lived on in Eva's memory as the "Francis Olympics" and larger-scale contests involving teams from other cities—as had occurred in the summer of 1929 with the visitors from Baltimore. African American teams from as far away as Philadelphia and New York traveled to the Francis facility to compete. Later, the Francis team reciprocated.

Here the hyper-competitive athlete and coach in Charlie took over:

> Neither of them (Charlie and Joe) competed in swimming events. They organized and coached the swimming and diving teams. Tough coaches.
>
> When we were in training for "The Francis Pool Olympics," Charlie would not allow the swimmers to eat sweets—candy.
>
> There were small licorice candies shaped like babies. They were called tar babies. We could eat those things. Today such a name for the jellied candy would be insulting. We had a curfew, too. Some of us tried very hard to do all the things he wanted us to do—not so much to win the races, but to please him. He was so enthusiastic about the whole thing.[32]

Sadly, these teams went largely unrecognized for their excellence. Joseph Drew later noted:

> In the late '20s, early '30s we had some terrific swimmers. We had a great program going on at Francis, but we couldn't get AAU sanction, American Athletic Union. We couldn't get sanctioned to get records. The only way we could get any recognition at all for about five or six years was to get a visiting permit and go up to New York. And if we did something up there, made a record, it would go down in the books. But in Washington we couldn't get this recognition. This was one of the nastiest things because we had some good swimmers in those days. This was one of the worst things that ever happened to me because we had some great guys and they weren't recognized.[33]

During these summer evenings the family would often gather and make music, as they had for Drew's entire life. Eva remembered:

> We had a radio and an upright piano. Television had not been invented. Papa played the guitar, Charlie played sax (awfully), Nora and Charlie played the piano. Papa sang bass and baritone, Mama sang alto, Nora was a soprano, Charlie and Joe were tenors. I could not sing. I still can't sing. They all sang together and they sounded good! When I tried to sing everyone would say "hush" or "shhh." Charlie loved music, loved to sing.[34]

One of Drew's favorite songs to sing was "Let the Rest of the World Go By," a sentimental Western ballad written in 1919:

Is the struggle and strife
We find in this life
Really worthwhile, after all?
I've been wishing today
I could just run away,
Out where the west winds call.

With someone like you, a pal good and true,
I'd like to leave it all behind, and go and find
Some place that's known to God alone,
Just a spot to call our own.
We'll find perfect peace,
Where joys never cease,
Out there beneath a kindly sky,
We'll build a sweet little nest somewhere in the west,
And let the rest of the world go by.

Is the future to hold
Just struggles for gold,
While the real world waits outside,
Away out on the breast
Of the wonderful West,
Across the great Divide?[35]

As the season of songs and swimming ended, it was time for Drew to prepare for the third year of medical school. He moved back into the familiar environs of 3580 Durocher Street in Montreal in time for the start of classes on September 17, 1930.[36]

The Second Division consisted of just three courses: pharmacology, pathology, and medical jurisprudence (which was considered a subsection of pathology, probably because the latter occasionally dealt with legal considerations). Pathology comprised both general pathology, a full-year, three-term course taught by Professor Horst Oertel, and a series of special pathology classes covering some specific anatomic structures and systems in greater detail. Only the examination for the general class had to be passed before the student could be advanced to the Third Division. Drew, of course, had already taken the pharmacology class in the spring of his second year. The medical jurisprudence class covered a variety of issues and must have been a fascinating, if rather grim, distraction from the routine of the medical curriculum:

> In this course the criminal and civil aspects of legal medicine are taken up and fully discussed, also lunacy in its medical legal aspects. Special attention is devoted to the subject of blood stains, the chemical, microscopic and spectroscopic tests for which are fully described and demonstrated, also the serum test for the detection of human blood. The modes of action of poisons, general evidence of poisoning and classification of poisons are first treated of, after which the more common poisons are described, with reference to symptoms, post-mortem appearance and chemical tests. The post-mortem appearances are fully illustrated by specimens. Injuries are fully discussed, with reference to their significance, under the Workman's Compensation Act and Accident Insurance.[37]

Fall in Canada also meant college track season. On October 17, 1930, the medicine team again prevailed in the McGill interfaculty meet, although the score was close. Rain had drenched the Molson Field track before the athletes began the competition, and there was still a mist in the air at the first starting gun. Drew won the high jump and the 110 high hurdles, but the final score of the meet was tighter than it should have been because, on the wet track, Drew knocked over three of the hurdles in his race and was disqualified.[38]

Drew was elected captain of the McGill intercollegiate track team that traveled to Queen's University the following week for the tri-meet with the hosts and the University of Toronto—surely one of the rare times in history when an individual held that prestigious position at two separate universities. He followed through, as well, taking home top prizes in the 120-yard-high hurdles and broad jump as McGill sailed to a team victory.[39]

In 1931 Drew's brother Joseph married Grace Ridgeley, a graduate of Smith College and the daughter of Dr. Albert Ridgeley, a physician and anatomy professor at Howard University. Aside from the happiness he felt for his brother, this affected Charlie from a practical perspective. On visits home he could no longer avail himself of the bedroom the brothers and their father had built above the kitchen; he was again relegated to the front room sofa as in the first years in Arlington.[40]

Sometime in the winter of 1931–32 Drew came to the melancholy conclusion that, despite his own efforts and those of his family and friends, especially the anonymous ones summoned to the cause by Coach Tuss McLaughry, he simply did not have the resources to finish medical school. As disappointing as this

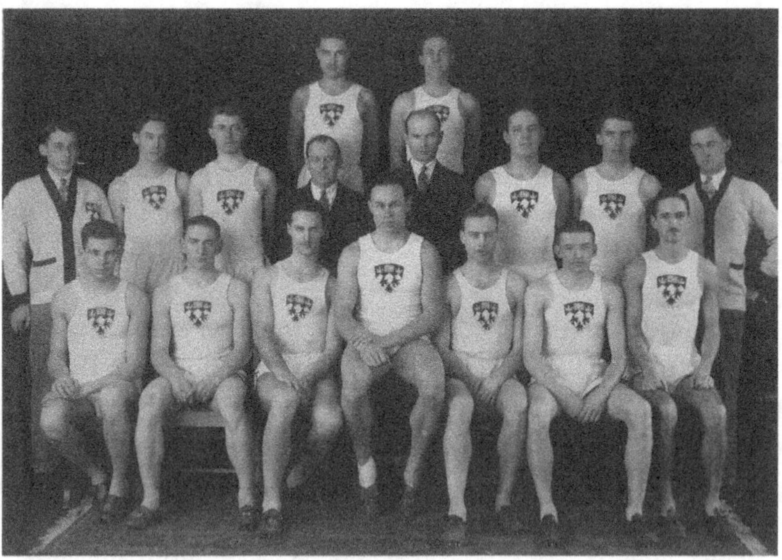

Figure 5.2 Drew as captain of the 1931 McGill track team

was on its own, the blow was doubled by the news that he had been nominated to Alpha Omega Alpha, the medical student honorary society that extended invitations only to the highest-ranked students. He made an appointment with the dean's office to explain his reluctant decision to withdraw, hopeful that he might be able to continue his studies at some future date when he had saved enough money.

Drew appears to have met with J. C. Simpson, secretary to the dean, at this time. Simpson had taught Drew's course in histology and, in his administrative position, would certainly have been aware of the young man's outstanding record both as a scholar and athlete. He encouraged the desperate youth to stick it out. More to the point, he provided what Drew described at the time as "personal assistance" that "made the finishing of this year possible."[41] In addition to his role in providing tangible, presumably financial aid, Simpson's office was also probably where Drew heard about another potential source of help—the Rosenwald Fellowships.

Julius Rosenwald was a wealthy businessman who had made his fortune in the clothing industry in New York City, including partial ownership of the Sears and Roebuck Company. In keeping with the philanthropic fashion among the well-heeled of the age, in his later years Rosenwald sought to give away as much of his accumulated largesse as possible, stating, "What I want to do is cure the things that seem wrong."[42] A meeting with Booker T. Washington convinced Rosenwald that neglect of education for African Americans was among the height of the wrongs in American society but, unlike many with good intentions, he had the wherewithal to do something about it. Rosenwald Foundation funds eventually helped finance the construction of over five thousand schools for Blacks, mostly in the South, where the need was most dire. In addition, the Foundation funded Rosenwald Fellowships for the cultivation of African American talents across the arts and sciences. Such luminaries as Marian Anderson, Gordon Parks, John Hope Franklin, and Ralph Ellison were among them.[43]

So was Charles R. Drew, who received one of the first Rosenwald Fellowships just four years into the program in 1931.

Drew filled out the application for the Fellowship on May 1, 1931. In it he stated that, at an even six feet tall and weighing 182 pounds, he was in good health. After giving a summary of his education and employment experience, such as it was, Drew listed his current expenses for the school year from September to June, estimating future costs based on an average of the expenses of his first two years.

Tuition at this time was $275, with books $60 and fees $35. Transportation costs he reckoned at $120 for the year, and "special equipment" at $40. His room was $5 per week, which totaled $175 for the 35 weeks in question. Board was $8 a week or $280 for the academic year. Laundry came in at $35, clothing $75, insurance $55, and Drew marked $50 for miscellany, in which he included haircuts and movies. The grand total was $1,200, of which he expected to cover $200–$400 from his family's contributions, summer work, and refereeing. Consequently, Drew requested $800–$1,000 from the Rosenwald Foundation for his next year at the McGill Faculty of Medicine—although he did not fail to point out that he had two years remaining.[44]

That summer he received a letter that began with the happy boilerplate, "I have the honor to inform you that you have been awarded a fellowship from the Julius Rosenwald Fund." Other Fellows that year included W. E. B. DuBois, Langston Hughes, and Drew's old friend from Dunbar High and Amherst College, Mercer Cook, who was then a professor of Romance languages at Howard University.[45]

This windfall did not mean that all was to be blue skies and smooth sailing in the year (or years) to come, but for a time the one overarching concern that generated inescapable anguish and worry was set aside and, for that time, Drew could expect to focus all his considerable energies on his classwork.

"O Essence of Negligence! Myriads of mystic tongues are made vocal in one speech, and myriads of hidden mysteries are revealed in a single melody; yet, alas! there is no ear to hear, nor heart to understand."—Bahá'u'lláh[46]

With this Bahá'í prayer, twenty-year-old Mary Maxwell began a thirty-two-page compendium of handwritten original poems, sketches, and scriptural quotes she called "Charlie Drew's book of thoughts about God and love and beauty." Mary, the strikingly beautiful daughter of a prominent Montreal family, compiled the book from July to December 1931.

Mary's father, William Sutherland Maxwell, was a native of Montreal and a highly regarded architect who had studied at the École des Beaux-Arts in Paris. He married May Ellis Boles, the sister of a prominent member of the Bahá'í

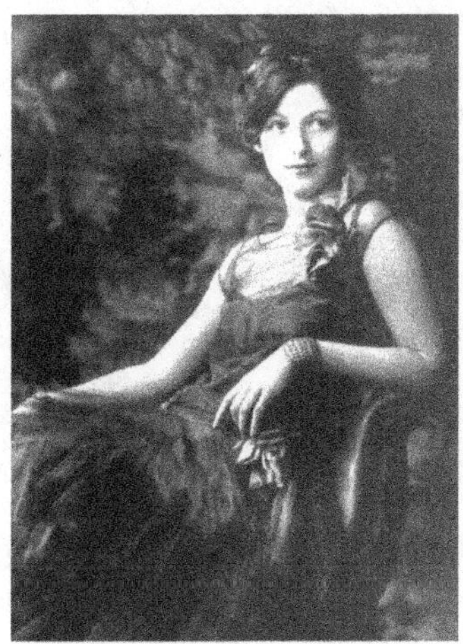

Figure 5.3 Mary Maxwell. Public domain; source: Worldwide Community of Baha'u'llah: 1926—Mary Maxwell (Ruhiyyih-Khanum) the year of her second pilgrimage (communitybaha .blogspot.com)

faith, in London in 1902. William converted to the faith himself not long before Mary was born in 1910, after meeting the worldwide leader, 'Abdu'l-Bahá, son of the founder of Bahá'í.

The Maxwells became leaders in the Bahá'í community in North America and raised their daughter Mary to be deeply involved, as well. By the time she met Charles Drew, Mary had—despite her tender age—risen to a place of regional prominence in the religion, having spoken eloquently on behalf of her beliefs across Canada and the United States, including on the topic of racial equality. The young lady could speak French fluently—not surprising given her upbringing in Quebec—but in a few years she would add Persian and German to the list as well.

The circumstances of Mary's introduction to Drew are not known, but, based on the intimate nature of the handmade book she compiled, the friendship was in full swing by the summer of 1931 and had clearly become a close one. In addition to many Bahá'í references, she included in the collection the majestic imagery of St. Paul's I Corinthians 13 and the unequivocal eroticism of the Old Testament *Song of Solomon*. Mary closed with three poems of her own composition, titled "Blessed," "A Love Song," and "Love," written late in the year:

Love
I would have my love for you
So strong that the flame of the flesh could not hide it
I would have my love for you
So bright that passion could not dim it
So that when I felt you on my heart
It would not take you from my heart
So that when you commenced kissing me

You would not have ceased kissing me
When my body is yours
My spirit, too
Must be yours
When our fleshes sing "we one wed"
It must only be the echo
Of our souls nuptials
When I see you beside me
It must be as strange as
As though I saw myself
As if I were disembodied
And when I say "I"
It must mean you
And when I touch you
It must be I
This would I have love to be
For us
I will not say I love you
I will say "love" and it will be you[47]

In 1932 Mary traveled to Washington, DC, to speak at Howard University on the subjects of Bahá'í and racial equality. It is likely that this event was inspired, if not actually arranged, by Drew. Mary and her mother May, who accompanied her, made a point to meet his family on this trip and together made a strong impression. Eva remembered:

> I met Mary—she brought me an exotic turtle which I lost the next day. Joe took her to an Omega Psi Phi costume ball. She draped herself in a white sheet and made a tiara of green leaves. Long blond hair—she was gorgeous.
>
> Mary's mother came to Arlington to meet Charlie's family. Mrs. Maxwell tried to persuade Mama to persuade Charlie to marry Mary. Mama, of course, refused and told Mrs. Maxwell that that decision was up to the children.[48]

May Maxwell was scarcely less enamored of Drew than her daughter. In one letter to him she revealed the depth of her admiration:

> Somehow, Charlie, courage and gentleness seem the keynote of you to me, and aside from your splendid intellectual attainments, these are innate qualities which have a peculiar appeal to my way of thinking, and I always love the words of Baha'u'llah and Speaking of the higher paths of service in life, such as your own, "Cowards have no place in these fields!"[49]

As in the case of Lelia Waller, another young lady of great appeal from a successful and prominent family, this romance was not destined to endure. As Eva recalled, "She (Mary) was in love with Charlie. I'm not sure what his deep feelings for her were."[50]

Obviously, there were enormous obstacles to overcome in terms of an interracial marriage in the 1930s, which was not an issue with Lelia Waller (whose youth, however, was likely a major concern). In both circumstances, though, it cannot be discounted that in his years of higher education Charles Drew was so utterly focused on reaching his aspirational goals to become a physician that, however much he desired true romance, with all its inscrutable machinations—the Montreal Testament being his plaintive expression—this most complex of emotions was, in his eyes, too great a distraction.[51]

Drew did compose a poem to Mary that survives; a reply to one she had written blaming the moon for her love for him:

> Your moon is horned and its points sink deep
> In my heart and let its life blood drip
> Drop by drop with a sad cadence,
> To the dark pool of comfortless doubt
> And longing in the depth of my being.
> Your moon crawls like an earthy thing
> In dark places, poking its horned head
> Into the shadows like an evil thing,
> Routing even love from its peaceful nest.
> But it brings no light, no cheer, no warmth
> To these dusky lanes of life, it only crawls
> And probes and goes on seeking things to route.
> My moon's points must be turned up towards
> The higher realms and not tipped down toward earth.[52]

Drew's fourth year of medical school began on Wednesday, September 16, 1931. The big change for this year, aside from the money the Rosenwald Fund provided, was a switch in curriculum from study of the basic to the clinical sciences. Reading, lectures, and laboratory work would not be abandoned, but the new focus was on absorbing the science of patient care through work on the wards.[53]

That fall, Drew continued his protracted career on the scholastic athletic field, although, nursing a sprained knee, he did not participate in the 1931 McGill interfaculty track meet that was held on October 9. Missing his contribution, the medicine team, a seemingly perennial winner, finished in second place.[54] Another star on the team had arisen, though. Phil Edwards, a twenty-four-year-old native of British Guyana who had already competed for Canada at the 1928 Olympic Games, broke the school's long-standing records at the meet in both the mile and quarter-mile running events. A week later at the intercollegiate event, the powerful McGill squad, led by a healed Drew and the new weapon Edwards, easily toppled its rivals from Toronto and Queens in the rain at Molson Stadium. Drew was beaten by a McGill Law student and teammate named John Hutchins in the 220-yard-high hurdles but rallied to take first place in the high jump.[55]

Unfortunately, to date Drew's full transcript as a medical student at McGill has not come to light. Consequently, given the wide latitude available to students in the Faculty of Medicine regarding course selection during their clinical years—as opposed to the more regimented terms of the basic science period—the classes he took during any particular session of his last three years of medical school are not known with precision. However, there are clues.

The final exams for Drew's courses in surgery have survived. They are dated from May of 1932 and May of 1933, suggesting that his two-year surgery course began at the start of the fourth year. Since this subject became his life's work, it bears further discussion.

The core of surgical instruction at McGill was the didactic lecture series, 120 one-hour morning sessions in all, spread over the two-year course. Augmenting this was, naturally, the required reading, which comprised selections from several texts. Theatre Clinics, demonstrations of cases with live patients where, frequently, actual procedures were performed, were offered twice a week at both the general hospitals affiliated with McGill, the Royal Victoria and Montreal General, and any student could attend them after completing their sixth term. The bulk of the learning would necessarily occur in the wards and outpatient clinics, where defined periods of clinical education during patient rounds were scheduled from 10:30 to noon, four times a week.[56] After the students had been properly exposed to the basics of general surgery, they could then proceed into exploration of the surgical specialties as they existed at the time (one of these, neurosurgery, was led in the 1930s at McGill by the world-renowned Wilder Penfield) as well as anesthesia, which was considered a surgical specialty in this era.

On May 14, 1932, Drew sat for the final exam of his fourth-year surgery course. Five questions were posed to the students, with three hours given to complete them. The questions were:

1. *Describe symptoms, signs and treatment of a perforation of a duodenal ulcer. What complications may occur?*
2. *Describe briefly the anatomy, and give the causes, pathology, common distribution, symptoms, complications, and treatment of varicosities of the great saphenous vein.*
3. *Describe the symptoms and signs of acute pyogenic osteomyelitis of the lower end of the femur in a child ten years of age.*
4. *Outline the changes in the kidney resulting from renal calculus; give the methods to be employed in making a diagnosis.*
5. *Describe very briefly—*
   (a) *Thomas's knee splint.*
   (b) *Whitman's position (neck of femur).*
   (c) *Colles' fracture.*[57]

Based on this exam, the results of which are unknown, Drew's Surgery course for his fourth year included topics related to intra-abdominal pathology and peripheral vascular disease, with extensive exposure to urology and orthopedics. However, in this era, surgical specialization had not advanced to the degree seen today, and, depending on the institution, these entities would have fallen more or less under the umbrella of general surgery. (Urology was a separate specialty in the Surgery Department at McGill at this time, as was orthopedic surgery, although inasmuch as the latter was a defined entity, it was then focused on issues related to deformities of the bones resulting from diseases such as poliomyelitis, rather than the treatment of fractures.)

Back in the District of Columbia for the summer, Drew continued with his pleasant paying occupation at the Francis Pool. As before, evenings were spent with the gathered family at the Arlington house. Although music was always at hand, Charlie could mix things up from time to time, even injecting some amateur stagecraft. Eva remembered one (literal) scene: "Charlie loved books. One he loved and shared with us was a collection of great plays. So, we were cast as different members in a play, the name of which I can't remember. Grace, Nora, Vashti, Charlie and I sat around the dining room table, passed the book from one to another to read our lines. It was fun. It was hilarious. It was awful!"[58]

In early August of 1932, Joseph Drew and his wife Grace welcomed their first child, a boy named Richard after the Drew family patriarch. The following day the brothers were at work at the Francis Pool as usual when Charlie made an inquiry of his sibling. As Eva recalled: "Charlie asked why he had not returned to the hospital to see his wife and new son. Joe said, 'That's not my son. He looks like a wrinkled-up monkey!' Charlie was disgusted with Joe. He then explained that all just-born babies are wrinkly and kind of ugly, but they are all (usually) beautiful the next day. Joe then became the "proud papa."[59] Drew's experience with newborns did not only come from his studies at McGill. Eva remembered another, very different event from around the same time:

> One night at home when Charlie was still in med school there was a loud, impatient knock on the front door. When I answered it there was this awful-looking man crying that his wife was dying and he needed the doctor. I knew the man. He lived in a shack across the field in back of our house. Charlie insisted that he was not yet a doctor, but the man insisted and Charlie went with the man.
>
> With nothing to work with and an oil lamp he delivered a fat, healthy boy. He instructed the man to pull down some dirty curtains, boil them, dry them and wrap the baby in the dry curtains. He named his son Mutsy. What a night. Mutsy was the strongest, healthiest boy in the neighborhood.[60]

Returning to Montreal for his fifth and final year of medical school, which happened to coincide with celebrations of the institution's centennial, Drew was accorded considerable recognition for his now consistently outstanding efforts in the classroom. He was elected to the McGill Medical Society, an association of top medical students (at least as far as the Society was concerned) that, in its sixth decade of existence, was venerable in itself. The Society had biweekly evening meetings at which refreshments were served and lectures provided on various interesting topics by both faculty professors and invited guests. Reports of intriguing cases were also a feature, and this was Drew's primary responsibility within the group. The Society was also involved in the planning and execution of a midwinter Medical Ball in December and a year-end Medical Dinner, at which visiting academic speakers of renown held sway.[61]

Drew's generation of interesting case reports for the Society dovetailed naturally with the student-run *McGill Undergraduate Medical Journal*, and in his senior year he also became a member of the editorial board in charge of writing up the reports.[62]

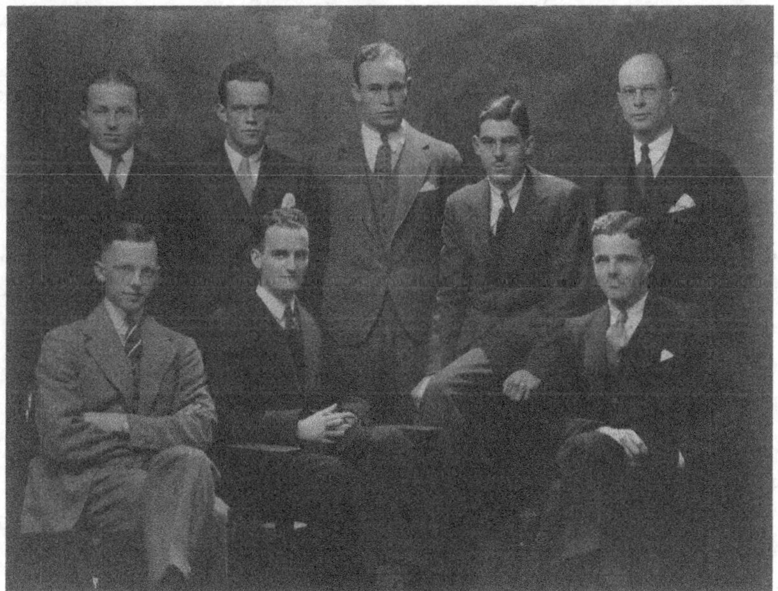

Figure 5.4 Drew and the staff of the *McGill Undergraduate Medical Journal.*

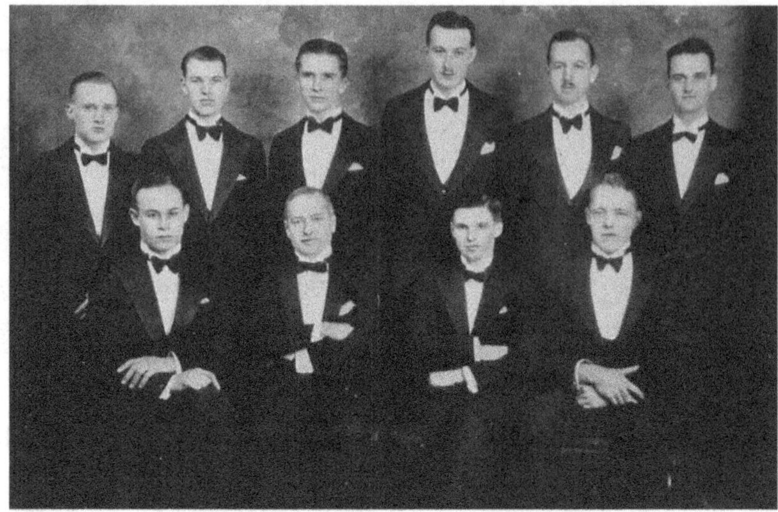

Figure 5.5 Drew with other members of the medical student honor society, Alpha Omega Alpha.

In addition to these laurels, Drew was elected vice president of the McGill branch of Alpha Omega Alpha, the international medical student honors fraternity.[63]

In his final year of medical school Drew lived at 3547 Jeanne Mance Street, three blocks north of his old place on Durocher Street. By this point in time the money from the Rosenwald Fund was long gone, and, as Drew himself put it, "I was broke again."[64] Fortunately, another cliffhanger period of financial turmoil was avoided when he won the Dr. J. Francis Williams Fellowship in Medicine and Clinical Medicine. This was a prize of $500, endowed by its namesake, available to students in their final year at the McGill Faculty of Medicine who were "in high general scholastic standing and approved by the Heads of the Department of Medicine."[65] The award was given based on the results of what Drew described as a "competitive exam, covering the whole of Medicine, for which only the top five people in the class were eligible."[66]

At the interfaculty track meet on Friday, October 14, 1932, Drew led the way as the Medicine team took home the top prize, making up for the previous year's anomaly. He won the 110 high hurdles with a time of 15 4/5 seconds, good enough to beat the meet record set by Howie Baker in defeating him three years before and equaling the Canadian national collegiate record. In addition, Drew triumphed in the high and broad jumps and took second in the 220 hurdles.[67]

A week later in Toronto, Drew again helped lead the red-and-white of McGill to an intercollegiate title, winning the 110 hurdles and placing second in both the long and broad jumps. He tied Phil Edwards with a meet-best 11 points as McGill thrashed Toronto and Queen's and took the Tait-Mackenzie Trophy back to its familiar spot on the shelf of honor at McGill Union.[68]

On Saturday night, March 8, 1933, Drew competed in his final intercollegiate track event, a most unusual international dual meet between McGill and the host Boston University. He went out on top with a win in the high hurdles and second-place finish in the high jump as the team from Montreal topped its American rivals.[69] Thus, Drew completed a remarkable college athletic career that dated back a full decade (including the two years at Morgan College when he coached rather than competed) to the spring of 1923, when he first donned the Amherst purple for Coach Nelligan's Lord Jeffs track team. Drew finished his career as one of the all-time top scorers in Canadian track and field history.

The final examination in Surgery for Drew's fifth year was given on May 10, 1933. It consisted of the following questions, representing a similar scope of clinical practice as the prior year's example but with more complex scenarios and requisite responses:

1. *Enumerate the conditions which produce swelling of the side of the neck, and discuss the clinical diagnosis.*
2. *Classify fractures of the tibia and/or fibula in the region of the ankle joint. Describe the mode of causation and the methods of reduction and fixation for each type.*
3. *Enumerate the benign lesions of the female breast which cause localized tumor. Differentiate between a benign tumor and a scirrhus carcinoma.*
4. *A man aged 45, in apparent good health, consults you saying that for several months he has been troubled with occasional "wind pains" felt here and there over the middle and lower half of the abdomen. These pains are gradually becoming more frequent. How would you handle the case, in respect of diagnosis and treatment?*
5. *Give the symptoms and signs of dorso-lumbar Pott's Disease. Mention three important complications and describe in detail the treatment of one of these.*

6. (a) *Enumerate the various conditions producing enlargement of the prostate gland.*
   (b) *Discuss their pathology, diagnosis and treatment.*[70]

Drew made notes in the margins of the test paper as he considered answers for the two parts of the fifth question regarding Pott's Disease, which is tuberculosis of the spine. As to the clinical manifestations (signs being elements identified on physical examination by the physician, symptoms being those reported by the patient), he wrote: "1 Pain 2 Rigid 3 Deform 4 Abscess 5 Paraplegia." For the second half of the question, apropos of complications, he marked "Deformity, Abscess Formation, Septicemia." On the question about prostatic enlargement he jotted, "Prostatism," "CA" (meaning cancer), and "stone." These are all reasonable responses, although we do not know how Drew wove them together into written answers.

There was also a bedside oral examination in the senior year surgery rotation, at which the primary objective of the student was evidently to determine the diagnosis, although treatment plan was also likely tested. It was described in this way:

> Each student will be assigned two cases for the purpose of his bedside examination. One hour will be allowed for the study of these two cases. The student must realize that he must study his cases carefully, and prepare himself for a thorough oral examination. He is expected to make notes of the history for reference, and as a help to his memory during examination, but not to write a complete case report. For this purpose he will be given, upon request, by the house-surgeon or by the Assistants in Surgery, who will be on duty in the Wards, the ordinary information afforded by routine laboratory investigations. He is not to be given such special information as would itself give the diagnosis, such as X-rays either of fractures or of the internal organs, X-ray reports, pathological reports, or other reports in which the diagnosis is mentioned. In this sense he may ask for such things as X-ray films (except of fractures), examination of the urine, the blood, faeces, serous membrane fluids, Wasserman tests, and such special reports as concern eye, ear, nose and throat conditions, bacteriological reports and gynecological reports.[71] Rectal examinations may be made by the student, but not gynecological.
>
> In cases of doubt he is to apply to those in authority in the Ward.

Details of dates, hours of examination and places, will be posted at the College and at each of the Hospitals.

Sgd. E. Archibald[72]

The results of this oral exam have again, unfortunately, not come down to us, but, based on Drew's final grade in surgery (see below), it may be fairly inferred that his performance was more than satisfactory.

In his senior year, Drew spent the months between September of 1932 and June of 1933 as an "externe/interne" on the internal medicine service at the Royal Victoria Hospital. The mixed terminology reflected the fact that he spent half of the rotation living in the facility. This position was roughly equivalent to what would now be called a "subintern" in US medical education. In this capacity, he worked as a "clinical clerk" (a concept that originated with Osler) "participating in the keeping of records, diagnosis and treatment of patients in the wards and Out-Patient Department, and the laboratory duties."[73] This was the official description in the McGill Calendar for 1934–35, although the reality was probably somewhat less glamorous.

The life of an intern in a large teaching hospital today differs little in the everyday sense from that of Drew's time, consisting almost exclusively of the performance of mindless tasks such as tracking down test results, placing catheters, and writing interminable chart notes: a thousand unappealing tasks collectively known from time immemorial by the grotesque term "scut." The extern/intern would act as the intern's intern and naturally be assigned the least appealing jobs of the whole litany. Nonetheless, these trying times were more than punitive hazing: they held practical value in permitting the tyro to understand at a grassroots level how a hospital functions.

It may well have been during this extern/intern period that a decision was made—both by Drew and the McGill faculty—about his further training following the completion of medical school.

A word about graduate medical education—internship, residency and fellowship programs following the completion of medical school—is in order since, despite the prosaic similarities noted above, there are significant differences between the institutions in the 1930s and the familiar ones of more recent times.

The first steps toward a recognizably modern form of postgraduate training in North America came in the late nineteenth century from the halls of the Johns Hopkins Hospital, where McGill's own William Osler and the great surgeon William Stewart Halsted, having observed the German system of residency firsthand, brought it with them to the new institution in Baltimore. From there the concept—newly graduated physicians learning the intricacies of patient care in a hands-on fashion while physically living within a hospital—spread across the continent as its many advantages and superior products became obvious.

Some elements of the new training regimens remained less than ideal for years, however. Perhaps of greatest concern to the trainee was the fact that the duration of internships and residencies was not only not standardized but could be treacherously nebulous—the length of time an individual was required to continue in a program was dictated only by the whims of the director, who made the decision when a physician was ready to leave the training nest. In surgery, in particular, the residency period could extend up to a decade.

By the 1930s, such ominous vagueness had been eliminated from most training scenarios: internships had, for example, been streamlined to a generally agreed-upon calendar year, although what subjects were covered were not regimented, as, indeed, is sometimes the case today.

At McGill in this era, an internship consisted of a year-long training program on the residency model, with "rotations" for a period of weeks on various clinical services within a major specialty such as surgery or internal medicine. The idea was to generate in the trainee experience and, hopefully, some expertise in caring for patients with the more common conditions and illnesses across the spectrum of that specialty.

Such a position was offered to Drew in surgery at the Montreal General Hospital for the academic year from July 1, 1934, to June 30, 1935, and he accepted without reservation.

Drew's final term grades are the only ones from his time at McGill that have come to light in documentary form as of this writing.[74] He scored A's in both surgery and medicine, with a B in obstetrics and gynecology. At the time, A's were reported along with a number representing the recipient's rank among his classmates in the subject. Drew's surgery grade was A2, thereby indicating that his was the second-best grade of the class, while his medicine place was A5. These sterling reports and what came before were good enough for an aggregate second-place standing in the final Faculty of Medicine rankings for the Class of 1933.[75] He had earned his MDCM.

Charles Drew's academic performance at the McGill University Faculty of Medicine was outstanding by any standard and, given the overwhelming obstacles in his way, a singularly impressive demonstration of both pure applied talent and unyielding force of will. These were attributes that he would need in ever greater proportion in the years to come.

In the early 1930s the McGill medical school boasted eight affiliated hospitals. In addition to the 680-bed Royal Victoria Hospital, adjacent to the medical school, there was a Royal Victoria-Montreal Maternity Pavilion, Children's Memorial Hospital, the Montreal Foundling and Baby Hospital, the Alexandra Hospital for Infectious Diseases, the Protestant Hospital for the Insane at Verdun, the Royal Edward Institute (a tuberculosis dispensary) and the Western Division of the Montreal General Hospital, an acute care facility.

The Montreal General Hospital, where Drew would spend the next two academic years, was then located at the corner of Tupper Street and Atwater Avenue, about two kilometers south of the medical school. The institution dated back to the 1820s, although it had twice moved locations as it outgrew earlier, smaller versions. In 1933 Montreal General had 404 inpatient beds, with about 7,500 annual admissions. The large, newly constructed outpatient department saw around 150,000 patient visits per year. Forty resident physicians called Montreal General Hospital home.[76]

The Surgery Internship in 1933 consisted of four three-month "rotations." In Drew's case, the first consisted of outpatient medicine clinic work in the morning and surgery clinic as well as emergency room coverage in the afternoon. The second stanza was "male surgery," and the third, predictably, "female surgery."* He spent the final four months of the internship on the eye/ear/nose/throat and neurosurgery services.

The strict time constraints and other unsavory rigors of an intern's life would stress the most diligent diarist's efforts. Drew, who rarely generated accounts of everyday activities anyway, left no written recollections of this period. Nevertheless a few tales exist, and some likelihoods can be inferred.

There is an old saying among practitioners of the medical profession who exercise their duties in a teaching hospital setting: "The intern who has made a decision has made a mistake." This aphorism underscores the low level of authority of the new graduate, who is assumed not to know enough to make a proper judgment regarding patient care or, indeed, anything else. Drew's internship year, if it conformed to the standards of his day (and the current one) consisted of a deep exploration of the seemingly limitless variations on the meaning of the spare, unattractive word noted above, "scut."

The typical daily scenario would have consisted of a routine, repetitive series of events. The morning began with early pre-rounding, at which the intern performed a general review of the overnight clinical course of the patients for which he was responsible. This included a limited physical examination, the gathering of vital signs and any available laboratory results, and a tallying of the volume of oral or intravenous intake balanced against the output from urine and other sources. This preparatory information-gathering was followed by morning Work Rounds. Here the entire "house staff" team—medical students, interns, and more advanced residents—would gather and move from bedside to bedside, discussing the particulars of each case and subsuming the results proffered by the interns from their pre-rounding. Sometimes nurses or other ancillary personnel would accompany the resident physician team.

---

* During this period there was an ongoing concern that white patients in teaching hospitals would not accept Blacks as their physicians or as observing medical students, particularly in obstetric and gynecologic scenarios. Indeed, this very point was mentioned by J. C. Simpson as a reason for not accepting Black medical student candidates in his 1938 letter to the University Counsel regarding racial quotas noted earlier. If such an issue arose with Drew, it has not been recorded and did not impair his progress. Conjecturally, his fair skin may have obviated any difficulty.

Work rounds were the setting where plans would be made, and orders given. The remainder of an intern's day consisted of fulfilling them.

The actual attending physician might also formally see the patients with the team on teaching rounds, which could be scheduled or ad hoc. On these, the residents' plans would be debated and confirmed or amended and nuggets of knowledge verbally tossed in the direction of the students and trainees—their didactic reward for services rendered.

At the close of the day, in the late afternoon or evening, yet another set of rounds would be performed, in which any results from the ordered tests would be reviewed and the patients' courses throughout the day discussed.

Although the details would change from rotation to rotation, this would be the general pattern of life for an intern (those on surgical services might spend some time in the operating room as an assistant, as well).

One of the enduring stories told about Charles Drew over the years involves a large, destructive fire that occurred at the Montreal General Hospital during his internship and resulted in numerous burn injuries. According to the tale, the young trainee Drew, inundated with patients suffering less from their thermal wounds than from attendant shock, is forced to come to terms with concepts of fluid resuscitation and blood transfusion, prefiguring the later work that would win him widespread acclaim that persists to the present day.[77]

It has not proved possible to identify such a discrete event from the record—the newspapers of the day and the records of Montreal General contain no mention of a fire with burned patients—but it is not at all unlikely that Drew was faced with burn victims during his postgraduate training period and that a realization of the era's inadequate therapeutic regimens for such injuries—the prevailing method of treating burns at the time involved tannic acid, which was later found to be not merely ineffective but actually harmful—stimulated an interest in improving the status quo. Whether he recognized at this early date the value of circulatory support through blood and fluid administration in burn cases—which was elucidated unequivocally a decade later within the crucible of World War II—is more dubious. Given his very junior status, it is unlikely that any novel therapeutic method Drew might have suggested would have been entertained, or that he would have had the autonomy to act himself, but he may well have internalized his observations and theories for later consideration.

Toward the close of his internship year, Drew successfully passed the National Board of Medical Examiners test, a prerequisite to licensing in the United States. He also decided, with the approval of the necessary administrative authorities, to continue his postgraduate training for a year as a resident at the Montreal General Hospital in 1934–35. In a modest departure from the norm, however, the residency position Drew took at this time was not in surgery but internal medicine.

For a future surgeon this was not an obvious path to take: although there is inevitable crossover between the patient populations of internal medicine and surgical services, the work of the surgical resident is bound up quite intentionally in acquisition of knowledge regarding the preoperative preparation and postoperative care of the surgical patient, not to mention honing of the manual skills so essential to successful surgical operations. None of these elements are inherent to internal medicine residencies. In Drew's case, however, the final choice of career had not yet crystallized in his mind, and he felt the need to test the waters of both ponds. Later, colleagues would report that he considered the year of training in medicine especially valuable to his becoming a well-rounded physician, a position with which most surgery training programs then or now would not concur.

Midway through this internal medicine year, as 1934 came to a close, Drew made up his mind to cast his fortunes in the realm of surgery. On December 7 he sent a letter to his old friend W. Montague Cobb, who had graduated from Howard University's medical school in 1929 and was now on that institution's faculty as a physician and anatomist:

> Dear Monty,
>
> . . . So far I have spent my 5th year as partly an interne partly externe. Last year a rotation included both medicine and surgery; this year I skipped a few pegs and was made resident in medicine here—seven years in all so far.
>
> Now, I want to make the final shift into surgery. Just where, I have not decided—at present I am working on several things. My big job is to visualize the final end result, if say, I spend 3 years more somewhere in surgery. . . . I'm starting to look around now.[78]

Having come to this conclusion, Drew determined to seek further training at the highest possible level. According to the reminiscences of others, he applied to the Mayo Clinic at that time regarding a position as surgical resident.

The Mayo Clinic was already famous in this era as the embodiment of a new form of what would later be called "health care delivery," the group multi-specialty clinic.

Most facility-based medical care in North America in the 1930s took place in local community hospitals, large city general hospitals, and university-affiliated teaching institutions. The new model that had been pioneered by the Mayo brothers and their associates in Rochester, Minnesota, some fifteen years before was built around the expert performance of surgical operations in concert with internist specialists providing perioperative medical care. The system was designed to generate excellent patient outcomes at high volume, and combine research and education in the process, too. By the mid-1930s the Mayo Clinic was spectacularly successful, and world-renowned. On top of that, the institution had been training surgeons in a formal residency program since 1915. With anticipation and high hopes, Drew reached out to the famous clinic. The response he received was a humiliating rejection.[79]

Reminiscences of a similar demoralizing response from the Howard University School of Medicine six years earlier must have weighed heavily on Drew. The Mayo rebuff, though, was worse. This was no application of an arbitrary rule about prerequisites—his academics were impeccable. The suspicion of more disquieting factors was inescapable. One of his future supervisors, Dr. Robert Jason, recalled the impact this had on the young doctor:

> Charlie had proven himself to be one of the top three if not the best student of his class. With this background he had every reason to believe that he would be accepted at the Mayo Clinics for a residency in surgery. He was turned down. . . . It was in this way that Charlie learned what he had had occasion only to suspect before. In the competition for a place at the top in his chosen field, merit alone was not enough. In this land of equal opportunity, he found that opportunity for him was not equal.[80]

It is not recorded whether Drew received similar responses from other American training programs or, indeed, whether he applied to any. In the same letter to Cobb quoted above, and nearly simultaneous with the bad news from Mayo, Drew inquired about the current possibilities at Howard: despite his sterling academic record at McGill, a predominantly Black medical center might be his only option: "I would appreciate a little dope on the workings of the surgery department at Howard—the way appointments are made—the chiefs, their rating, opportunity for new blood in the future. . . . I would appreciate it a great deal if you in a spare moment would lay out for me a sketch of the ground plan there now."[81]

Cobb provided what information he could. Later, he reflected on Drew's position at this critical juncture: "He was highly esteemed in Montreal and had good opportunities for a Canadian medical career, but as he had learned at Amherst something of the subtler limitations on the Negro in the United States, so he came to sense the invisible lines under the British system."[82]

Indeed, the limitations on Drew in Quebec were not as subtle as Cobb believed. A few years later one of Drew's surgery professors, Albert Bazin, observed, "We would have wished him to stay with us longer but felt it would be unfair to him as he is quadroon and there would have been no future for him in practice in Montreal."[83]

There was one interested individual who had no illusions about the sort of obstacles Charles Drew was facing, whether in Canada or the United States, regarding placement in a surgical training program. He knew because he had spent several years coping with those challenges in the lengthy and uphill process of raising the institution he ran to a higher level. That individual was Numa P. G. Adams, dean of the Howard University School of Medicine. Drew may have begun thinking about Howard as a place for surgery residency in December 1934, but Howard—and Adams—had already been thinking of him.[84] Informed of Drew's availability, Adams reached out with an offer.

To put a troubling exclamation point on a difficult season, in January 1935 Drew received word that his father, Richard, was gravely ill with pneumonia. Speeding southward on the train from Montreal, Charles arrived just hours before his "Pop" succumbed on January 14 at age fifty-six.[85] The family, which had not endured the passing of a nuclear member since Elsie fifteen years before, was crushed. If there had ever been doubt that he must return to Washington, it was gone forever.

Charles Drew was now head of his family.

Part Two

6

A Young Man of Ability and Promise

Howard University, 1935–38

In the 1930s the Howard University School of Medicine occupied two buildings on the edge of campus at Fifth and W Streets NW. One of these dated to 1869, not long after the opening of the school itself, although it had been renovated in the intervening years. By the 1930s, this unnamed premises housed only the affiliated colleges of dentistry and pharmacy. The other structure, known simply as the Medical School Building, had been completed in 1927 at a cost of $500,000 and contained the other classrooms, laboratories, and essential facilities that constituted the requirements of medical education in the era.[1] A third necessary edifice was Freedmen's Hospital, which was affiliated with Howard as a teaching institution but owned by the United States Government and administered by the Department of the Interior. Freedmen's stood between the medical school and the main campus and predated both, having been founded in 1862 to provide care for the influx of former slaves emancipated by the activities of the Civil War, many of whom came to Washington, DC.

The university was established in 1867. It was named for Oliver Otis Howard, an abolitionist and, in the Civil War, a Union Army general who had lost his right arm in combat.[2] At the time of the university's founding, Howard was commissioner of the Bureau of Refugees, Freedmen, and Abandoned Lands, commonly known as the Freedman's Bureau. This organization was responsible for the "supervision and management of all matters related to refugees, freedmen and lands abandoned or seized during the Civil War," a mighty charge if ever there was one, particularly during the chaotic time of Reconstruction. In 1869 Howard became the president of his namesake institution and held the office for five years.

Although Howard University admitted students of any race, it was, from the start, primarily focused on the education of African Americans. It was technically a private institution, but the main source of funds for the school (for many years almost exclusively) was the federal government. Tuition provided additional support, of course, as did philanthropy, depending on the vicissitudes of the era. From its inception Howard was also a provider of graduate and professional degrees—a university. The medical school held its first classes in 1868.[3]

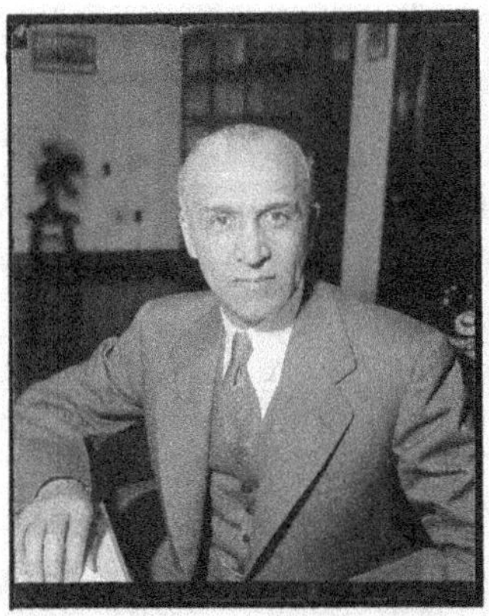

Figure 6.1 Numa P. G. Adams, Dean of the Howard University Medical School. Harris & Ewing, photographer—Library of Congress Catalog: https://lccn.loc.gov/2016875808Image download: https://cdn.loc.gov/service/pnp/hec/26800/26852v.jpgOriginal url: https://www.loc.gov/pictures/item/2016875808/, Public Domain, https://commons.wikimedia.org/w/index.php?curid=67554230

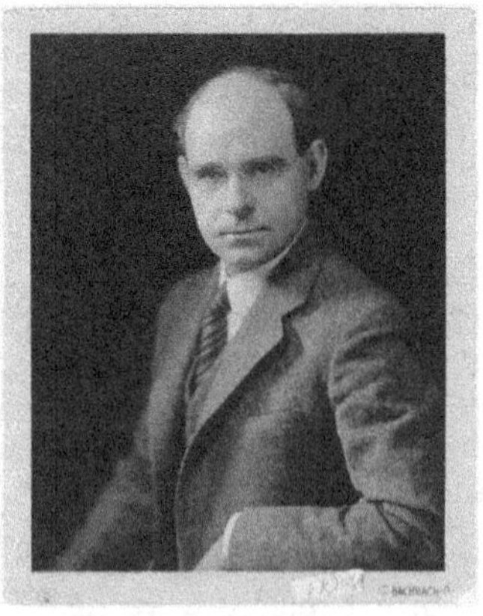

Figure 6.2 Mordecai Johnson, President of Howard University. Schomburg Center for Research in Black Culture, Photographs and Prints Division, The New York Public Library. "Portrait of Mordecai W. Johnson, first African American president of Howard University" New York Public Library Digital Collections. Accessed June 12, 2024. https://digitalcollections.nypl.org/items/69b00ec0-59bd-0130-1511-58d385a7bbd0

The dean of the Howard University School of Medicine in the 1930s was, as previously noted, the impressively named Numa Pompilius Garfield Adams, a native of Delaplane, Virginia. Adams was a graduate of Howard with both bachelor's and master's degrees. He had attended Rush Medical College in Chicago and was practicing in that city when *alma mater* came calling again in 1929. Despite the grandeur of his name, the man who became at age forty-four the first Black dean of an approved medical school in the United States was quiet, shy, and unassuming. Behind the peaceful exterior and kindly visage, however, dwelt a deep and incisive intellect, as well as a powerful spirit. Some felt that his gentle nature would serve him poorly in the shark-infested waters of academic medicine, but Adams returned to the university with a well-conceived plan to bring the Howard medical school up to par with other institutions in the country. Vitally, he had the support of the university administration in his efforts.

That administration was personified by the university president, also a relative newcomer to the scene named Mordecai Johnson, who was installed as the first African American in that important position in 1925. Johnson's powerful personality, broad vision, and indifference to stepping on toes would, in time (and there was much of this—he served until 1960) thrust the entire school into modernity and prominence. One of his first clear moves in this direction was the deliberate hiring, for the first time, of a Black physician to head up the School of Medicine. That turned out to be Numa Adams.

For decades before Johnson and Adams arrived, the medical staff of Freedmen's Hospital had been composed of both Black and white physicians, although most of the positions of authority were held by the latter. The motivations of these white physicians were generally honorable, but concessions that had to be made to accommodate their sources of revenue, private practices, wrought some hardship on the Howard medical students and Freedmen's patients. As an example, classes and clinics were often held late at night or early in the morning so as not to interfere with the white doctors' other, higher-priority responsibilities.[4] For this reason—and in a more general move to infuse the school and community with doctors who were the same race as their patients—Adams made a conscious effort to recruit and train Black physicians and scientists to assume as many positions on the faculty as possible.

Before tackling the more politically complex issues of the clinical professors, Adams began the systematic introduction of basic science instructors with a greater academic bent; individuals with PhD degrees who were doubly focused on teaching the medical students and producing the kind of research that would broadcast the name of the school into the academic community through publications and presentations. In most cases this required obtaining temporary, advanced training positions at other institutions for the putative professors.[5]

Once this effort had taken hold he pivoted to the issue of the clinical faculty, those practicing physician educators who did the actual instruction of the nascent doctors in the arts of patient care.

Adams's plan was ambitious and would require years to unfold, but the concept was sound. Improving both the preclinical and clinical faculty would, however, depend on the cooperation of outside resources, a fact intertwined with the most significant upheaval ever to occur in American medical education.

At the turn of the twentieth century, medical schools in the United States comprised a dizzying spectrum of adequacy, with a few institutions of relative excellence counterbalanced by many fly-by-night ones of stunning deficiency, and all manner of proprietary "trade" schools in between. Most were for-profit enterprises, often accepting students without even high school diplomas, provided they had the cash. These schools' courses frequently offered little or no laboratory work or practical teaching. Eventually moved to action, energetic leaders in the legitimate segment of the field called for a systematic review of medical education across the country.

Here entered Abraham Flexner, middle-aged master of a private school in Louisville, Kentucky, who brought no experience to the task but possessed a crusader's zeal and reformer's heart. Over several years, under the auspices of the American Medical Association's Council on Medical Education and the Carnegie Foundation for the Advancement of Teaching, Flexner visited every medical school in North America (155 in total) and rendered his opinion on their value.[6]

When the Flexner Report was published in 1910, a flurry of publicity and action resulted, roughly analogous to the effect of the muckraker Upton Sinclair's exposé of the meatpacking industry in his stomach-turning work of the same era, *The Jungle*. The American medical education community swiftly enacted a brisk tightening of standards, based on the model of the Johns Hopkins

School of Medicine, which Flexner considered the closest to ideal. This reform came at a price: within a decade nearly half of the country's medical schools had closed.

One of the serious consequences of the Flexner Report was the elimination of five of the seven Black medical colleges in the country, which left only Howard University's and the one at Meharry College in Nashville still standing. The nation's supply of African American physicians was already limited; the effect of closing these medical schools had the potential to be devastating.

Another important result that had a more ameliorative impact was the nascent involvement of the Rockefeller Foundation and its affiliated General Education Board (GEB) in addressing the resultant new medical education landscape via philanthropic donations (massive government funding from the National Institutes of Health and other agencies was still in the future[7]).

The GEB, which installed Abraham Flexner himself as its secretary, became an important supporter of the "new," more scientifically based medical schools, including the two surviving African American medical schools at Howard and Meharry.[8]

In 1920 the GEB pledged $200,000 to the Howard University School of Medicine in matching funds. It took seven years for the school to raise that amount, but, in that same year, the Board gave $130,000 toward the construction of the new medical building (the federal government ponied up the remaining $370,000).[9]

Aware and involved in all this, Adams wisely sought the support of the General Education Board in his efforts to enhance the Howard medical school faculty, by obtaining funding for advanced fellowship training. This was initially focused, as noted above, on the preclinical members—specifically anatomy, public health, pharmacology, and pathology—and the effort met with great success.* By 1935, with a new GEB grant, Adams was ready to apply the same methods, with a key variation, to the issue of clinical professors.

His initial idea called for bringing to Howard accomplished Black physicians to head up the clinical departments of internal medicine and surgery, but he faced the twin difficulties of identifying suitable candidates and "local

*Drew's longtime friend W. Montague Cobb was among these, in the field of anatomy.

professional jealousies" that were sure to arise. Reluctantly, Adams was compelled to alter the plan, instead recruiting established white academic physicians to serve as temporary chiefs of these services. Also supported by GEB funds, these men would guide their respective programs for five years, shepherding their departments into the modern era of academic medicine—including intensive residency training, which had not been present at Howard—while grooming their own successors from new, young Black faculty that would be brought on board. Part of the grooming process would involve GEB-sponsored clinical fellowships at other institutions for promising Howard trainees.

For the surgery part of this temporary position Adams selected Edward Lee Howes, a brusque but steady Yale man who had been a surgical resident at Columbia University in New York City. Howes had already established a reputation at the tender age of thirty-three with important research into wound healing as well as excellent clinical work.[10]

For the surgical trainees, the Dean selected three young physicians: J. Richard Laurey, a graduate of Wayne State University in Detroit; John B. Manly, a native of Tuskegee, Alabama, who had finished medical school at Howard in 1935; and a Washington, DC, native who already had two years of postgraduate training in Montreal, Canada, named Charles R. Drew.[11]

Although he was hired by Adams as a surgery trainee, Drew's initial year at Howard was dedicated to teaching pathology to medical students.[12] The pay was $1,800 per year, only ¾ of what Drew had received to be a lecturer and athletic director at Morgan College eight years before, but physicians in training have rarely been well compensated.

In the autumn 1935 term (his first at Howard) Drew was assigned to teach Pathology 170, a general introduction to the subject not much different from what he had studied under Professor Horst Oertel in the Second Division at McGill.[13] The Howard University catalog described the class this way: "A laboratory course in general pathological histology supplemented by lectures, recitations, and the study of gross specimens. Lectures and recitations, thirty-three hours; laboratory, seventy-seven hours."[14] Howard was on the semester system, the school year beginning in mid-September and finishing in June, and the class spanned both terms. All the members of the Pathology Division—including his direct supervisor, Robert Jason—pitched in, but as low man it was Drew's responsibility to shoulder most of the burden of teaching the class.

Although he must have harbored annoyance at the interruption in his clinical training, Drew approached his pathology work with the same zeal that had marked all his academic pursuits since his senior year at Amherst College. As an initiation for his students, he composed a comprehensive memorandum that detailed his perception of the subject. Not all pathologists would concur with the views he expressed in this document, but it provides unique insight into the structure and organization of Drew's thought processes, as well as the gathering core of his philosophical approach to medicine:

Pathology #170 CR Drew

Pathology is the study of disease producing constellations and their effect on living organisms. It has reared itself since the time of Virchow to the status of a science, if any field in biology may be truly called a science, and as such has and can divorce itself from its previous servile position as the hand maid of medicine; yet, for us its greatest raison d'être is the part it plays in elucidating the processes of disease in man.[15] *It is well to remember from the very beginning however that the purpose of any science is to reconstruct physical experience into a system of law and order; To bring natural phenomenon closer to our comprehension.*

The domain of science is one of causal explanations. Purpose, as such, lies outside of this realm; teleology must find its proper scope elsewhere. The moon was not hung aloft in the heavens to keep our gas bills down, neither does blood clot to prevent a man from bleeding to death. The formation of the clot may be the saving factor, but its formation is the result of a definite series of genetically related processes or steps, the absence of any one of which precludes the possibility of success, the presence of them all is tantamount to its completion. So again, bacteria, per se, are not the cause of disease, but rather are they but a single link and a long concatenation of causally connected events which include such other links as hereditary background, and environment, age, sex, mental attitude, previous state of health and the variable factors such as type, morphology, mass, and virulence of the bacteria themselves.

What is disease? It may be considered as the reflection of a pathological process or lesion upon the organism as a whole. What is a pathological lesion? It may be defined as a morphological expression of disproportion of values between stimuli and living cells. All living processes may be considered as a resultant of the interplay between various stimuli and the response of living tissues to these stimuli. If the stimulation is of short duration and of mild intensity and the activated tissue returns quickly to a state of equilibrium then the process may be considered as physiological. If on the other hand the stimuli are of greater intensity and prolonged in time, than the result may usually be considered as pathological. To state this in another way—irritants are environmental factors which are responsible for the emancipation of organismic potentialities. The degree of disproportion between the stimulating effect of an irritant and the response on the part of the Organism determines Physiology or pathology. A cloth dipped in water heated to 55 degrees Celsius and applied to a part causes a physiological increase in activity of a part with a pleasing effect and a rapid return to its previous state when the mild irritant is removed. Increase the temperature of the water to 100 degrees Celsius and it stimulates just a bit too much, and on removal there is no rapid return to the status quo ante because actual damage has been done to the tissue and this "burn" is pathological.

As beginning pathologists let us take a part of our early guidance from that great pathologist, Virchow, who said many years ago:

(1) all knowledge of disease must be based upon objective, anatomical experience.
(2) conclusions as to the nature of disease must be based on this experience and be made strictly according to natural laws of cause and effect.

There may be many exceptions to these rules at the present time that they still may serve as a sure foundation for accurate, restrained, scientific thinking and pathology. At times, perchance we shall leave our special field and indulge in theorizing and interpretation and where facts fail to us take the perfectly legitimate heuristic, somewhat circuitous route to truth, but when so doing we knowingly leave the sphere of pure sciences and enter the domain of philosophy and metaphysics.

With these few introductory the remarks let us begin our work.[16]

In the spring of 1936 Drew also taught Pathology 171, one of the medical school's required special pathology courses that met three times a week on the third floor of the Medical School Building. The 171 class covered infectious granulomas (inflammatory masses), tumors, and similar lesions.[17]

In January 1936, barely four months into his stint at Howard, Drew underwent a performance review by Dean Adams. The depth of evaluation was understandably limited, but Adams indicated a growing esteem for his youthful protégé in some of his answers to the standardized questions (in addition to revealing what traits he valued in his subordinates):

Evidences of competence as a teacher: "A young man of ability and promise."
Evidences of competence in research: "None so far. His duties have been routine laboratory work and teaching."
Evidences of increasingly able publication: "None"
Value as a counselor and guide to students: "Very limited."
Increasing administrative ability and contribution to the welfare of the university through committee services, etc.: "None."
Enhanced standing among his professional associates as evidenced by their demand for his services as speaker, counselor, consultant, committeeman or leader: "Very limited."
Any other considerations which you may wish to advance as offering illumination regarding the abilities of the teacher concerned: "He is a steady worker, intelligent, confident, and commanding. He has a very good mind and a good use of language."

Given lists of adjectives to describe the personal qualities of the individual in question, under the category "personality," Adams chose such words to describe Drew as "congenial," "polite," "reserved," "assured," and "refined." He eschewed "boisterous," "crude," and "supercilious." In the categories of "character" and "scientific aptitude" Adams saw fit to characterize the young man as "original," "independent," "reliable," and "versatile," but not "self-centered," "stubborn," "muddled," or "careless."

Summing up his promising surgeon-to-be, Adams remarked, "A very high type of man. Intelligent, forceful. Willing to work." *Recommended rank:* "On one year tenure. Would be glad to recommend him as Fellow in Surgery."[18]

Adams's final comment is of particular significance. Only a few months into his time at Howard, Drew was confirmed by his dean as a candidate for one of the important Rockefeller Foundation / GEB Fellowships—a fast track to prominence in the Department of Surgery and the university faculty. With only two years of clinical training under his belt, though—and none of it at Howard or in surgery—Drew was not yet ready for any advanced program. When his year as a journeyman pathologist ended, he would move on to his first work dedicated to learning the art and science of surgery, with the title of assistant in surgery at Howard University. He was officially offered this position in a letter from Adams dated April 29, 1936:

> Dr. Charles R. Drew
> Rosslyn, Virginia
>
> Dear Doctor Drew:
>
> I am pleased to inform you that at its meeting on April 14, 1936, the Board of Trustees of Howard University took the following action:
>
> "That Charles R. Drew, Rosslyn, Virginia, be appointed to the position of Assistant in Surgery, full time, at a salary of $1,500.00 per annum, for the year 1936–1937, with the understanding that—
>
> 1. The appointee shall be available for duty for eleven months during the period of this appointment;
> 2. During the period of this appointment the appointee shall not engage in the practice of medicine;
> 3. This appointment shall expire automatically on June 30, 1937."
>
> I shall appreciate it if, on or before May 15, 1936, you will notify this office of your acceptance of the above appointment.
>
> Very truly yours,
>
> Numa P. G. Adams
> Dean[19]

Although it must have been alarming to see his income continue to diminish while his status within the medical community ostensibly rose, particularly since the Great Depression was still underway, Drew scarcely had any alternative at this stage and gladly accepted the offer.[20]

After the death of Richard Drew in January 1935, the family had been forced to stay with friends and relatives in Washington for several weeks due to the laying of city utility pipes, which rendered the streets nearly impassable. It was during this time that Joseph and Grace's second child, a boy named Jay, was born on February 25. When the street work was finished, Mrs. Drew, Nora, Eva, Joe, Grace, and their two children returned to the Arlington home. Shortly afterward Charles, having completed his internal medicine residency year at Montreal General, joined them.[21]

With so many people living in the relatively small house, structural changes were necessary (although, assisted by his sons, Richard never really stopped making improvements after the family moved in back in 1920). In the coming months, a side porch and pantry were added, and a wall between the dining room and hall was removed. It added no space, but Mrs. Drew also planted a small spruce tree—originally intended for her husband's grave—along the side porch. Since they were both new additions at around the same time, this became known as Jay's Tree. For a while the boy kept pace with his namesake spruce as it grew, but in time the tree left him far behind. It continued to tower over the house for decades.[22]

The surgery residency at Howard would evolve in coming years under E. L. Howes, but, for Drew and his colleagues Manly and Laurey, the academic year from July 1, 1936, to June 30, 1937, consisted of three clinical blocks of four months each. These rotations were dedicated to general surgery, orthopedics, and urology. In July 1937 another trainee, Burke Syphax, joined the team (technically he was the second resident after Manly). This required a fourth rotation, and obstetrics and gynecology was added to the bill; the blocks necessarily diminished in length to three-month periods.[23]

No longer relegated to the scutwork of the intern or junior resident, Drew could focus on mastering the essentials of the surgeon's task: developing operative skills. Much of his time was now spent in the operating room, assisting Dr. Howes or the other staff surgeons in their cases.

Although obviously possessing physical capabilities of the highest order—in addition to skills in sewing imbued by his mother—Drew would require, as do all who aspire to the goal, many hundreds of hours of practice in the operating room to achieve proficiency as a surgeon.

Despite its great age as a tool of the healing arts, surgery only entered the modern era at the turn of the twentieth century. Many practitioners contributed to the process that coalesced at that time into a handful of deceptively simple rules to maximize safety in surgery, but credit for codifying them into a system has generally devolved on William Stewart Halsted, the great surgeon who worked alongside Osler in the halcyon years of the Johns Hopkins School of Medicine. During the time of Charles Drew's training, the "Halsted School" was paramount in the education of surgeons.

In the Halstedian view, careful technique on the part of the surgeon was of utmost importance to the success of the operation and well-being of the patient. Although this may seem self-evident, in the late nineteenth century anesthesia was still a relatively new arrival on the scene and, before its advent, *speed* was the most essential of the surgeon's skills. Relatively little concern was given for other technical attributes. With the luxury of time the new anesthetics provided, attention to subtler aspects of the surgical operation, and the surgeon, increased.

Halsted advocated for surgeons to adhere to four basic principles: asepsis, hemostasis, adequate exposure, and the gentle handling of tissues.

Asepsis refers to the elimination of microorganisms from the operative field. An essential aspect of this is, of course, the surgical team's pre-procedural hand scrub and donning of sterile gowns and gloves. Of equal significance is the proper application of sterilizing materials to the patient's skin, which is the main source of contaminating bacteria in wound infections. Even today, the seemingly ceaseless scourge of this surgical complication remains largely avoidable if asepsis is scrupulously achieved.

Hemostasis refers to the control of all bleeding in the operative field. The advantages of this are many, including the obvious reward of minimizing the patient's blood loss. In addition, meticulous hemostasis can minimize further wound complications that result from subcutaneous collections of blood called hematomas.

Adequate exposure refers to the need to open the operative field sufficiently to see all the affected or targeted tissues and thus exercise appropriate intraoperative judgment.

The gentle handling of tissues is perhaps the most obvious of the Halstedian precepts but the easiest to overlook and most difficult to impart to the neophyte.

In the late 1930s, these were the four cornerstones of surgical teaching, precepts that extended to every case and every form of surgical pathology. Charles

Drew would have been immersed in them by Howes and his other instructors every day.

The spectrum of procedures that the assistant and resident surgeons at Howard would have learned in the 1930s can be surmised from a classic textbook of that era, written by professors Elliott C. Cutler and Robert M. Zollinger of Harvard Medical School and the Peter Bent Brigham Hospital, the *Atlas of Surgical Operations*. It was first published in 1939.[24]

In addition to invaluable material on pre- and postoperative care of the surgical patient, Cutler and Zollinger's *Atlas* provided the step-by-step details of operative procedures that community surgeons would be expected to perform in their practices.

The *Atlas of Surgical Operations* was divided by systems.

The first section, "Neck," described the procedures of tonsillectomy, thyroidectomy, and tracheotomy. This was followed by a chapter on chest surgery, which in the 1930s—properly defined—was in its infancy. Thoracostomy ("chest tube" placement) was illustrated, along with minor breast procedures and mastectomy. Under "Abdominal Wall," the authors grouped hernia repairs (umbilical, femoral, and inguinal) as well as a detailed presentation on the closure of abdominal wounds—an indication of the significance placed on this vital, but often overlooked, aspect of abdominal surgery.[25]

The chapter titled "Gastro-Intestinal" system illustrated operations on the stomach, gall bladder, small and large intestines, spleen, and appendix. The stomach procedures included gastrostomy ("stomach tube"), gastrectomy (several variations depending on the pathology involved), and gastrojejunosomy (connection of the stomach to the small bowel in special circumstances for ulcer or cancer cases). Gall bladder operations included two methods of removal of the organ (cholecystectomy) as well as the more esoteric connection of the gall bladder to the stomach (cholecystogastrostomy) used in some very unusual cases of bile duct obstruction. The bowel procedures comprised resection for benign or malignant processes and various means of reconnection or diversion of the intestinal contents (e.g., colectomy, enterostomy, abdominoperineal resection for colorectal cancer). The appendix and spleen chapters covered only removal of these organs.

The next two chapters of the *Atlas* discussed gynecological procedures such as total abdominal hysterectomy, removal of the ovaries and fallopian tubes (salpingo-oophorectomy), and various vaginal and cervical resections and reconstructions. Such operations were considered in the domain of general surgery at the time.

The final chapter, "Extremities," illustrated methods of incision and drainage of infections in the hand; injection and excision of the saphenous vein of the leg for venous stasis disease including varicose veins; skin grafts; and amputations.

These, then, represented the techniques and methods of general surgery in the 1930s that Drew and his fellow trainees were expected to master during their years of residency.

On June 26, 1937, Drew's sister Nora, now twenty-four years old, married Francis Gregory at the Arlington house. Nora had graduated from Dunbar High School and moved on to her mother's alma mater, the Miner School (her fiancé was, in fact, the son of one of her college professors). She was now teaching at the Giddings School in southeast Washington, DC. Nora's brothers set to work creating as idyllic a setting as they could for the ceremony. Eva remembered: "Charlie and Joe made our home absolutely beautiful. They cleaned and painted, manicured the lawns, trimmed the hedges and shrubs and planted flowers. They wound vines and leaves around the posts on the porch. Everything was beautiful."

Unfortunately, nature took a hand and a cloudburst opened just as the festivities commenced. Undaunted, the brothers engaged in damage control: "Joe and Charlie moved the piano and sofa in the living room (when it stopped raining) and took the carpet outside. They made an area where the wedding party could stand like an altar."[26]

Later in the year, with the completion of the new Arlington Boulevard, streets in the area were named (or renamed) and numbered. From this point on, the Drew house was officially 2505 First Street South.[27]

Although the long hours at Freedmen's Hospital sometimes made it seem as if he still were living at some distant place, Drew and his family cherished the opportunity to spend more time together after so many years apart (Joe and Grace lived in the Arlington house with their two boys; Nora and Francis moved in with the Gregorys after their wedding). Eva's recollections of this period paint a vivid picture of the brother who was both a friend and father figure to the young girl. As a mentor with impeccable scholastic credentials, he gave the teenager affectionate but strict instructions on how to study properly:

> I was told that I did not study correctly. To study more profitably, to have better retention (his words), to be more comfortable, and to be successful with my classwork I should follow these specific directions.
>
> 1. Sit in a straight backed chair.
> 2. Have my reading material or other work on an uncluttered table or desk in front of me.
> 3. Keep my feet flat on the floor with legs uncrossed.
> 4. Sit up straight—don't slouch.
> 5. Since I am left-handed always have light coming from my right or over my right shoulder.
>
> It's hard to nod off with these directions. I guess they worked.[28]

Eva remembered that Charlie always wore black socks, often with white linen knickers and a navy-blue jacket. One of his favorite foods was a cold baked bean sandwich. Although Drew did indulge in tobacco, he did not drink alcohol. This fact sometimes led to amusing conflicts with his sense of propriety: "Charlie didn't drink alcoholic beverages. He smoked zillions of cigarettes and pipes, but he didn't drink. At parties when he was offered drinks he didn't always refuse them. He didn't want to be too different. So, during the course of a pleasant evening, if there were a house plant available he would sneakily water it with his drink."[29]

It was around this time that Drew acquired his first automobile, a necessity given his long hours at Freedman's and the responsibility to be prompt. Eva remembered this as well:

> Charlie's first car was a two-seater. It had a rumble seat. You had to climb up on the back fender, then step into the rumble seat. I wonder what you did if it started raining. It had no roof.
>
> Charlie tried to teach Nora how to drive in that car. What a disaster! She backed it out of the driveway next to the house, on to the street. She kept backing—in a

circle—right into Joe's and Charlie's precious hedges that they had nurtured and groomed from little sticks.[30]

This memory coincided in Eva's recollections with one of the few areas in which her very accomplished older brother did not excel: driving. On one occasion he rear-ended a streetcar while distracted by an animated conversation with his mother, and on another he fell asleep while driving and struck a trolley car station. Luckily, no one was injured in either circumstance. As Eva recalled, "He wasn't the best driver."[31]

As a member of the resident staff, Drew was not only expected to learn surgical care and take care of patients but also teach the rudiments of the subject to the medical students—just as he had been taught while in Third Division at the McGill Faculty of Medicine. He had general instructions for his students typed up, and these have survived, providing special insight into what life was like for a tyro on the service of the rising Dr. Drew in the late 1930s at Freedmen's Hospital:

Routines for Students on General Surgical Wards:

1. Students must report for duty on the Surgical wards promptly at 9:00 A.M.
2. Leave telephone numbers on Bulletin Board in Ward 6 for emergency calls.
3. History, physical examination and initial laboratory work must be handed to Dr. Drew 48 hours after the case is assigned. Initial laboratory work consists of urine examination, complete blood count, Hgb., and sputum examination when present. Also write your laboratory findings on the progress sheet of the official history. Sign your name and in brackets, (Student).
4. Extra laboratory work required is also to be written on the same sheet with the same notation. This work must be on the charts before ward rounds the next day. Staff rounds are held daily at 10:30 except Thursday when they are held at 9:00 A.M. Observe the Bulletin Board at all hours until 6:00 P.M. for the assignment of required laboratory work.

5. A post-operative urine examination must be done on each case and recorded on the progress records.
6. All students both Juniors and Seniors are to scrub on their cases. Students must observe the operative schedule in MOR each morning to see if their case is posted.
7. Ward conferences for students will be held Monday, Wednesday and Friday at 10:00 A.M. Watch Bulletin Board for the ward assignments as to where the Senior and Junior group will meet. Please report promptly at 10:00 A.M.
8. All students are to attend staff dressing rounds Thursday at 9:15.
9. All students are to report Tuesday morning at 9:30 to Dr. Laurey in the west side pathological laboratory for Surgical Pathology. Bring microscopes.
10. Students are not to be absent from ward conferences, surgical pathology and dressing rounds for any reason except to scrub in MOR. If need be, histories, physical examinations and laboratory work must be done at times other than the 9–11 hours assigned.
11. Surgical Diagnostic and Follow-up Clinic is held Tuesday and Thursday at 4 :00 P.M. in the Medical Clinic. Attendance at those sessions is optional, but it is hoped that both Juniors and Seniors will avail themselves of this opportunity.
12. All students must know the history, physical findings and progress of his case at all times and be prepared to present this data at ward conferences or surgical clinics. All new cases will be assigned in rotation and all old cases will be divided among the group. Summaries of the old cases assigned not over two pages in length must be handed to Dr. Drew not later than one week after beginning work on the wards.
13. Assume that the assigned cases are your cases and do not hesitate to do extra laboratory work. Check all positive findings with a second examination. Cooperate with the interne in charge of the case and report to him any developments observed. Write your own progress notes on the official ward history & sign your name with "Student" in brackets. The interne will be glad to have you see the dressings, assist at

giving clyses, transfusions, and taking Wassermans. Look at the X-rays taken as well as reading the reports.

14. Have the staff check any clinical signs you are in doubt about and do not be afraid to ask questions, or solicit aid for any procedure.[32]

In the spring of 1938 Drew finished his second year of surgery residency—technically, as noted above, assistant in surgery—at Howard University and his fourth year of postgraduate clinical training, including his internship and year of internal medicine residency at Montreal General Hospital. He had developed a good working relationship with his department chief Howes (who was only a year older than Drew), learning a great deal about operative surgery in addition to the key elements of pre- and postoperative patient care. He was now deemed ready to proceed with the General Education Board clinical fellowship.

Likely on the recommendation of Howes, Drew was given a two-year assignment as a fellow in surgery at his chief's former training ground, the Columbia University College of Physicians and Surgeons in New York City. His salary there would be $1,800 per year.[33]

Charlie Drew was headed to Manhattan.

7

Naturally Great

New York City, 1938–40

The chief of surgery at Columbia University in 1938 was fifty-seven-year-old Allen Oldfather Whipple, a slim, graceful man with luxuriant gray eyebrows and the bespectacled appearance of a New England schoolmaster. Whipple had, however, been born in the more exotic location of Urmia in far northwestern Persia, the son of missionaries. A fine education at Princeton and then Columbia's medical school had produced in Whipple an adult of considerable intellectual capacity and breadth of interests, contained in a persona of uncompromising standards and integrity. By the time Drew encountered him, Whipple had attained a place of prominence in the world community of surgery commensurate with his contributions; later that would magnify as he became famous for devising a *magnum opus* of general surgery: the operation known as pancreaticoduodenectomy that would ultimately bear his name.[1] Whipple had run the surgery program at Columbia for seventeen years and elevated it to one of the most rigorous and well regarded in the land; the residency he founded was New York City's first.[2]

The Medical Center of Columbia University—comprising the College of Physicians and Surgeons, the Presbyterian Hospital, Babies Hospital, Neurological Institute, Institute of Ophthalmology, Harkness Pavilion, Vanderbilt Clinic, the New York State Psychiatric Institute, and the Schools of

Nursing and Dental/Oral Surgery—was located in the Upper West Side of Manhattan along the Hudson River, on the blocks between Riverside Drive and Broadway between 165th and 168th Streets. The main campus of Columbia straddled 116th Street and Broadway well to the south.

When Drew arrived at the Columbia Medical Center in mid-June 1938, he went straightaway to Presbyterian and the office of his new chief. Dr. Whipple took the measure of this unusual charge who, at thirty-four years of age, was no longer a youth by appearance or mien. He was, however, in Whipple's words, "of colored extraction, but this is only slightly evident."[3] Columbia and Presbyterian Hospital had never had a Black surgery resident, evident or otherwise, because the same sort of preemptive reasoning that Drew had encountered in Montreal held sway in New York City: *white patients will not accept a Black physician.* Not coincidentally, by this time Presbyterian had developed something of a nose-in-the-air reputation as one of the health care institutions preferred by the Manhattan upper crust, even though it had been founded to serve the poor of the city "without regard to Race, Creed, or Color" (all races were still admitted).[4]

When the issue of his race arose in the conversation, Whipple noted that Drew, undoubtedly aware of the importance of this opportunity not only for his own future but that of his home institution, Howard University, "very frankly said that he did not wish to cause any embarrassment and would be glad to confine his work to the laboratory."[5]

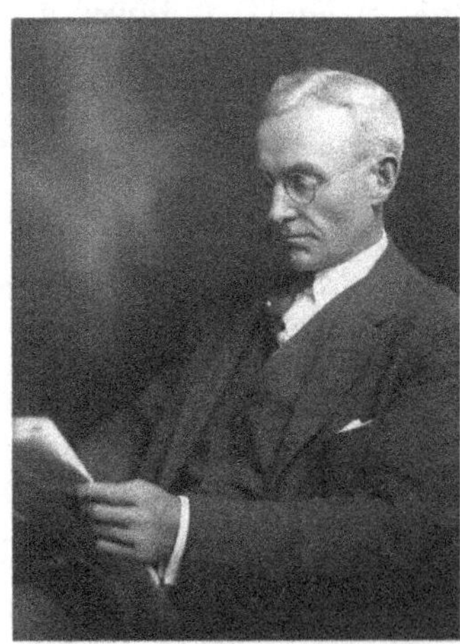

Figure 7.1 Allen Oldfather Whipple, Chair of Surgery at Columbia University College of Physicians and Surgeons.

Academic programs—strictly speaking, those affiliated with universities, although some large community hospitals share similar characteristics—have long had a tripartite mission: to care for patients, to educate students and residents, and to perform meaningful research. The last of these was the element still missing from Drew's curriculum vitae. As things evolved, he would have ample opportunities to apply himself in the clinical realm at Columbia, but from the start the laboratory was his New York City home, and the place he would spend the most time.

Whipple assigned Drew to the tutelage of one of the Department of Surgery's important faculty research men, Dr. John Scudder.

Like Whipple, Scudder had been born abroad—in his case, in Villore, India, in 1900—and was the son of missionaries. In fact, generations of the Scudder family had served as medical missionaries in that country, and their ties went correspondingly deep. For this reason, after finishing medical school at Harvard and surgical postgraduate study in Cleveland and New York City, Scudder returned to India to work in the hospital his namesake great-grandfather had founded in the city of Ranipet in the southeast portion of the country in 1819.

Scudder spent several years in India, practicing surgery and developing an interest in shock and its treatment that would last for the remainder of his career. He later summarized this period and its evolution into work on blood transfusion:

> My interest in blood stemmed from the treatment of surgical shock in India, in the '30's. The shock seemed associated with dehydration of cholera and similar states which responded varyingly well to the correct administration of salt solution in sufficient quantities. However, from the magnitude of surgery which had to be performed, the effectiveness of salt solution was insufficient and one would need blood to bring the patient out of shock, especially in those cases associated with post-partum hemorrhage.[6]

When he returned to the United States in 1936, Scudder joined Whipple's Columbia surgery faculty as an instructor and established a lab in the Surgical Pathology section to study the physiology of shock as well as potential methods of its treatment. He also began working toward an advanced degree that Columbia offered called doctorate in medical science. Drew arrived on the scene two years later, and, at Whipple's behest, Scudder "put him in the 'shock lab' where he soon mastered the tests and became very useful to the hospital."[7]

Only a few days after arriving in New York City, Drew wrote to his mother from his new dormitory, a medical school residence building on the northwest edge of the medical campus.

Bard Hall
50 Haven Ave.
Columbia Presbyterian Medical Center
June 18th 1938

Dear Mother,

Here goes the first of a new series—Salem—Amherst—Morgan—McGill—Montreal General, now Physicians and Surgeons of Columbia and Presbyterian. Each new step has marked growth in 1000 ways, yet through it all I have seemed to have remained the same; the people and things dear to me from a very long time ago retained, and probably always shall retain first place in my thinking and feeling, so much so that though separated from them, never estranged and the living force in this intangible bond which holds so tightly is you.

This place is so immense and has so many ramifications that I haven't even found my way around it yet. I've had a good fast start, a pleasant time, and expect to enjoy it a lot. At the present time I am working all day (and a good part of the night) in the laboratory making determinations of the components of blood in very ill patients under Doctor John Scudder of the Scudder Memorial Hospital, Ranipet, India. He has been carrying on experimental work here for three years and is to continue his work at the Rockefeller Institute on July 1st and I shall carry on the work here.* He gave me two days instruction and techniques and then left on a short vacation and I've been stewing ever since. This morning at 1:00 A.M. I was called in to interpret the blood findings on a very sick patient with reference to the best therapy. Four days and a consulting specialist already (but between you and me I haven't the slightest idea about what all these figures mean in terms of living or not living).

Later on I hope to be able to do some work in the clinics and at least make the big weekly grand rounds. What I get out of this year will depend to a large degree on the amount of work I do and the ability to get along with people and get them to give out what they know. I believe I'll do both without too much strain.

* Scudder appears to have continued his work at Columbia while, as will be seen, engaging in separate but similar research at the Rockefeller Institute.

There are some grand people here, it's good to feel the impact of new ideas and the surge of creative activity.

Love to all, Charlie[8]

In a short period of time Drew became well acclimated to the lab and, in addition to performing blood tests on the inpatients, began to apply himself to research projects.

Early in 1939, the first two of Drew's published papers appeared in the medical literature. These were "Anhydremia in Appendicitis" in *Surgical Clinics of North America* and "Plasma Potassium Content of Cardiac Blood at Death" in the *American Journal of Physiology*.[9] Both these articles were coauthored with Scudder, as well as assistant professor of surgery Lawrence W. Sloan on the appendicitis paper and fellow "shock lab" colleague Margaret E. Smith on the potassium one. Neither of these papers was a particularly outstanding contribution to the profession's fund of knowledge, but they marked Drew's entry into the field and clearly indicated the emerging focus of Scudder's laboratory: fluid and electrolyte balance in health and disease ("anhydremia" is an archaic term for relative paucity of water in the blood, roughly synonymous with the modern term hemoconcentration). As the world of surgical bench research entered a golden era in the years to come, these fields would prove to be of abiding interest and import.

In April 1939, Drew made the long trip from New York City to Alabama to attend an annual free clinic and medical conference at the John A. Andrew Memorial Hospital in Tuskegee. This was the twenty-eighth consecutive version of these gatherings, which had long since become, as honorary president Walter Gray Crump, MD, observed, "the greatest teaching clinic for Negroes anywhere in the world today."[10] That was only part of the story, though. The Andrew clinic was a weeklong affair, and included physicians (mostly Black, but many whites, as well) from across the country, offering their expertise in medicine, surgery, radiology, otolaryngology, ophthalmology, dermatology, cardiology, orthopedics, obstetrics and gynecology, pediatrics, anesthesia, and neuro-psychiatry. In addition to the patient care services, which were offered at no charge and attracted the indigent population from across many states of the deep south, conferences were held in which the latest developments in these many fields were presented and discussed. It was one of the main items on the calendar of every African American physician who was able to attend.

Drew took the train to Washington and had a brief stay with his family before setting out for Tuskegee by automobile. He and two physician co-travelers planned to drive as far as Atlanta before stopping for the night. One of his fellow physicians on the trip was Lowell Cheatham Wormley, a graduate of the Howard University School of Medicine who was practicing in the Harlem Hospital at this time.[11]

In this era, and for many years, motor hotels in the south typically did not accept Black guests.[12] Knowing this, the men had made plans accordingly. One of Drew's longtime friends from Dunbar and Amherst, W. Mercer Cook, was at this time a professor of French on the faculty of the University of Atlanta. He offered to put them up.

One afternoon during his brief stay, Drew caught sight of a strikingly beautiful young woman at the Bessie Strong residence hall of Spelman College, a liberal arts school for Black women adjacent to Atlanta University.

The woman was Minnie Lenore Robbins, a twenty-seven-year-old teacher of home economics at Spelman. Originally from Philadelphia, Robbins had been educated at State Teacher's College in Cheyney, Pennsylvania (the same school Drew's excellent 1927 Morgan Bears football team defeated to start their renaissance season), Columbia Teacher's College, and Cornell University, earning a master's degree in home economics education.[13]

Hearing of the encounter, Mercer Cook arranged to have Miss Robbins invited to an impromptu dinner party at his home, where she and Drew were introduced. The two spent much of the evening dancing and conversing, and Drew later walked her back to her dormitory. By the time he had to continue to Tuskegee, Drew was spellbound in a way that was entirely novel for the deeply grounded young man. He was utterly unprepared to be so affected and confessed the fact to his companions.

At the close of the conference on the night of Wednesday, April 5, Drew sent a startling telegram to the object of his newfound obsession, referring to her by her middle name, as he would for the remainder of his life:

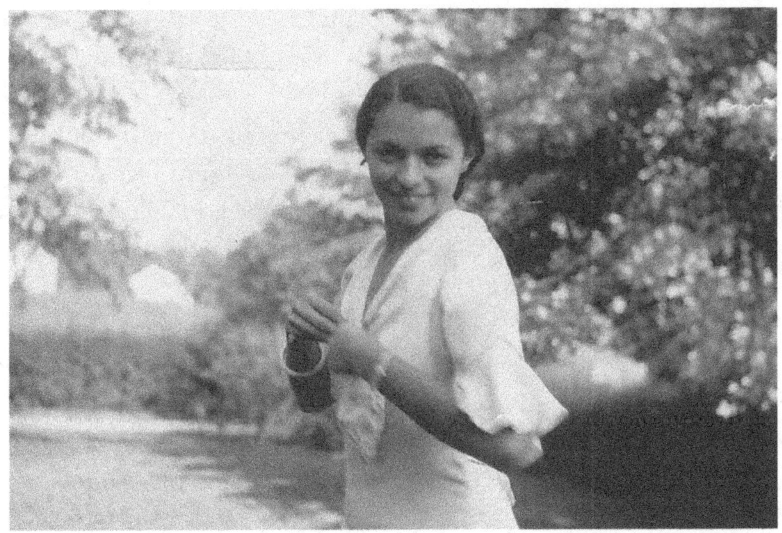

Figure 7.2 Minnie Lenore Robbins. Personal collection, Charlene Drew Jarvis.

TUSKEGEE, ALA 1939 APR 5 948P
MISS LENORE ROBBINS
SPELMAN COLLEGE ATLANTA

ARRIVE ABOUT ONE A.M. PLEASE STAY UP COMING TO MERCER'S

CHARLIE.[14]

Atlanta is 130 miles from Tuskegee, but Drew was as good as his word, covering the distance in rapid form, apparently accompanied only by Wormley, to arrive on Thursday in the early morning hours. Speed was key because the need to act was great. After half a lifetime of carefully thought-out decisions, some accompanied by unbridled joy and enthusiasm, others coupled with frustration and regret, this most circumspect of men was breaking every prior tendency in a rapture of romance. He had made up his mind while at the Andrew Clinic to ask this exquisite Minnie Lenore Robbins to marry him.

Her response to what must have been a shocking turn of events was measured, a kind of *definite maybe*. In later years Lenore remembered her first impression of Drew: "The moment I saw him I knew he was a man to be reckoned with. He seemed to be from another—a more old-fashioned and courtly—time and place."[15]

Drew and Wormley stayed the night at the home of Mercer Cook and his wife, then left Atlanta the following day with a last visit to Lenore. When he took his leave of her, Drew let the memory linger in his mind's eye: "I left you standing in the window as we pulled out—a lovely picture that completely filled my vision as the miles sped by."[16]

Drew and Wormley drove as far as Charlotte that day, "hardly a word having been passed" between them. They spent Friday night with a physician friend of Wormley's, then the next day in Oxford, North Carolina. Wormley's grandfather had founded a Black orphanage there, and his widow proudly took the young physicians on a tour. The next day they made the 230-mile leg to Washington, DC:

> We arrived at my home about 10:00 P.M. to find things in an uproar my brother having just been brought back from the hospital with a broken leg which he sustained earlier in the afternoon when the ladder on which he was standing to give the roof a spring coat of paint broke and dropped him about 30 feet. Lowell spent the night with us, then pulled out for New York early in the morning. I stayed to see how my brother was going to make out. During the morning I took my mother to church and then spent two hours with the Dean of the medical school.[17]

Undoubtedly Drew told his mother all about his new infatuation; the conversation with Dean Adams probably steered toward more practical issues such as how well things were going at Columbia. In the afternoon Drew went to see the great vocalist Marian Anderson perform before a gigantic multiracial crowd at the National Mall (like Drew, Anderson was a recipient of the Rosenwald Fellowship). He described the memorable scene to Lenore:

> I went down to the Lincoln Memorial to hear Marian Anderson sing. In all my life I have never seen such an impressive thing. With the soft rays of a pink sun

gleaming against the white marble beauty of that magnificent structure and reflecting itself in the long still pool of water that stretches off toward the Washington Monument she raised her exquisite voice in song and lifted with a sweep of melody a whole race to higher levels of thought, feeling and hope. Countless thousands paid her the tribute of almost reverent silence when she sang her songs of joy and sorrow. She held them beneath her magic sway, making them laugh or sigh at will and when she finished with "Nobody Knows the Trouble I've Seen" many eyes were moist with unashamed tears and hearts too full for words. Filled with a strange pride and awed by the loveliness and significance of it all my thoughts went out to you and in the beauty of the moment I communed with you and found my happiness increased. Oh how I wish that you might have been there with me.[18]

These thoughts were recorded a few days later, after Drew had returned to New York City. That Sunday night, after the concert and while still at home in Arlington, Drew sat down to pen in his immaculate handwriting the first of what would become a host of love letters. Other than his New Year's Eve Montreal Testament of 1930 these are the existing writings that best reveal the inner workings and vulnerable aspects of this very private, confident, and driven man:

Easter Sunday
At Twilight

Lenore,

With a heart that's full with a newfound joy my thoughts turn to you as the day closes, and a sigh rises as an evening prayer to ask whatever gods there be to keep you safe for me. Since first seeing you I have moved through the days as one in a dream, lost in revery, awed by the speed with which the moving finger of fate has pointed out the way I should go. As the miles of countryside sped by on our return trip I sat silent and pondered on the power that lies in a smile to change the course of a life, the magic in the tilt of a head, the beauty of your carriage and the gentleness that struck so deeply.

Later, when I become more coherent, I shall say perhaps many things but tonight this one thing alone seems to ring clearly, I love you.

Charlie
Washington, DC
April 9, 1939[19]

If there had been any doubt as to Drew's sincerity, on the way back to New York he stopped in Philadelphia to spend two hours with Lenore's family: "Your mother was sweet, your dad tolerant, courteous and kind, your brother puzzled but decent."[20]

Although he dove back into his laboratory work at Columbia, Drew made a point to take the few opportunities his heavy schedule offered to continue corresponding with Lenore, nurturing what was finally, for him, a serious romance. He professed his love in a dizzying parade of variations:

> Sunday morning 2 A.M.
>
> April 16, 1939
>
> My sweet . . .
>
> When I first kissed your hand it was almost reverently done for even then I felt an inward surge that was inexplicable. When you walked I felt lifted by the graciousness of your carriage, when you talked it was your gentleness that struck so deeply, when you smiled there was sweetness that only a fortunate few can carry over from an unspoiled childhood to full glorious womanhood; poised but vibrant, there was something which responded in me and left a glow which still suffuses my whole being and warms my heart. It's a grand feeling Lenore. The only rash, unplanned, unpremeditated thing I've done for years is already paying dividends in 1000 delightful ways.[21]

In this same impassioned missive Drew revealed, for the first time, what was and would continue to be the main focus of his life and career, even after the plaudits of a grateful world gathered around work he considered of lesser import:

> For years I have done little but work, plan and dream of making myself a good doctor, an able surgeon and in my wildest dreams perhaps also playing some

part in *establishing a real school of thought among Negro physicians and guiding some of the younger fellows to levels of accomplishment not yet attained by any of us* (emphasis added). I have known the cost of such desires and have been quite willing to do without many of the things that one usually regards as but natural. Then I met you and for the first time mistress medicine met her match and went down almost without a fight. Life suddenly widened its horizons and took on new meaning. I know clearly just how lonely I had become, first how badly I needed someone rather than just something to cling to, someone to work for, rather than just a goal to aim at, someone to dream with, cherish from day to day, and share the little things with, the smiles and if need be the tears that will sometimes come.[22]

For her part Lenore was more reserved in her affections, or at least displays of them: after all, she had only known Drew a few weeks, and for only a few hours in person. After receiving several letters in the month of April, most of a similar theme, in one of her replies Lenore observed, "Frankly, I'm not sure a wife would help you."[23] Aghast, Drew responded by calling her attention to the contrast of the passionate present with his stoic past, the names and faces of Lelia Waller, Mary Maxwell, and others undoubtedly crossing his mind:

May 3, 1939

Dear Lenore,

. . . It's not just a wife for the sake of having a wife that's important to me, Lenore. I've ducked, dodged, and squirmed away from would-be wives for a long time, it's almost become an art.[24]

Drew then went on to reveal the inner doubts he kept hidden from all, the true emotional needs he felt, and what he saw as—despite their brief acquaintance—Lenore's unique ability to fill them:

My headstrongness would listen to your council, my fears I'd tell you, my weaknesses confess. This must sound silly but these are the things I don't do. . . . People have expected me to be strong, when I would much rather would be weak. I'd not

> be ashamed to admit my weakness before you, for there is no place for vanity in the presence of those we love, and in the presence of those who love us even weakness becomes strength.[25]

Lenore's answer to this has not survived, but events confirm that it must have been supportive—not to say that were no further hazards to negotiate in the early relationship of two individuals who were highly intelligent but navigating new emotional waters.

Drew's next letter, from May 7, contains no declarations of love or maudlin musings on its vanity, instead being a report of a day-long effort to quell a small forest fire. Drew had been invited to spend the day with John Scudder and his wife at their property on Shelter Island. There, Scudder inadvertently ignited the surroundings while burning trash. Instead of enjoying a relaxing Sunday, the two men spent the next hours extinguishing the flames. When their work reached a successful conclusion there was finally time for reflection:

> I like this place because from the house there is nothing but water in front and rising wooded hills on the other three sides. One comes here and it seems strange that people persist in living over and under and around each other so densely in the city. Tonight we climbed to the highest point on the island to be sure no new fires were not breaking out from sparks carried by the wind and the heavens seemed so close—the work a day world so far away.[26]

The following Thursday was May 11, 1939. In preparation for the day—and beyond—Drew composed for himself a typewritten memo titled "THINGS TO DO," which sheds some light on the scope of his laboratory efforts under Whipple and Scudder, as well as other practical aspects of his Columbia experience during this period:

1. Call Mrs. McCurdie about printing of labels.
2. Make up outline for Blood Bank record book.
3. Write Miss Stoddard and tell her to report for work on June 15th.[27]
4. Find out from Mr. Bush when ice box is likely to be here.
5. Types of container:

a. Bell jar (see Dr. Rosenthal about purchase)
b. Type in use at Belleview
c. Blueprint of plan for narrow neck type
d. Erlenmeyer flasks

6. Types of anticoagulants
   a. 21.5% sodium citrate
   b. Citrate with sufficient glucose make pH of 7.0
   c. Citrate with sufficient CO_2 to make pH of 7.0
   d. Determine the toxicity of isotonic ozalic acid in quantity sufficient to prevent clotting for use in cases of hemophilia and the bleeding of pregnancy.
7. Ask Dr. Bull if volunteer worker will be available June 15th.
8. See Dr. Whipple about living in hospital after June 15th.
9. See Dr. Rose about studies in agglutinins, antigens, fibrolysins, and malarial parasites in banked blood.
10. Check cellular changes in citrated blood and compare with the immune quantities.
11. Note to Dr. Barbour.
12. Note to J. Biol. Chem. to use falling drop chart.
13. Finish series of normal hematocrits.
14. Finish series of normal specific gravities.
15. Legend for Hematocrit-Protein patterns
16. Note to Hugh Simmons. Cannot speak.
17. Appointment with Dr. Sloan.
18. Check qualifications with American Board of Surgery.
19. Do series of normal rabbits.
20. Help finish x-ray series.
21. Placental bloods. Do next.[28]

Drew sent a copy of the list to Lenore along with his May 11 letter. He went on to discuss plans for her to visit him in New York, meeting his family in Washington along the way, as well as his misgivings about the old specter—money. By this time Drew seems to have become inured to the personal impact of what was once the overriding issue of lack of funds, though finances were as bad as ever with the growing family at the Arlington house and the vagaries of day-to-day events (Joe was out of work recovering from his broken leg and Nora took a hiatus from teaching for the birth of her son, Frederick). Subjecting Lenore to poverty for the sake of love, though, was quite a different thing:

> Dear Lenore,
>
> Tonight I've sat a long time, just sitting, very little more, wondering why it seems so difficult to make definite plans and tell you about them concerning the thing I most sincerely desire—to have you near me—to have you with me—always.
>
> In contrast I look at a sort of schedule I jotted down this morning as a memorandum for the day. There are plans, some of rather long range, yet I seem to have no trouble. Looking at it now a great deal of it is built around you. 3. Miss Stoddard was to report next week but if the blood bank starts next week I will not be free to be with you should you come between June 1st and 15th. 7. If the volunteer worker comes during that time I'll have to train her. 8. If a new rule goes into effect June 1st I may have to live right in the hospital at all times and go back to intern uniforms. This I must find out. 16. Obviously if you are here I can't speak in Washington on June 8th.
>
> There are other things. At present this is all I can say. My intentions are honorable. I too have many things to talk over with you; My mind and heart are sure, only the details have to be worked out. . . . I think you should take a look at the rest of the Drews too on your way up. I've told you all I know or can find out at present about my immediate plans unless I rob a bank or something comparable. When I started South I had no more idea of changing my way of living than I had of flying. I therefore had made no preparations. Even at that time there was no particular drawback. Both my brother's injury and the announcement of my sister's retirement from teaching have sort of stymied me for the moment. All three events are the sort of things that are relatively unpredictable, the warp and weave of life.
>
> This I ask, that you trust me to do all I can to, as speedily as possible, bring about the things which I'm sure will bring me happiness greater than I've ever known and you some of the joy I wish for you.
>
> For the moment may it not suffice that your heart is no longer empty and that I love you with a love that grows deeper and surer and warmer each day.
>
> Charlie[29]

The May 11, 1939, letter to Lenore is also significant because it is the first mention Drew is known to have made of the Columbia University Presbyterian Hospital Blood Bank.

While he was in the surgical research lab at Columbia, Drew took on several different projects simultaneously, neatly summarized in Whipple's annual report to the dean of the School of Medicine for 1939: "Dr. Drew and Dr. Scudder have been working on a wide variety of problems concerned with surgical shock, fluid therapy, plasma proteins, the role of potassium in surgical conditions, and blood preservation."[30] Although these topics might appear superficially distinct, they were all deeply related within the pathologic condition mentioned by Whipple and chosen by Scudder as the unofficial moniker of his lab: shock.

Even today the word "shock" used in the medical context engenders confusion, not least due to its many definitions outside the field. Most modern physicians and scientists would likely accede to the definition of shock as *a mismatch between the oxygen supply and demands of tissues caused by circulatory failure*. The causes can be many, although they fall within a few reasonably well-defined categories. Cardiogenic shock, for example, arises when the heart fails, and the circulation follows suit. The term hypovolemic shock refers to the state wherein blood loss, as from trauma, causes the circulatory collapse. Infection and severe allergic reactions can initiate shock not from loss of blood from the body but sequestration of the fluid component in the tissues, the result of a disastrous increase in permeability of blood vessel walls. In neurogenic shock a loss of muscular tone in the vascular walls causes circulatory failure. In all these situations the flow of oxygenated blood to the tissues is disrupted and injury ensues. If allowed to progress unabated the result is a spiraling course with severe injury and, ultimately, death. If properly treated and the underlying cause addressed, the process can be interrupted with restoration to health.

In the 1930s the severity of the problem of shock in clinical medicine, especially in surgery, was well appreciated, but the many mechanisms by which it arises were poorly understood. Effective therapy was consequently elusive. For this reason, labs across the world, including Scudder's at Columbia, were dedicated to studying the phenomenon in all its manifestations and physiologic complexity.

The derangement of the conceptually simplest shock scenario—blood loss—seemed clear enough and the most amenable to existing therapies (although even this, in time, would prove to involve far more complex mechanisms than there being, simply, "not enough blood"). Blood replacement via transfusion was the obvious solution.

The removal of blood from a healthy individual for infusion in one suffering from blood loss had a long history. Unfortunately, it was mostly one of failure.

The technique of transfusion was the least problematic of the issues involved with the concept, but even that was a protracted exercise in calamity. Things had gotten better by the 1930s, but the procedure remained far from elegant. With very few exceptions, transfusions were performed directly from donor to recipient, frequently in the operating room, for practical reasons. Each patient had a needle placed into an arm vein, then the donor's blood was either pumped directly into the recipient via a syringe and rubber tubing or, in more sophisticated circumstances, into an intervening bottle containing sodium citrate and saline solution, which would inhibit clotting (imperfectly). In even more primitive versions of the operation, a syringe was simply filled with donor blood and injected into the recipient. These alternatives were all messy and prone to failure—needles were frequently dislodged; blood inevitably spattered over patients, staff, and surroundings; and clotting mid-transfusion was a frustrating likelihood.

Beyond the unsatisfactory technique, though, there were worse problems with transfusing blood between individuals.

Chief among these was the specter of sometimes-fatal transfusion reactions. Although the ABO blood groups had been discovered in 1901, the Rh factor would not be elucidated until 1940, and, in any case, typing and crossmatching techniques were anything but perfect: as a result, adverse reactions were a common and serious threat in transfusions, ranging from mild symptoms like itching and fever to the catastrophic circulatory collapse called anaphylaxis—ironically, a form of neurogenic shock. Death was a legitimate and terrifying possibility, usually due to crossmatching errors. There were other poorly understood if less dire concerns, too, such as a tendency for recipients to become jaundiced after transfusions, their urine to turn dark with the breakdown products of blood cells, and the unclear threat of elevated potassium levels in the donor blood (which appeared to be caused by the trauma of the transfusion process).

Despite these drawbacks, the concept of transfusion held enormous appeal as a ready-made solution to the problem of blood loss, if the cited issues could somehow be overcome. However, there was another obstacle: the availability of donors. When a patient was in hypovolemic shock, they needed help immediately. Even if the issues of the transfusion procedure itself and the adverse reactions could be mitigated, it meant nothing if there were no donors at hand. This is where the idea of *indirect* transfusion—and the blood bank concept—arose.

If blood could be donated, then kept in a storage facility until it was needed, the problem of having immediate, on-site donors would vanish—at least in theory. Blood that could be stored could be transported, too, to places where donors might be wholly unavailable. Dr. Allen Whipple's purpose in hiring John Scudder in 1936 was, in fact, to spearhead investigative efforts in this direction. Scudder later remembered that "the dramatic deaths of a boy who died from a ruptured spleen and the postpartum death of a staff member's wife only too vividly brought to mind the necessity of having blood on hand."[31]

For all these reasons, by the late 1930s the concept of a *blood bank*—where blood could be collected, carefully typed, and stored for elective crossmatch and infusion at any necessary time—was beginning to muster widespread support. Indeed, the concept had begun to be realized in actual physical facilities. Bernard Fantus founded the first such unit in the United States in 1937 at the Cook County Hospital in Chicago (he also coined the term "blood bank"). Within a few months, others had appeared in medical centers in Philadelphia, Minnesota, and at Mt. Sinai and Bellevue Hospitals in New York City.

This progress came despite daunting obstacles that still stood in the way, beyond the risks of transfusion itself. The entire concept was severely constrained by poorly understood but undeniable limitations on how long blood could be safely stored, not to mention whether it would retain its all-important physiologic functions. Although these questions remained unanswered, by the summer of 1938 the reality of hospital-based blood banks was well afoot.

As usual, it would be up to the medical scientists in the laboratories to solve the problems that vexed the doctors in the clinical setting.

In the spring of 1939, the Drew-Robbins long-distance romance saga seemed to embody the expression, "One step forward; two steps back." Lenore's reply to the May 11 letter has not survived, but it appears to have been a change of heart about visiting Charles in New York. He was forced again into impassioned pleas:

> May 17, 1939
>
> Dear Lenore,
>
> . . . Why did you decide not to come to New York? I really have looked forward to this as the high spot in what promised to be a hectic summer. Can't you come? I'd like so much to have you see and get the feel of the setup so that you'll know what you're getting yourself into, to see if you like it or could get used to it. . . . I've just about got everything clear between June 1st and 15th so that I can cut work. The blood bank has been purposely delayed, a chap will do my emergency work, Miss Sergeant will do the lab work. . . .
>
> . . . I'd meet you in the afternoon up here—then a show or so, a bit of chatting, the world's fair, a bit of planning, a swim perhaps and a bit of scheming, a bit of music and perhaps a kiss as we said good night and when your time was almost up and each knows better what the other is really like and what the future holds we could go back by Philadelphia together and announce the results of our findings.[32]

This letter accomplished its desired goal, and the New York visit was reinstated. The last sentence also reveals that, even though Drew's visit to Lenore's family in Philadelphia must have raised suspicions, the pair had not by this time informed anyone, kinfolk or friend, of their tentative wedding plans.

In his next letter, written on Sunday, May 21, Charles recommended that Lenore leave Atlanta the following Saturday and spend a day or two with the Drews in Washington before heading up to see him.[33] To prepare her for this, he provided memorable descriptions of his family:

> Each Sunday at 4 they eat together. They consist of Joe, my brother, usually not too bad but mean as a bull now since he's laid up with a broken leg, no spring cleaning done, the yard in shambles, a couple hundred dollar bills, unable to work

and likely to go in debt during the summer. Well I guess he's got a right to be blue. Grace, his wife, never says much, knows a lot, seems a little aloof, but really is a swell person. Their two brats, Richard and Jay, bad, a little smart alecky, just two boys of six and three—that always means trouble.

Nora my older sister, 26, married, teaches school, exuberant but sincere. About to have a baby, at least so she thought when I was home, which looms as a personal item for it was our plan for her to teach and give a lift until I finished, but then one can't regulate everything and I hope she is going to have a baby. It will make her very happy and Francis her husband is one of the finest.

Eva, my kid sister, has just reached the jitterbug stage, a senior in high school. I think you'll like her. You see I think they're all pretty swell. I'm the prodigal, the wanderer, the black sheep of the family. Yet strange enough I fear a bit of the pet because I'm never there.

The whole thing revolves of course around my mother.[34]

Also in this letter, Drew revealed the results of his important meeting with Dr. Whipple:

> First, he has permitted me to formally register for the degree of Doctor of Science in Medicine, a thesis to be turned in next April, the rest of my work to be completed by next June. There is more here than meets the eye. There are no such Negroes at present, Lambert of the Rockefeller Foundation is opposed to it, attempts have been made before by others to no avail.[35] It's much more than a degree I'm after. There are those in high places who feel that Negroes have not yet reached intellectual levels which will permit their attempting the very highest reaches.[36]

Drew's anger at the prejudice of "those in high places" who would stifle the opportunities of others based only on their skin color is palpable in this letter, but equally obvious is his intent to use this emotion to fuel his efforts at proving the ignorant powerful wrong. On another level, Whipple's offer was precisely what Numa Adams had intended when he championed the GEB fellowships for Howard's clinical faculty leaders: an advanced degree to add to the MD they already possessed. Columbia's doctorate of medical science was not a PhD, but it was in the ballpark. "Second, on June 15th I will be eligible, I believe, to take the examination of the American Board of Surgery. I shall apply as soon as I'm eligible and Dr. Whipple has assured me that he will back me in my right to take it and push the thing until it's over with."[37]

The American Board of Surgery was a new body, just incorporated in 1937. It was established by leaders in the surgical community, mainly professors at university hospitals, to set minimum standards for physicians who presented themselves to the public as surgeons. If a candidate had completed suitable training, he could become eligible to "sit for the Boards." The examinations were in two parts: a written test called the Qualifying Examination and, if this were passed, an oral one known as the Certifying Exam. Whipple played a major role in the establishment of the American Board of Surgery. "Thirdly, to be sure that I won't be stale in actual operative technique, beginning on June 15th I go back into the wards as a member of an operating team to stay until such time as I have brushed up a bit after a year in the laboratory doing research."[38]

This was a piece of unexpected good luck. Although Drew's GEB Fellowship was for "graduate training in Surgery" he had, of course, spent nearly an entire year doing research only and would have had no reason to expect that to change. Moreover, the lab scenario was adequate for the greater purpose: Dean Adams's hope was that his clinical fellows, future faculty members, might bring back to Howard knowledge of advanced research techniques and thus launch the institution into the academic forefront. Now, in addition, Drew would spend time in clinical activities, even take part in the operating room. The surgery residency at Columbia was one of the most prestigious in the country, certainly on par with the program he had been denied at the Mayo Clinic four years earlier. Some of the most advanced procedures in the world were performed in the Presbyterian ORs. Drew's obvious intelligence and work in the lab had impressed Whipple sufficiently for him to be offered an extraordinary opportunity to learn the operative techniques of the Columbia surgeons: "He demonstrated his ability so outstandingly," reported Whipple, "and was so highly approved of by his associates in the hospital."[39]

The lone obstacle that Drew had no control over, his "slightly evident colored extraction," had been overcome by his performance in the shock lab.

As it happened, and as was the case at McGill, the stern admonitions regarding the rejection of a Black physician by white patients appear not to have had much validity when put to the test—no stories of Drew's rejection by white patients have come down to us, and the only recollections of racial prejudice relate to its summary rejection by the Columbia medical staff.

One of these tales involved a white resident from Mississippi named Octo Lee. Since a Black resident physician was a new phenomenon, the administration evidently thought it prudent to inquire from Drew's peers whether they would permit him to dine with them in the hospital cafeteria. Lee, who considered Drew "just great," took public offense to the question. He was "appalled that they would even ask."[40]

Lenore followed through on the visit to New York in early June. Writing to her parents after her return to Atlanta, she described the trip, including a short stay in Washington (on which Drew accompanied her after the New York stay) in the briefest of terms:

> I had an exciting time in New York. We went everywhere. Charlie must have spent about $75 in all—my room, meals, and other expenses together.
>
> Charlie and I arrived in Washington about 9:00 and were met by Nora his sister and Francis her husband. They took us to Arlington (a 10 minute ride) to his mother's house. There I met his mother a very kind, and cordial but quite informal woman; his brother Joe who is still incapacitated because of his broken leg; his wife, Grace, a Smith graduate and a very fine woman. They have a large, very simple home there in Arlington, and they made me very welcome in it.[41]

At the tail end of this matter-of-fact correspondence, Lenore let slip the big news that had been kept so carefully hidden up to now: "There was so much else to talk about when we got home that there wasn't a chance to say what we had wanted to say—that we will be married in the early fall—very quickly."[42]

Any second thoughts she may have had about the marriage appear to have been erased by the June visit. On his return from accompanying her to Washington, Drew sent Lenore a short, glowing note. The salutation told the story:

June 9, 1939

My Wife,

I love you, I miss you, I want you; the whole place is empty without you.

Charlie[43]

The month of June is an awkward time in academic medical centers for many reasons. It marks the end of one scholastic year and the beginning of another: responsibilities change up and down the roster. New trainees and students are setting out on their educational journey, their senior counterparts are in the process of departing, and even for those who are staying on it can be a time of unnerving personal and professional flux as duties shift. It is also a popular time for vacations.

These issues affected the surgical research labs at least as much as the clinical services. Not long after Lenore had left, a nearly idle Drew confessed to her in writing that "I truthfully haven't done a great deal since you arrived in town a little over a month ago."[44]

Since he was unable to accomplish much lab work, Drew amused himself with the social events he could manage on his limited income, lately even more depleted from Lenore's visit. One evening he went to a prize fight at Yankee Stadium in which heavyweight champion Joe Louis knocked out challenger Tony Galento. "In spite of his reputed low IQ," Drew reported to Lenore, Louis had all the appearances of "a true thoroughbred."[45] On another night Drew found himself seated for a Wagner concert, wishing Lenore had accompanied him since, aside from some of the opera *Tannhauser* that his father had sometimes sung at home, he was—unlike his future wife—not much of an aficionado of the composer. He also attended a soiree for one of his medical students from Howard, a night on the town with Lowell Wormley and other friends, and the Fokine Ballet at the Lewisohn Stadium of the City College of New York. These were all in one week. As the calendar turned, though, the time for frivolity came to an end.

Whipple's generous offer to allow Drew's candidacy for the doctorate in medical science degree carried with it additional responsibilities. The onus of composing a doctoral thesis was the greatest of these but, in the end, he would also have to sit for an examining committee, both to defend the dissertation and to submit to general testing in his field.

Drew had to apply formally to Columbia's Graduate Studies in Clinical Medicine dean and committee for all of this, too, which turned out to be a sizable undertaking. From a practical perspective he had to enroll for the winter and spring terms, at $20 tuition per session. The process began in September 1939. In addition to Drew's own completed application, the school required letters of recommendation, for which the administration reached out to the faculties of both Howard and McGill in early October:

> Dr. Charles Richard Drew has made application for admission to graduate studies in Surgery leading to the degree of Doctor of Medical Science in Columbia University.
>
> Any information regarding the quality of Dr. Drew's work, his character, industry, reliability and personality will be appreciated. Such information will be held in confidence.
>
> Sincerely yours,
>
> Vernon W. Lippard, M.D.
> Assistant Dean
> Graduate Studies[46]

Naturally, Dean Numa Adams at Howard was happy to respond with a glowing endorsement:

> I am pleased to recommend Dr. Drew as a man of good moral character who so far as I have been able to ascertain has formed no undesirable habits. He is a young man of pleasing personality who is intelligent, industrious, and reliable.
>
> I hope that you will be able to accept him as a graduate student in Surgery. I believe he is the type of man of whom your institution will in the future be proud.[47]

Members of the McGill faculty and Montreal General Hospital staff wrote on behalf of Drew in their capacity as institutional leaders. Their assessments echoed those of Adams. John C. Mackenzie, general superintendent of the hospital, wrote:

> Our opinion of Dr. Drew was that he was a man of unusual ability, far and away above the average. He was thoroughly responsible in every way, absolutely dependable, of sound judgment based on knowledge and ability and all in all we feel he can be recommended for his character, industry, reliability and personality in the strongest terms possible.[48]

Albert Bazin, who was a staff surgeon at Montreal General when Drew was an intern and resident, had by this time become chair of the McGill Department of Surgery. In his letter Bazin observed: "He is a hard working and brilliant student, has a good demeanor without forwardness, an excellent physique and bearing. We found him entirely trustworthy and reliable."[49]

Both the Canadians felt the need to provide additional remarks on Drew's race. Bazin's comments on Drew's inability to practice in Montreal due to being a "quadroon," noted earlier, appeared in this letter, and Mackenzie also added, "I would mention, confidentially, that Drew has some coloured blood in him, but in some parts of this Continent, I would opine he could pass for white. Despite the above, he was entirely persona grata with us and we had absolutely no regrets."[50]

Any one of the broader ideas on fluids and electrolytes that had been developed in the shock lab over the previous year would have been reasonable topics for a doctoral dissertation, but Drew chose to pursue, at Scudder's recommendation, the subject he found most compelling: all of the experiments, clinical data-gathering, and administrative decision-making that attended the establishment of the Columbia Presbyterian Blood Bank.

As required by the school, Drew outlined his research problem and thesis:

> **<u>Studies in Blood Preservation</u>**
>
> 1. The fate of cellular elements in preserved blood.
> 2. Electrolyte changes in preserved blood.
> 3. Protein changes in preserved blood.

4. Cell disintegration as a function of the interface between the cells and plasma.
5. Hemolysis as an index of toxicity.
6. Trauma as a factor in the toxicity of preserved blood.
7. The effect of pH on the preservation of red blood cells.
8. Changes in the electrocardiograph of patients during transfusions.
9. The establishment of an "Experimental Blood Bank" at the Presbyterian Hospital.
10. Clinical observations and conclusions.[51]

Although the work involved in assembling such a thesis would be enormous, Drew would have the advantage of watching the development of the blood bank unfold, in the language of a later era, in "real time." When it was finished, this effort would also put him in the first rank of medical scientists in the rarefied field.

Although he had mentioned the date of June 15 in his letter to Lenore, it was on July 1, 1939, that Drew began his clinical work in the Department of Surgery at Presbyterian. After some fourteen months away from the lifestyle of a surgical trainee, the reality of his new schedule was, at first, nearly overwhelming. "I have to be in the wards at 7:30," he told Lenore, "And usually do not leave until 10:30–12."[52] He "had just sort of forgotten my way around. Assisting a half dozen surgeons I had never assisted before, trying to remember all the routines, how to get things done and by whom."[53] As if this were not enough, he was still obligated to ramp up work on the new blood bank, including performing and writing up the experiments planned to underpin its scientific basis and solving any operational problems that arose. Everything, of course, needed to be summarized in his all-encompassing doctoral thesis, due in nine short months. "It's good perhaps that you were not here," he wrote Lenore after the first two weeks in July, "for I would have been good for nothing when I got home but being put to bed, yet I do wish that you were here. We're facing a difficult year, Lenore, but if our hearts keep right I'm sure we'll come out of it strong and shining like glimmering steel."[54]

Preliminary discussions about a blood bank at Columbia had been taking place on a sporadic basis even before John Scudder arrived from India in 1936. After the advent of the Cook County unit, and those that followed, the level of urgency rose. On November 28, 1938, the hospital medical board, at the request of its chair, a prominent urologist named J. Bentley Squier, formally called for a committee to investigate the advisability of initiating a Presbyterian blood bank. The committee was composed of three senior physicians who set about their task in a studious and logical fashion. They approached six facilities that were already operating blood banks: the University of Pennsylvania, the University of Minnesota, the Mayo Clinic, the two area facilities—Mt. Sinai and Bellevue Hospitals—and, of course, Cook County. The committee composed a questionnaire for the authorities at these banks, inquiring about the length of time the units had been operational, the number of cases, the source of the donor blood, the incidence of adverse reactions and deaths, and other information about the day-to-day functioning of the programs. The results were uniform: each of the facilities had performed hundreds of transfusions of banked blood, most donors were family members or friends of the recipient, adverse reactions were in the 10 percent range, and deaths were unusual, if not rare.[55]

Based on these findings, the committee recommended that a Presbyterian blood bank be initiated on a trial basis but noted that ongoing experiments into the potential dangers were necessary. Scudder was appointed "to direct the laboratory and experimental aspects of the project and Dr. Charles R. Drew to manage the bank and direct clinical investigations."[56]

The experimental blood bank went into operation for a four-month trial period (later extended to six) on August 9, 1939. It was headquartered in Room #43, Ward L—East of Presbyterian Hospital, with the donor unit located on the north corridor of C unit in the Vanderbilt Clinic. Drew composed a memorandum for the resident physicians to guide them in use of the new facility, which was necessarily constrained by the ongoing investigations into its feasibility, safety, and best method of functioning.

Adopting a rule from other blood banks, and banks in general, at Presbyterian a clinical service could not "withdraw" blood unless it had accumulated credit by means of having provided donated blood (temporary debit status was allowed). Forms were made available for both donation and withdrawal, both of which had to be done according to a rigid schedule. Emergency usage was discouraged at first since this would interfere with careful study of the cases—the primary focus of the experimental bank. Any adverse reaction—"rise in temperature, chill, nausea, vomiting, urticaria (an itching rash), shock or convulsion" was to be reported to the blood bank staff at once.

In the laboratory proper, away from the evolving chaos of the provisional bank, experiments were underway into the basic science of the storing and transfusion processes. Drew described the rationale behind these efforts:

> The advantages of having on hand at all times bloods of each group are obvious, especially in case of dire emergencies when there is insufficient time to get voluntary or professional donors. Certain disadvantages, however, immediately come to mind: the blood is older; changes may be taking place which make such blood less desirable, even undesirable. Is such blood dangerous? Is it capable of normal function when used for transfusion? Are the advantages of speed and utility in its use offset by decreased therapeutic value for the patient? Are reactions increased or decreased? This series of studies was begun in an attempt to answer the first question: Is blood which has been kept in a preservative of some kind for varying periods of time dangerous? If so, in what quantities and in what conditions? Finally, what is the toxic factor?[57]

Thus, Drew and Scudder focused their work in the surgical research lab on studying the potential toxicity of banked blood.

Eva Drew graduated with honors from Dunbar High School in the spring of 1939. As a present, amid his busy ward and lab work, Charlie invited her up to visit him and she gladly accepted. Since he was living in the hospital at the time, Drew had to make special arrangements for his sister's lodging. The economical solution turned out to be a room in the nurses' quarters. The only drawback for the young girl, excited for her first trip to New York City, was that the room had no clock so she could not tell when to get up. Her brother's doting solution was to buy her a Mickey Mouse watch.[58]

During Eva's stay Charlie took what time he could to show her the sights of Manhattan—on the shoestring budget tour. On Broadway near Columbia, they dined at an Automat, a popular forerunner of fast-food restaurants in which patrons put nickels into slots and selected plates of premade food from glass compartments. He took Eva for a ride on the elevated train, where she was shocked to see that "one could look right into people's bedrooms and see whatever they were doing." Next was a trip to the World's Fair, where the teenager gawked at the "famous Trylon and Perisphere, exhibits and people from all over the world," and enjoyed the spectacular Aquacade, a gigantic pool featuring a water ballet and the celebrity swimmers and Hollywood stars Johnny Weissmuller and Esther Williams. A ride on the Ferris Wheel was interrupted when the machine broke down. For a half hour Charlie and Eva were stuck in their carriage, which was a replica airplane. "Naturally I panicked," Eva later remembered. But "Charlie calmed me down. We had great seats to look all over the fair. He explained so many of the things we observed in great detail. . . . Almost everything we saw, anywhere we were, was an opportunity for him to teach me."[59]

Charlie also spent time convincing Eva, against her wishes, that she must attend the Miner Normal School, like her mother and sister. Cash-strapped as he was, he still would pay her tuition.

No one who was aware of the concerted effort to establish fully functional blood storage facilities in the late 1930s doubted the value of the effort, but events on the world stage drove the point home with the sharp violence of a bayonet thrust when, just three weeks after the Presbyterian blood bank opened, Hitler unleashed the Wehrmacht against Poland, inaugurating World War II in Europe.

Transfusions on or near the battlefield for traumatic, hemorrhagic shock had been attempted in World War I, with predictably dire results. More recently, though, the value of stored blood in the treatment of battle casualties had been demonstrated during the Spanish Civil War, when a physician named Frederic Durán-Jordà in Barcelona developed a large-scale transfusion service that included citrated blood and refrigerated trucks for its delivery.[60] Individuals and groups aware of this work hoped that, as a much larger conflagration enveloped the globe, some similar system might be deployed that harnessed the rapidly advancing knowledge of the scientific issues in play.

One such organization existed in New York City and was already familiar at Columbia: the Blood Transfusion Betterment Association. Founded back in 1929, this group—entirely focused on Gotham—had spent most of the past decade recruiting donors and bucking up transfusion facilities through the city, in addition to providing some funds for research (including support for John Scudder's work). When the war broke out, even though the United States was not involved, the leadership of the association began to contemplate a bigger role.

While the conflict unfolded in faraway Europe, Drew and Scudder mapped out a series of experiments to be performed over the coming months in the shock lab, designed to find answers to the many questions that attended the issue of safely storing blood for a reasonable period. Much of this was contained in the ten points Drew outlined as his "research problem" for the Graduate Medical Committee at about the same time.

This research focused nearly exclusively on the use of *whole blood* in transfusion. There were, however, naturally occurring alternatives.

If whole blood is allowed to sit in a container, the cellular elements will clot and settle at the bottom, leaving a protein-rich, amber-colored fluid above them known as *serum*. If an anticoagulant is added to the whole blood the cells will settle but not clot. The fluid above the cells, which in this case contains unused coagulation proteins such as fibrinogen, is called *plasma*. The use of plasma or serum instead of whole blood had been contemplated almost since the concept of transfusion became a practical reality, and Scudder even received funding from the Blood Transfusion Betterment Association to explore the possibility in early 1940. Soon the Columbia team would cast a definitive lot in the debate, but for now the focus for Drew was on whole blood.[61]

The first set of the blood bank laboratory experiments revolved around the presence and concentration of potassium in stored blood (it will be recalled that one of Drew's first papers at Columbia, submitted for publication in March 1939, was an investigation into the concentration of potassium in the cardiac blood at death).

Potassium is an elemental mineral that is nearly ubiquitous in the body and an essential component in an impressive array of physiologic functions. For the purposes of the Drew/Scudder experiments, the most significant characteristic of potassium was that, in the normal state in the blood and tissues it is almost exclusively *intracellular*—that is, found inside cells (this is in direct contrast to potassium's otherwise very biochemically similar elemental mineral cousin, sodium, which is almost always found outside the cells). For this reason, any time potassium is found freely in the blood in significant concentrations, it is an indicator that something drastic and detrimental has happened to the cells—either their walls have become pathologically permeable or been disrupted entirely (some of Whipple's own research had shown this).[62] In the case of stored blood, this means injury to the red cells. Bad enough as this is, since the donor red cells contain the hemoglobin necessary for oxygen exchange—a major physiologic function of blood—high levels of potassium in the blood are *themselves* dangerous—particularly to the electrical system of the heart. If the potassium concentration in blood gets high enough, fast enough, it can cause disruptions in the electrical cardiac rhythm, even cardiac arrest (it is one of the components of the "lethal cocktail" in executions by injection).

Not all of this was perfectly understood at the time, but Drew and Scudder certainly recognized that a high level of potassium in banked blood might be a threat to the recipient and needed to be investigated.

Their first experiments in this series confirmed that potassium begins to leak from red cells in stored blood almost at once, and the concentration of ion in the fluid portion (serum or plasma) rises continually as time passes. Some preservatives slowed the process down, but not much; the same was true of anticoagulants. The next tests demonstrated that trauma to the cells (as from shaking their container or even the process of drawing the blood through a needle from the donor's vein) enhanced the potassium leak, an effect that was greater the longer the blood had been stored. The size of the interface between the plasma and the cells (which were driven to the bottom of containers by gravity and/or the centrifuge) was also important: narrow cylindrical flasks with a smaller interface area had less free potassium than wide ones.

This last observation led the team to develop a specialized flask for storing blood. Spherical at the top, with a wide cylindrical base but narrow waist, it somewhat resembled a dumbbell set on end. The idea was that the flask would be filled only to the waist, so that the cell/plasma interface area would be minimized, but the volume of blood held would still be substantial and the flask easy to handle.[63]

Since the breakup of red cells was known to increase the plasma potassium concentration, Drew and Scudder examined whether the connection could be exploited for clinical purposes: measuring potassium in blood was not easy, but hemolysis caused the plasma in centrifuged blood to become discolored in a predictable and reproducible manner. If that could be extrapolated to reflect the potassium content, albeit indirectly, a clever shortcut would be identified. Alas, such was not the case: potassium levels did not correlate with color of the fluid.

The last test in this series was an unsuccessful effort to determine the lethal dose of potassium in animals.

Next, on a different tack, the team examined the effect of ammonia on the potassium leakage phenomenon, hypothesizing that the presence of this toxic chemical from protein degradation might influence the course. This thread did not, however, generate useful conclusions.

Placental and cadaveric blood had been championed as possible donor sources by some, especially in Russia, but each of these exotic alternatives, although not eliminated as possibilities, was found to harbor significant drawbacks (the Columbia exploratory committee had already ruled them out for the Presbyterian blood bank before any lab work was done).

In other experiments, blood stored near body temperature (38 degrees Celsius in the studies) was found to degrade at a markedly faster rate than that kept at low, though not freezing temperatures; 3–5 degrees Celsius seemed to be ideal.

White blood cells, responsible for important immune and microorganism defense functions, deteriorated rapidly. Some had considered the possibility of transfusion to bolster the natural white cell effects in cases of infection or immune dysfunction, but the results did not support this application. Others wondered if transfusion might buttress the coagulation system in disease states where it went awry; however, the stored blood concentration of platelets, key initiators in the clotting cascade, diminished quickly. On the other hand, prothrombin, a protein also important in clot formation, remained at stable concentrations for up to ten days.

Finally, having explored potassium in the setting of stored blood to the limit of their technological capacity, Drew and Scudder shifted their efforts to considerations of other ions known to be present in blood and the possible implications of storage on their fate. Calcium, magnesium, sodium, and phosphorus were subjected to their experimental scrutiny. Although the findings of these studies were of scientific interest, they did not rise to the level of practical significance.

When the experiments had reached their conclusions, Drew summarized the investigators' findings:

> Blood preserved for periods not exceeding ten days, insofar as could be determined in these investigations, is safe and for most purposes should give results when used for transfusions comparable to those following the use of fresh blood. Its rapid loss of white cells precludes its use in cases where bactericidal properties or antibodies usually associated with white cells are desired. It would seem less effective in cases of thrombocytopenic purpura and bleeding due to prothrombin deficiency. Its use in large quantities would seem contraindicated in patients suffering with diseases associated with hyperpotassemia but even in such cases its moderate and intelligent use should lead to no untoward effects.[64]

Amid this avalanche of important work, and with the Nazi blitzkrieg in Europe on the front page of every daily paper, Lenore and Charlie were married in her hometown of Philadelphia on September 23, 1939. They moved into apartment 2D at 230 West 150th Street, which they rented for $59.50 per month.[65] The building was in Harlem, about twenty blocks southeast of the Columbia Medical Center. Here the Drews began their married life, an island of fragile domestic peace in a surmounting world of tumult.

Back in the blood bank, the cases began to add up. One of the part-time secretaries, Margaret Nelson, had to take some time off and Lenore filled in for her, which may have added some well-received income to the little Drew home.[66] By February 1940, the end of the experimental period for the blood bank, the makeshift facility had accumulated four hundred transfusion cases. At this juncture Drew began to analyze the data.

More than 90 percent of the donors were male, ranging in age from fifteen to sixty-eight (the average age was thirty-four). Ten percent of the potential donors were rejected, mostly because they were in ill health themselves or had known or suspected communicable diseases. Nearly 2 percent had positive Wasserman reactions—suggestive of syphilis. More than 90 percent donated blood for a friend or relative in Presbyterian, although only 8 percent of the donations went to that individual.

Recipients fell into six pathologic categories: hemorrhage, anemia from chronic disease, primary blood disease, prophylactic or therapeutic transfusion for operations, infection with anemia, or malnutrition states such as cancer or certain gastrointestinal disorders. The transfusions generally resulted in appropriate responses in terms of increased red cell counts and hemoglobin concentration in the recipients.

Fifteen percent of banked blood transfusions were accompanied by adverse reactions, although the lion's share of these were mild: slight fevers, itching rashes, chills. There were four cases of jaundice. No one died.[67]

At this point Drew sent a memo to John F. Bush, trustee of the hospital and president of the Blood Transfusion Betterment Association, giving some thoughts on the outcome of the six-month trial. "Blood preserved for a few days is not markedly different in cellular contents, chemical make-up and biological properties from fresh whole blood," he wrote, adding, "Certain limitations in is use have been shown to be wise." There was no doubt, however, that "the presence of blood of all types, serologically tested and from healthy donors speeds up the efficiency of the hospital, reduces the cost of transfusions and greatly increases the insurance against fatalities in great emergencies."[68] Drew went on to outline the salient needs of a permanent blood bank, as if the certainty in establishing one were not even in question.

With the completion of the laboratory experiments and the compilation of the clinical blood bank data, Drew had the information he would need to write his monumental thesis. He labored over it for endless hours, parsing the data and honing the language. He also made a point of referencing as many of the major papers and research that had been done in the field of blood transfusion throughout history up to that time, an important contribution in itself. When the dissertation was finished it would encompass 245 pages of text, including forty-eight graphs and twenty-one illustrations, spread over five chapters (by some accounts the first draft was as much as twice as long, but, on reviewing it, Whipple returned the manuscript with instructions to condense it to a more digestible size).

Drew submitted the completed thesis, finally titled *Banked Blood: A Study in Blood Preservation,* to the doctorate of medical science committee in early

April 1940. On April 15, this group, composed of five physicians and chaired by Whipple, reviewed the paper and also conducted an oral examination of Drew on advanced medical subjects. The following day Whipple sent a memorandum to Assistant Dean Lippard of the graduate studies office that read in part:

> The committee after examining Dr. Drew, not only on the subject presented, but on the pathology and physiology of other conditions and a discussion of the chemical changes in body fluids, agreed unanimously that Dr. Drew should be granted the degree of Doctor of Medical Science. In fact it was their conviction that the thesis presented and the examination of Dr. Drew were of a very much higher order than most of the other candidates coming up for the degree.[69]

Scudder later referred to this thesis as "beautifully executed . . . one of the most learned ever submitted for the degree."[70] He went on to call Drew "naturally great," and remark that "Of all the pupils I have trained, I would place Drew at the top of the list."[71]

In early May 1940, a paper by Drew and his colleague from the lab, David Bull, was presented at the prestigious American Surgical Association annual meeting in St. Louis. In fact, the talk, "The Preservation of Blood," opened the conference (Scudder followed with his own presentation along similar lines). Whipple was president of this organization at the time, and another luminary from American surgery, Owen Wangensteen of the University of Minnesota, contributed to a spirited discussion on the topic.[72]

A few days before his Columbia graduation, Drew set aside time to compose a long letter to his old high school basketball coach, Edwin B. Henderson. Drew's sister Nora and her husband Francis had sent him as a present the previous Christmas an autographed copy of a book Henderson had written called *The Negro in Sports*.[73] At five hundred pages in length, this was a comprehensive, encyclopedic work that was destined to become a classic. Drew appeared in the book for his multisport exploits at Amherst (the McGill years were not mentioned). Now, at another crossroads, he reached back to congratulate and thank an important influence from his past:

Dear Mr. Henderson:

Through great want of time I have put off too long congratulating you on the splendid book you got out on Negro Athletes. It is a grand job. I want to thank you for autographing the copy Francis Gregory and my sister sent me for a Christmas present and express my appreciation for your generosity in the amount of space you allotted to me.

I doubt if anyone has really told you how big a part you have played in the lives of a lot of the men you wrote of in your book, not so much by the things you have said, or the things you have done or the lessons in physical education but rather by virtue of the things you have stood for and the way you have lived throughout all these years. The big thing is that in these days of fallen idols of all types it is particularly refreshing to know a few people whom we thought were just about tops when we were kids and when looked at in the sober light of more mature years to find that they still are tops, that they have consistently been the things which they have said other folks should be, that they have tried to do the things which they have said should be attempted. I personally feel a very great debt of gratitude to you. I owe you and a few other men like you for setting most of the standards that I have felt were worthwhile, the things I have lived by and for and wherever possible have attempted to pass on.

Drew went on to point out the value of Henderson's book to African Americans from coast to coast:

Some few always have to set the pace and give the others courage to go on into places which have not been explored. We have so few things to be really proud of that the presentation of so much that is good in one book is sure to have results far beyond your farthest dreams.

Warming to his topic, Drew then expressed to Henderson, in a kind of manifesto, the goals he had shared earlier with Lenore, goals that would define him over the decade to come and on into posterity:

My work here is about finished. I've gone as far as I can go in formal medicine so I guess I'll have to go to work now. It has been good fun. Chiefly

I suppose because it has never been done by a Negro before and it is felt that the higher realms of medicine are not the place for him. On Tuesday I get the degree of Doctor of Science in Medicine. Now that all is over but the shouting it feels just about like the day after a big race that is won. One wonders why all the excitement before the race was run, the anxious days of training, the striving for form, the all too slow increase in speed, the fine edge on the day of the meet, the gun and then the whole thing is over. The only thing in medicine is that it takes so much longer. When it is all over it is just another medal in the box and we begin looking forward to the next season's competition. My next big meet is at Howard in the Department of Surgery. There the situation is comparable to the sport situation when I took over at Morgan College. They were playing high school teams and getting licked. In two years they had won three college Championships and had a nucleus for one of the best series of teams ever seen in the colored colleges. Those boys who made that first great team for Morgen on the football field were the men I started as freshmen and seniors in the Morgan Academy. I count it as one of the most pleasing experiences I have had. In medicine we still are in the scholastic class. Whether I can do anything about that or not is a challenge that is well worth taking on. Seventy years there has been a Howard Med School but still there is no tradition, no able surgeon has ever been trained there, no school of thought has been born there, few of their stars have ever hit the headlines. In American surgery there are no Negro representatives, in so far as the men who count know, all Negro doctors are just country practitioners, capable of sitting with the poor and the sick of their race but not given to too much intellectual activity and not particularly interested in advancing medicine. This attitude I should like to help change. It should be great sport. If at the end of another 25 years I can look back over my steps and feel that I have kept the faith in my sphere of activity in a manner comparable to that in which you have carried on in yours I shall be very happy. Again I congratulate you.

Very sincerely yours,

Charlie Drew[74]

The degree of doctor of medical science was officially awarded to Charles Drew by Dr. William C. Rappleye, dean of the College of Physicians and

Surgeons, at the 186th annual Columbia University commencement on June 4, 1940.[75] Drew was the first African American to earn this degree.[76]

The tasks of the GEB fellowship were now complete, and then some. In addition to absorbing the advanced laboratory methods that would enable him to direct his own independent research programs at Howard in the future, Drew had learned cutting-edge surgical technique from one of the world's masters and advanced the science of transfusion along its tortured but inexorable path. And there was more.

The Charles Drew who departed New York City for Washington in the spring of 1940 was a different man from the one who had appeared in Allen Whipple's office two years before. Any physical or emotional semblance of the journeyman doctor was long gone. He had left Howard University as a trainee but was now fully qualified to join its faculty; a position as assistant professor of surgery awaited him there. The interminable hours of his chosen profession were beginning to etch themselves on his freckled visage, his hairline was rising, and, at thirty-six years of age, the physique of the sprinter was giving way—if gradually—to the spread of middle age. Drew's lifestyle and status had changed, too. He had left Washington an unattached bachelor with no serious prospects but was now a married man and, as it happened, soon to be a father: Lenore was expecting in August.

The dues had been paid. It was time to go back home. But fate, blood, and New York City were not yet finished with Charles Drew.

8

Playing at Bigger Games

Blood for Britain and the Red Cross, 1940–41

A big part of John Scudder's research time was spent at the shock lab he had built at Columbia—but not all of it. As noted above, he also worked at the Rockefeller Institute on the upper East Side, funded by the ubiquitous Rockefeller Foundation. One of the benefits this extramural research afforded Scudder was the opportunity to see what sort of work was being done by other scientists at the prestigious institute. Many of these researchers, attracted by the foundation's deep pockets, were among the world's finest. One of these was a Swede named Arne Tiselius.

Tiselius was already well known in scientific circles for his work in chemical analysis. Much of this was focused on blood plasma, which was more than enough to attract Scudder's attention. Tiselius had developed a method of analyzing the molecules in a solution by a method called electrophoresis. Prior to this discovery, about the only way to separate out component molecules in a solution was by centrifuge, taking advantage of differences in the size and weight of the solutes. If, however, the molecules were similar in these properties—as, for example, the proteins in blood plasma—the centrifuge method did not work: everything of interest clumped together. Tiselius had the insight to realize that individual proteins would have unique electrical properties based on their different chemical compositions. He developed a device to exploit this phenomenon, consisting essentially of a sheet of paper impregnated with the test solution and set within an electric field. The proteins in the solution would migrate to different points along the paper according to their response to the electric field, separating themselves from one another and allowing identification.

The development of electrophoresis would eventually earn Tiselius a Nobel Prize, but the more immediate impact it had for Scudder related to studies he performed at the Rockefeller Institute using not just Tiselius's method but the Swede's actual equipment. When Scudder looked at plasma samples of varying ages, it turned out that the proteins did not significantly change over time: for weeks or even months after harvesting, the composition of the plasma remained the same, even if it were not refrigerated. In other words, unlike the whole blood he and Drew had worked on for months, plasma was remarkably stable for a significant period under less-than-stringent conditions.[1]

As early as the First World War, with its multitudes of casualties, plasma had been considered as a possible substitute for whole blood in the treatment of hemorrhagic shock. An editorial in the *British Medical Journal* from 1918 pointed out the possible advantages, although focusing mainly on the likely reduction or elimination of transfusion reactions: "Surely this difficulty might be avoided by not transfusing the corpuscles at all, but only citrated plasma, which would be easy to keep and easy to give. . . . A man apparently dying from haemorrhage is not dying from lack of haemoglobin, else severe cases of anaemia would die long before they do, but from draining away of fluid, resulting in devitalization and low blood pressure."[2]

This editorial oversimplified the problem of hemorrhagic shock, but the other reasoning was sound. The end of the war later that year diminished the urgency of studying the problem, but into the 1930s investigators such as Max Strumia in Bryn Mawr, Pennsylvania, and John Elliot in Salisbury, North Carolina, continued to evaluate plasma in the context of transfusion.[3] Scudder's discovery of the stability of the substance over time materially added to its promise.

One of Louis Pasteur's many memorable quotes relates to the role of luck in great moments of science: "In the fields of observation chance only favors the prepared mind."[4] So it was that in early June 1940 Scudder, keenly aware of the practical implications of plasma's newly appreciated lengthy shelf life, happened to be attending a luncheon at the Rockefeller Institute with a number of high-ranking members of the organization's administration. The issue arose in conversation of how the American scientific community could assist those in Europe under attack and threat of attack by the Nazi regime. One guest at the informal gathering was Alexis Carrel, a French surgeon-scientist and Nobel laureate who had made many groundbreaking advancements in the nascent field of vascular surgery. For Carrel, the problem was not hypothetical: he had just arrived from his home country, which was then being overrun by the Germans in the tragically brief Battle of France. He indicated to the group that casualties were high and expected to mount as the French and British forces were pushed toward what became their last stand at Dunkirk.[5]

An inspired Scudder brought up the possibility of gathering blood in the United States, converting it into plasma on a large scale, then sending the product to the beleaguered Allies. He pointed out that new results suggested that plasma, unlike whole blood, could survive the time and trauma attendant to traversing such a great distance.

Among a group of learned and powerful men like those at the Rockefeller Institute, such statements were capable of inciting real action, and before he knew it Scudder was making a formal presentation on the subject at the New York Academy of Medicine in a hastily called meeting of the Trustees and Medical Control Board of the Blood Transfusion Betterment Association. If any confirmation of the degree to which the suggestion was taken seriously were necessary, the presence at the meeting of representatives from both the US Army and Navy, as well as the National Research Council, would have sufficed (in fact, the NRC had initiated its own committees on blood transfusion, including blood substitutes, in May, and would never be far from the major work in this arena).[6] Also invited to the June 12th conference were representatives of the Rockefeller Institute and several sizable pharmaceutical companies. As a newly minted expert in the field, Drew also attended. Scudder's talk on the latest advances in plasma research was one presentation; the attendees also heard an encouraging report on the topic from a Captain Douglas Kendrick, who represented the Surgeon General of the Army, as well as an impassioned plea for swift action from Carrel (unfortunately no effort could be swift enough; France surrendered less than two weeks later).[7]

The result of this meeting was an endorsement of the concept by the Association and a tentative commitment to proceed: "Although the use of plasma was still in an experimental stage, enough knowledge was available to justify an effort at quantity production to save lives of war casualties in the emergency then existing."[8] Two overarching goals were planned: to relieve the suffering of the Allied casualties in France and England and, with a nod to the presence of the representatives of the armed forces and the NRC, to provide a model for any large-scale blood procurement drive that might be necessary should the United States, as it seemed increasingly likely, go to war.

Immediately after this meeting, a special ad hoc assembly of the association's board of trustees was held, at which several steps were taken. Foremost of these was the decision to involve the American Red Cross, which was, after all, the organization historically most involved in war relief. The association also earmarked $15,000 of its own money for the project and voted to survey the New York City–area hospitals as to their willingness to participate. Lastly, the board opted to proceed with liquid plasma rather than dried because, although dried plasma would be easier to transport than liquid in glass bottles, and probably last longer, too, the drying apparatus was expensive, the process time-consuming, and the data regarding dry plasma efficacy was not considered adequate.[9]

While the brass of the association's board, President John F. Bush (the same Presbyterian Hospital trustee to whom Drew had sent the January memo on establishing a permanent blood bank), Medical Board of Control chair DeWitt Stetten, and attorney Tracy Voorhees prepared a presentation for the Red Cross, a small but important committee composed of Scudder, Drew, and a public health physician named E. H. L. Corwin was formed. These three immediately went to work on a vital and comprehensive report "covering the subjects of personnel, requisite floor space, supplies, preparation of equipment, serology, bacteriology, supervision, routines for non-centrifuge technique for the preparation of pooled plasma, and criteria for the selection and protection of voluntary donors."[10] This report, essentially a blueprint for the operations of what came to be called the Blood for Britain project, was presented to the Blood Transfusion Betterment Association's trustees on July 1.

Amid all this Drew, of course, was expected back at Howard to begin his new duties as a staff member in the Department of Surgery. His start date was August 1. As if there were not enough going on, Lenore was in the final weeks of her pregnancy, too. Although Drew was forced to split time between Washington and Columbia for a few weeks, she stayed in New York City, which may have reflected a reluctance to subject her to travel. In the meantime, her husband found and rented an apartment in the capital city at 3324 Sherman Ave NW, a few blocks north of the Howard University campus. The financial burden of duplicate rents would only last a short time, but it was felt sharply while it lasted—particularly with the costs of moving and the fact that the couple had no income in the months of June and July.

The Drews' first child came into the world on August 8 at Presbyterian (thankfully, the hospital wrote off the costs of Lenore's confinement).[11] It was a girl, and they named her Bebe Roberta in a deliberate nod to the fledgling institution that had dominated their lives for much of the previous year—the Columbia blood bank ("BB"; Lenore's father was named Robert). Less than a week after Bebe's arrival, Drew was back alone in DC, digging into his new role as assistant professor of surgery and trying to set up house in the apartment while Lenore recuperated from childbirth. Leaving Lenore at such a time cannot have been a popular move, and, overall, it was a highly stressful time for the young couple, as a surviving letter indicates:

> Wednesday, August 13, 1940
>
> Dear Lenore,
>
> To get the business of the house over first. It had been my hope to have a place at least pseudo-home-like when you got here so that you could spend your time learning to be a mother and I could spend my time proving that I am a surgeon during the day and resting and basking in the evenings in the warmth and joy of a lovely wife, a darling baby and a comfortable home. You have won, I shall ask only a bed to lay my head on. The rest of the job is yours. At your direction I shall help as much as I can, but remember I have gone back to work.
>
> As to seeing eye to eye on the affairs of the home: I have been willing, I am willing and more than anxious to turn the whole running of the house over to you, but since being home and finding that the pump is broke, the bathroom hopper doesn't work and nobody seems worried, the kitchen floor is worn and dirty I am and shall be increasingly adamant in my attitude toward the type of place I will live in.
>
> I think we see eye to eye well enough—only in the fourth dimension—time—do we strike a snag in our symphony of ideal home making.

> As to the care of the baby: I have seen Warick Cardoza and talked with him about a plan for watching and recording the health and progress of Bebe in great detail for a year.[12]
>
> As to your "fanning" up enthusiasm to come down here: I am disappointed that you find it necessary to work up enthusiasm "in starting and building a home there." I am more enthusiastic about it than anything I've ever done. I had assumed that you would be, too. Sometimes perhaps I am presumptuous.
>
> I am sorry to write like this because until I got your letter I had spent six happy hours roaming the stores visualizing various pieces in various places as trimming for you and Bebe. I am not too happy tonight but I am glad to know that you and the baby are doing so well. In spite of the fact that your letter has had me mad as Hades for the last two hours, I love you both very, very much.[13]

Periods of bliss and strife would come and go for the Drews, as they do in any marriage; the long-sought day of "warmth and joy" was not yet at hand.

As Drew took up his new duties at Howard, one of the men who had done the most to make his advancement come to fruition was not there to greet him: that summer, medical school dean Numa Adams had taken sick and returned to his previous home, Chicago, for specialist treatment. Sadly, on August 29, three weeks after Bebe's birth, Adams died of pneumonia. He was only fifty-five. In his eleven years at the helm of the Howard University School of Medicine, Adams had accomplished what many deemed impossible: the establishment of an excellent modern clinical, teaching, and research facility. He would be missed, but the foundation Adams had laid provided the leaders to come with a firm footing on which to build still higher.[14]

By September, Lenore and Bebe joined Drew in Washington and a new routine was established, based around the needs of the new mother and infant as well as the teaching and clinical duties attendant to a professor of surgery. No sooner had this pattern been established, though, than it was suddenly and fatefully interrupted. As if in a scene from a contemporary melodramatic film, the portent announced itself with a knock at the door on September 3, followed by the surprising presence of a Western Union delivery man.

The messenger's telegram was from, of all people, John Beattie—Drew's old professor of anatomy from McGill. Beattie had left Canada just as Drew was beginning his postgraduate training at Montreal General Hospital, returning to his home country of England to take a position as director of the research laboratories with the Royal College of Surgeons. In the ensuing years, Beattie had done yeoman work in this position, including collaboration with the great American neurosurgeon Harvey Cushing. As war broke out in Europe he was, with the rank of colonel, put in charge of the British Army's Blood Transfusion and Surgical Research Service, in which the labs of the Royal College of Surgeons were instrumental. When London itself began to be bombed by the Luftwaffe in mid-August 1940 and civilian casualties became a reality, the already robust urgency of this work ramped up considerably.

Beattie's telegram read, in part, "Could you secure five thousand ampoules dried plasma for transfusion work immediately and follow this by equal quantity in three to four weeks? Contents each ampoule should represent about one pint whole plasma."[15]

At the same time, Beattie wired the Blood Transfusion Betterment Association in New York City: "Uniform standards for all blood banks of utmost importance. Suggest you appoint overall director if program is to continue. Suggest Charles R. Drew if available."[16]

These two telegrams raise intriguing questions.

From a practical perspective, Beattie's request of Drew was unfeasible. In early September 1940, Drew was not in a position to acquire 5,000 ampules of dried plasma. He was not involved in the Blood for Britain program at the time, and even if he were, not only was there no such volume of dried plasma anywhere in the world but, as noted above, the decision had also been made by the Blood Transfusion Betterment Association back in June to eschew the dried form in favor of its liquid version.

Why did Beattie contact Drew regarding this? It is likely that the Englishman, ensconced in his role as a leader in his beleaguered country's transfusion work, immersed himself in the literature of what was, to him, a new field. There, he found Drew's name featured prominently (even though his Columbia dissertation was not published, much of the experimental work that went into it had, as we have seen, appeared in respected physiology and surgery journals). Beattie would also have been aware of the Blood for Britain Project and seen Drew's name featured in leadership positions among its medical committees. Thus, he may have made the logical, if presumptive, inference that Drew oversaw the program and reached out accordingly.

The recommendations Beattie made to the leadership of the Blood Transfusion Betterment Association were bold but, as it happened, on point. How seriously they influenced those leaders is unknown.

Since Drew had left for Washington the Blood for Britain project had been highly active. Even before he departed, Bush, Stetten, and Voorhees had gone to Washington to meet with the chair of the American Red Cross, Norman H. Davis, where they succeeded in obtaining a pledge of $25,000 to the effort, as well as the aid of both the New York City and Brooklyn branches of the organization. While there, these three also met with members of the National Research Council, who put them in touch with that agency's Blood Substitutes subcommittee—an important liaison for the project's role as a pilot program in any national blood drive to come.[17]

A central office was established in donated space at the New York Academy of Medicine Building at East 103rd Street and 5th Avenue and what was soon a burgeoning staff—volunteer physicians, administrators, clerical and stenographic teams—went to work. John Scudder, who continued with his research at both Columbia and the Rockefeller Institute, was made assistant to the Board of Medical Control.

Six hospitals immediately offered their services: Presbyterian, Mount Sinai, New York Post-Graduate, New York, Long Island College, and Memorial. Most of these either already owned or had purchased the necessary equipment: centrifuges, pumps, iceboxes. The association provided whatever was needed for the other institutions as well as transfusion sets (and mission-specific objects like forms, labels, and record books) for all.

In the big picture, the plan was simple: the Blood Transfusion Betterment Association would collect as much blood as possible in the metropolitan area and convert it to plasma. The Red Cross would provide publicity for this to aid in attracting donors, then take the collected plasma and transport it overseas (now, with France having fallen, to England alone). The particulars, on the other hand, turned out to be extremely complex. As Stetten wrote at the time, "We received the impression that preparing plasma would not be much more difficult than mixing a cocktail, but we soon learned, much to our distress, that such was not the case."[18]

A host of scientific and wholly practical questions plagued the Association's physicians and investigators, taking up large swaths of time:

Should the blood be collected by an open or closed method? In a closed system the drawn blood would go from the donor vein into a sterile bottle without being exposed to the air. All agreed this was best.

What type of bottle should be used—dumbbell, square straight-sided, or cylindrical? What is the best size for the bottle? This related to the issue of the cellular/plasma interface. Drew and Scudder had designed the dumbbell bottle but not all were convinced of its superiority.

Should vacuum, suction, or just venous pressure be utilized in drawing the blood? The concern here was trauma to the cells resulting in high potassium concentration and accelerated breakdown of the product.

The list stretched on:

How should the blood be mixed with the sodium citrate solution? How should these bottles be corked or capped after filling? What is the best way of drawing off the supernatant plasma into the pool bottles? What should be the age limits, the minimum blood pressure, and the minimum hemoglobin percentage for the volunteer donors? Should the blood be taken only from fasting donors to avoid turbidity of the plasma from fat globules? What serological test for syphilis should be used? Should the blood of the donors be grouped? Was sedimentation or centrifugation the better method of separating the plasma from the blood cells, from the standpoints of yield, sterility, speed, and economy? How much and what strength sodium citrate solution should be used? Merthiolate was the antibacterial chemical recommended by experts, but what strength Merthiolate solution should be used? What was the best type and size of pool bottle? How much normal saline solution should be added to the plasma to keep it from becoming too viscous and to prevent the precipitation of the fibrinogen? What system should be used for transferring the plasma from the pool bottles to the final bottles so as to expose the product to the least danger of contamination, and what type and size of this bottle was the best for the packing and shipment of the solution? At what temperature should the pooled plasma and the plasma saline solution be kept until shipment abroad? How should the final bottles be labeled, what kind of record card should be kept at the hospitals, and how should the release signed by the donor be worded? What size carton should be adopted for shipment?

Some of these issues were prosaic, others convoluted, but each of them—and many more—required a definitive consensus answer, and "innumerable" conferences and meetings were held in the late summer of 1940 as the association struggled to move forward. Whether Beattie's telegram had any influence or not, in late September the decision was made that progress by committee was glacially slow and inefficient at a moment when speed was paramount. A single medical supervisor possessed of knowledge and experience in the specific technical details and armed with decision-making power was necessary. According to Stetten, "On October 1, we engaged a full-time, salaried Medical Supervisor to help us solve the technical problems, to formulate a standard, uniform technique and to coordinate the cooperating hospitals. The unanimous choice of the Board of Medical Control fell on Charles R. Drew."[19] President John Bush himself sent Drew the proposition by telegram:

> The Board of Medical Control of the Blood Transfusion Betterment Association at its meeting this afternoon decided to create a position of full-time Medical Supervisor to act as a liaison officer between the Board and the hospitals engaged in procuring plasma for shipment to the British Red Cross. I am requested to offer you this position and all it involves to you as being the best qualified of anyone we know to act in this important development. I'm sure your university will feel under the wartime circumstances it will grant you a leave of absence at least until the first of the year to help us in our efforts with the American Red Cross and establishing this vital medical relief. Will you please wire or telephone me if you can arrange the matter and in so doing just how long you can remain and what you feel under the circumstances would be the proper monthly compensation to be paid you. I cannot tell you how much depends upon your university and yourself giving us a favorable reply. I await your answer with the utmost interest.[20]

One of the questions the association put to itself early in the process—and settled before Drew was assigned the supervisor role—was whether to accept blood donated by African Americans. In January 1941, Stetten wrote, "This was answered in the affirmative but with the proviso that the plasma therefrom should be specially labelled as to its origin."[21] This policy was apparently put into place to assuage what was assumed to be the British preference.[22]

Another decision made early in the Blood for Britain project was to proceed as rapidly as possible even though all the clinical questions had not been answered. The Red Cross mobilized its considerable publicity prowess through the advertisements in the press, on the radio, and via posters and pamphlets. The response of the public, clearly motivated by an altruistic sense of wanting to do *something* to help those suffering overseas, was enthusiastic. The first donor appointments were scheduled for August 15 at Presbyterian. By the end of the month, 1,044 appointments had been made. In September that number rose to 3,822. On August 27, Sir Edward Mellanby, the secretary of the Medical Research Council of Great Britain, sent a letter to the association reporting that the first batch of plasma had arrived, been found in good condition, and, after passing sterility tests, was forwarded to the Royal Air Force.[23]

His job as medical supervisor may have officially started on October 1, but Drew went to New York City in late September to get a jump on what were obviously considerable responsibilities. He and Lenore had given up the 150th Street apartment when she moved down to Washington with the baby, so he took a room at the YMCA. Howard University gave Drew four months' leave to work on the project. Other than the clerical workers, Drew was the only salaried staff member on the Blood for Britain team. He earned $400 per month plus expenses.

The first task he took on, and the greatest concern to all involved, was the specter of bacterial contamination of the plasma, which could turn the fluid from a lifesaving panacea to a vehicle of sepsis and death. In individual hospitals it was comparatively straightforward to minimize this problem, but with so many steps spread across multiple institutions, the opportunities for breakdown in proper sterile technique were manifold. At the outset, the association had adhered to existing standards of the National Institutes of Health (at this time known mainly as a branch of the US Public Health Service and not yet the federal monolith it would become). Despite this, some samples became contaminated. One of Drew's first acts as medical supervisor was to call a meeting about the problem, inviting bacteriologists from the participating hospitals as well as representatives from the City Health Department and the Eli Lilly pharmaceutical company, manufacturers of the antiseptic Merthiolate.[24]

The result of this consultation was a reiteration of the existing precautionary measures, which mainly consisted of careful sterile technique in all handling of samples, then culturing the blood at its drawing point and again when it was pooled at the hospital. Drew then added a crucial final step of testing the pooled plasma by means of aerobic and anaerobic cultures taken at a new Central Lab (it was understood that the British would do their own testing when the plasma reached them, too). The proper use of Merthiolate, introduced into the plasma (in this era before widespread antibiotic availability) to retard the growth of any bacteria that escaped the sterile techniques, was also finalized.

There was a scare in November when reports came back from England indicating that some of the shipments had grown out bacteria from their on-site testing, but it turned out that these had been drawn in August before the new, more stringent criteria were initiated.

Many of the other problems and questions that led to Drew's assignment as medical supervisor he had already solved or answered during the preparatory experiments for the Columbia blood bank or could be found in the references he had included in his thesis. Not every answer was immediately clear, though, and support from his superiors (he answered directly to the association's Blood Plasma Committee) and colleagues would be essential as the job unfolded. Drew's approach to the contamination problem—definitive and uncompromising but incorporating the component of consultation necessary to any consensus building—was the first demonstration in his new role of what Scudder meant when he described Drew as "an indefatigable worker, a man who took infinite pains . . . a genius at detail and an outright first class organizer."[25] From this point on, support was unwavering and Drew's judgment and authority as medical supervisor were unquestioned.

Although Drew's work on the Blood for Britain project was "hectic," he made the mature and caring point not to lose sight of his family back in Washington, keeping in touch and in the moment regarding the many practical concerns and costs of the new baby and home. That autumn he faced another daunting professional hurdle, too: the American Board of Surgery qualifying exam—the written section of the two-part test—which he was scheduled to take at the end of October. The night before the bacteriological consultation meeting, he penned a letter to Lenore:

Sunday, Sept 29, 1940

Hello My Sweet,

. . . I sit now in the 11th floor of the YMCA and thank my stars that this is only a transient abode, that I have a home of my own, that you are there and Bebe is there and it is cheerful, bright, happy and comfortable. A single little room always seems to hem me in so tightly.

I'll be busy here but I have just been thinking how terribly busy you are there and after payday, even more so. All the bills to pay, the curtains to fix, the covers to make, the studio couch frame to get built, another chair to find, scatter rugs to find, a baby carriage to get, new clothes to purchase, your abdominal muscles to tighten up by daily exercise, your food to get (enough of it) and the thousand other details of running the house you wanted to be absolute boss of. Of course you'll spend some time missing me, as I told you.

During the month of October I may not be able to get to Washington for I must pass the bloody examination on the 28th. But after that I think we ought to plan to be together at least every other weekend, first you up here then me down there. By that time Grace will be home and about and mother can keep BB.[26] It should be great fun, especially your trips up here for then we can do some of the things together we haven't had a chance to since your first visit in June a year ago. I look forward to it with all the eagerness of your first visit.

Until tomorrow,

Charlie[27]

In October the program generated 4,690 donor appointments spread over the participating hospitals (there were now eight of these with the addition of the Lenox Hill Hospital and the Hospital for Joint Diseases). With built-in delays from the sterility tests and quarantines, 576 liters of plasma were realized in the month.[28]

Feedback from the British as to the results of the plasma program, much to the frustration of the Americans, came only intermittently. On October 8, though, A. N. Drury, chairman of the Committee on Traumatic Shock and Blood Transfusion of the Medical Research Council of Great Britain, sent a letter to the association stating that seven cartons, or forty-two liters, of the plasma saline solution had arrived safely and was "proving very useful."[29] Two weeks later, a second letter came from Sir Edward Mellanby, urging for continued shipments at least until the end of January 1941. It was thought by the British team that their own blood substitute program would be up and running by that date.

Earlier in the month, the association's president Bush, along with Stetten and Voorhees, had again traveled to Washington to meet with Red Cross chairman Norman Davis. These men anticipated the information about progress by the British that came in Mellanby's note but decided to continue with the Blood for Britain program funding because of its usefulness as a precursor to what all anticipated would be an American national blood drive effort soon.

Late in October Drew wrote to his mother back home in Arlington, touching lightly on specifics of his work but revealing the personal and professional stress he was under: the plasma program was running at full tilt, Lenore had temporarily moved to Philadelphia to be with her mother (who had come down with pulmonary tuberculosis and been admitted to a state hospital), and the American Board of Surgery qualifying exam loomed. There was also evidence, though, of an equanimity that, like the maturity evident in his September 29 letter to Lenore, had been lacking in earlier missives:

> October 25, 1940
>
> Dear Mother,
>
> Your first born has been neglecting his very lovely mother too much these days and he is very sorry for it. I miss you all very much, especially after the very pleasant time at home this summer. The pace is so fast here there simply is no time for anything. . . . By coming up here I had hoped to increase my income for a short while and get out of a hole. . . . I did not anticipate Lenore's move which means I am now running three places. Yet I suppose her mother's illness is the type of thing one cannot anticipate and has to do the best one can under the circumstances. Mrs. Robbins is in pretty bad shape and I am not at all certain about the proper or perhaps the kind attitude to take in regards to Lenore and her staying in Philadelphia. There have been other tough nuts to crack in the times that have gone by and I suppose that I will handle this one too before very long.
>
> At this time it is difficult for the job here is big, hard and important. Mistakes will have international sequelae and must not be made. To add to the present rush

of events I am supposed to take the American Board of Surgery exam on Monday. I have been getting ready for it for five years and just now that I wish that everything should be most serene, it is most upset. I shall take the exam and hope for luck. I am not prepared and all I can hope is that the general rating will not be so high that my unpreparedness will not stand out in bold relief.

Give my love to the family. In these times of such swift action when everything seems so uncertain and rather unstable, in my heart I cling to you more than ever before.

Charlie

P.S. Find enclosed $20[30]

Drew took the qualifying examination of the American Board of Surgery in New York on October 28, 1940. This was an all-day written examination in two sessions, with essay questions intended to measure the candidate's knowledge about common diseases across the spectrum of the practice of general surgery. When it was finished, Drew and the other candidates had to wait six weeks for the results.

With the word from England that further shipments of plasma would not be necessary after the end of January, the Blood for Britain program, which was operating at peak efficiency and prepared to expand to more hospitals, was intentionally leveled off in November 1940. The job was far from over, though. As John Bush wrote, "The project for England has ended before certain vitally important questions which have arisen affecting any work in this general field have been answered."[31] Anticipating that the US armed forces might soon be engaged in combat activities, an aggressive research program was put into action to answer some of the lingering questions from the project and to pave the way for the full-scale American effort on the horizon. Drew was put in charge.

For one thing, the ideal container question was still unanswered (the "dumbbell" design advocated by Scudder and Drew after their work on the Columbia blood bank turned out to have serious drawbacks).[32] In fact, the entire closed-system apparatus was not yet foolproof, and improvement was required in the process of separating the plasma from the cells, too.

Everyone recognized that dried plasma would be a better option than the liquid form from the perspective of transport and storage, if the technical and safety issues could be resolved. Work on this had never really stopped, as in the still-unsettled bigger question of plasma versus serum (the British advocated for serum, mainly because it could pass through very fine filters used to remove bacteria—plasma, containing the clotting proteins, tended to gum them up).

Drew and his team developed comprehensive lab and clinical experimentation protocols to address all these issues and more in both university labs and industry settings.

In early December Drew received his results from the board written exam. Any misgivings about preparedness—if they were genuine—turned out to be unfounded, as he easily passed with an excellent score of 86.5 percent.[33] This meant he was qualified to proceed to the oral certifying exam, which was to be administered on March 14 in Baltimore. He sent Lenore the good news, as well as an update on the impact he had made on the Blood for Britain project:

> Hello My Sweet,
>
> Just got word that I passed the American board of surgery written examination. That is quite a Christmas present.
>
> To make this day very happy we just received a cable from England stating that since the standardization of techniques (that's when I took over here) no more infected material has arrived in England.
>
> See you Saturday
>
> Love, Charlie[34]

After a brief weekend with the visiting Lenore, Drew returned to work as the focus of the project shifted to the future:

> Monday, December 9, 1940
>
> Dear Lenore,
>
> I enjoyed being with you over the weekend very much. Hope you found everything O.K. on your return home.

> Today I have attended three meetings in a row, the first down on Wall Street, the second at the Commodore Hotel (swell lunch) and the third at the American Red Cross. Quite a busy day.
>
> It was decided to bring this work to a close on the first of February. That is the answer as to when I shall be home for good. Before that time I shall have to write up the experiences of this association in this work in order that they may be available for other groups which might undertake such an adventure. It has been great fun.[35]

Drew realized that, from a purely professional standpoint, his experiences on the Blood for Britain project had been some of the most valuable he could have imagined. He had crossed paths with some of the most important men in American medicine, either in person or through correspondence, and the impact this would have on his career was incalculable:

> I have made contacts that I may have waited a lifetime to make in the ordinary scheme of things.[36] One cannot tell what the future of anything is going to be in times as turbulent as these but up to now fate and chance have been very kind to me. I have gained insight into so many things that I did not clearly understand before I started this job.

He then took the time to reflect on how his experiences would affect his new role at Howard, as well as the more settled family life that was, hopefully, in store:

> When I get home a whole new world will have to be readjusted in terms of recent events. It too will be fun. While not on so large a scale, there is much work to do, many problems to be settled. We should have fun working out things together once our lives have settled down a bit. We'll make a go of it I know, but some of the spots are not going to be easy. As I see it the making of a real home is just about the biggest and most important job ahead of us and unfortunately most of this load will fall on you. Honest, I'll help all I can and promise to try to get away from some of my bachelor ideas and you must try to get out of your decoration classes in school into the swing of real life off campus.
>
> Love to all,
>
> Charlie[37]

In the last week of January, Drew labored over the report he mentioned in his letter to Lenore. He finished it in the remarkably short time of ten days and submitted the completed work on January 31, 1941. After some editing, in which Drew did not take part, the text was published under the title, *Report of the Blood Transfusion Association:*[38] *Concerning the Project for Supplying Blood Plasma to England, Which Has Been Carried on Jointly with the American Red Cross from August, 1940 to January, 1941. Narrative Account of Work and Medical Report.* Association president John Bush wrote the narrative and Drew the medical section. Two weeks later, in a letter to Lenore, Drew called this report "to date . . . my greatest single writing effort . . . I believe that it is a good piece of work and will in years to come prove of greater value to all concerned than anything I might have done at Howard during the period just being brought to a close." He then added, "I think that I was wise to come."[39]

When the final numbers were established for the project, it was determined that 14,556 donations had been made, resulting in 5,272 usable liters of plasma (475 liters were contaminated or otherwise unsuitable). Costs of the project were nearly exactly met by the original estimate: $15,000 was provided by the Association and $25,000 by the American Red Cross. Based on the commercial price of plasma, it was calculated that the monetary value of the product generated by the program was $400,000.[40]

In a later reflection, Drew wrote, "This project . . . had two objects, the first, to aid England in a very dark hour, the second, to make available increased information in the field to our own government and its armed forces. Both, we believe, have been at least in part achieved."[41]

Drew did not have to wait long either for the new, nationwide blood drive to begin or to find out his own role in it. Soon after the coming of the new year, well before he was set to return to Howard University on February 1, 1940, rumblings were evident. On January 9 he wrote Lenore:

> My dear Mrs. Drew,
>
> You will be pleased to hear that the State Department has considered your husband too valuable a citizen to allow to expose himself to the rigors and dangers of the European scene at this time, therefore they will not issue a passport.[42]

From word we have received in this office today there is some evidence that the word has been passed down to have certain of our armed forces ready for war if need be by the first of April. To that end we have been asked to prepare to start collecting blood for plasma for the U.S. Navy. Things do happen fast do they not? I do not know what the next step is at this time but whatever it is I am pretty sure, I believe, that your hubby will be in the middle of it. The first chance that I get I will come down and discuss the future of this rapidly increasing little band of Drews.*

Your devoted but wayward husband,

Charlie[43]

Drew had good reason to believe that he would be involved in any expanded effort, both because he had been the medical supervisor of the Blood for Britain antecedent program and because he himself had been one of the advocates working toward such a sequel.

At the Blood Transfusion Betterment Association and Red Cross meetings he attended on December 9 (the busy day of three conferences and a "swell lunch" he had written about to Lenore) DeWitt Smith of the Red Cross "requested that this Association suggest a program which might be quickly carried out for the bleeding of 100,000 donors in six months, should this amount of blood be asked for by the United States Navy."[44] In preparation to answer this request, Drew reached out to key officials in twelve major cities from coast to coast regarding their blood and plasma collection operations, much as J. Bentley Squier's committee had sought the experience of existing facilities when starting the Columbia Presbyterian Blood Bank back in November 1938. The clear implication was that these twelve would also be the centers around which the national effort would be built.

Even more to the point, Drew, in conjunction with the association attorney and trustee Tracy Voorhees, had followed this up in late December with a proposal to the Red Cross for a three-month pilot program for the mass production of dried plasma—felt now by all to be the blood substitute of the

* Lenore was now pregnant with what would be the Drews' second child, daughter Charlene.

immediate future. As it happened, the NRC and its "clients," the armed forces, had been planning such a thing for months, also utilizing the auspices of the Red Cross.

On January 9, 1941, the Board of Medical Control of the Association met. The work of the Blood for Britain project was essentially complete, and it was time for all still aboard to pivot to the new project. Replies had been received from nine of the twelve queried officials, and—with a few exceptions—confidence in a successful operation was high. Protocols were discussed, largely based on the proven successes of the past several months, and the location of a central national laboratory considered.[45]

As the calendar flipped to February on the accelerated prewar schedule, the Red Cross/Blood Transfusion Association national pilot program was set to commence, with Drew as the assistant director. The director was Cornelius P. Rhoads, medical director of Memorial Hospital and chairman of

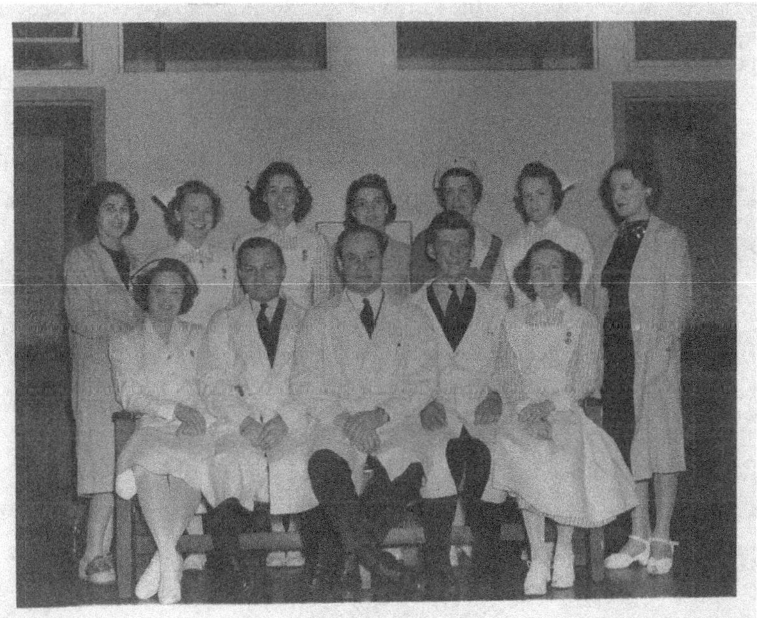

Figure 8.1 Drew and other staff members of the American Red Cross blood drive in early 1941. Earl Taylor *(front row, second from the right)* succeeded Drew as leader of this organization. Personal collection, Charlene Drew Jarvis.

the Blood Plasma Committee of the Blood Transfusion Association, to which Drew reported as medical supervisor of the Blood for Britain effort. Drew was essentially serving the same role for this new, national program—leader of the medical and technical work. He was also put in charge of the New York City Red Cross blood bank, which turned out to occupy most of his time and was, in fact, the source of his salary. This was the first site for the program, which would expand to encompass the entire nation in the years to come.

Conspicuously absent from the list of medical scientists working on the new drive was the name of John Scudder. On February 10, Drew wrote Lenore with an update on his work and, after giving particulars about the current tasks, explained the omission of his colleague from the current lineup:

> Dear Lenore,
>
> It has been one week today since we started the new project of collecting blood for the American Red Cross. It seems ages ago. So many things seem to have taken place that it does not seem possible that only seven days have passed.
>
> We have a full time staff of 12 people: 2 doctors, 4 nurses, 2 technicians, 1 bookkeeper, 1 secretary, 1 shipping clerk and 1 handyman.
>
> The bleedings are done from 1:00 to 8:00 P.M. daily on Tuesday through Friday, from noon to 8:00 P.M. on Saturday and from 10:00 A.M. to 3:00 P.M. on Sunday. For everyone but the secretary, Monday is a day of rest.
>
> I, as usual, have no special hours and no particular day of rest.
>
> At present we are bleeding 60 donors a day. At the end of about 2 weeks we shall be doing 100 a day and try to work out the details of such a system on this level of activity. To date the whole thing has worked very well with no hitches of any importance.
>
> Scudder, of course, was very hurt when the job which he has felt that he was creating for himself was not offered to him. I truthfully felt very badly for him. There is no doubt about his knowledge of this subject and his deep interest in it but he has antagonized so many people that his nomination for the job became almost an impossibility. I tried to save some of his face by adding his name to my report to the board of medical control. I feel that I have now paid back in work and favors any debt I might have owed as a result of his early kindnesses to me here in New York. Our relationship will never be entirely cordial for there is enough

> of the Nietzschean about him to feel that "man is but to be surpassed" and he will not ever take kindly to the idea that I started under him and gradually took over.

Drew went on to lament, once more, his frequent and lengthy absences (Lenore cannot have been overjoyed when her husband announced that his February 1 return date was to be postponed for three months). This time he cast himself in the grandiose role of an intrepid scientific martyr-explorer. Though quickly recognizing the comic overreach, he reserved a moment to reflect on the mysterious impetus that drove him onward:

> For you I know it has been a disappointing. Our separation has caused us to miss much that we may have shared together. For this I am sorry. Many of the days and nights have been lonely here for me. I know that they were much more lonely for you, but from time immemorial, men who have beat out new paths into unknown regions have had to strike out alone, leaving all that was dear behind. These have been new paths that I have been treading, Lenore, as new as the uncharted seas that the early sailors defied, as strange as the new lands early explorers mapped while good wives waited in fear and loneliness lest the wandering ones failed to return. Yet it has always been true that there are where one man dared to go, others would follow, and me these, the ones who followed after, often brought their whole families along and knew more joy than those who first came that way, and some of those who came along later, were the children of those who had gone before, and their joys were a recompense to those who had gone ahead., the lonely ones. Maybe Bebe will someday live and laugh and work under conditions which will make you glad that during long, apparently useless days you pushed back the tears and lived alone while I found new places in which to grow.
>
> I know that you think that all of this is just a little bit heroic, sometimes I do too, and laugh at myself. But most of the time I am deadly serious about it, as though I had nothing to do with it but simply carried out commands given me by some inner force which never wants to play. I should play more, we should play more, not separately, but together. Sometimes, I forget that no woman is all woman, totally grown up and self-sufficient, but that each and a large measure is a little girl who needs the loving, the understanding, the tolerance and even guidance that little girls need. Sometimes, you forget that all men are just little boys grown up and playing at bigger

> games, that they too need understanding, encouragement and even and help even when they seem to be going along at a great pace. We both forget at times that the essence of life lies in making two blades of grass grow where one grew before, and bringing a smile where there was a tear, and giving and sharing as much as we can.[46]

The olive branch contained in the final paragraphs of this letter spotlights the challenges the Drews were clearly having in early 1941 with the protracted long-distance nature of their marriage, so soon into its course. Two weeks later, having evidently received what he felt to be an unsatisfactory response, Charles sent another note. This time his tone was distraught and combative, the text packed with unflattering observations. Only at the close does the language soften in a self-conscious and unconvincing effort to ease the blows that came before:

> Sunday, February 24, 1941
>
> Dear Lenore,
>
> You are a lovely but sometimes strange person. You complain that my letters no longer make you feel that without you I could not live, that the place you fill is one which no one else can possibly take, that they are so philosophic anyone could read them etc., etc.
>
> I do not know how to answer such a letter. Warmth is engendered, not demanded; compliments are never lacking when compliments are due; indispensability is an acquired estate, not an inherent one and true devotion is built on something more real than repeated protestations.
>
> Undoubtedly I lack many things which one should have to become an ideal husband, but lack of appreciation of you is not one of them, nor do I minimize the part you now play in my life. I have tried in indirect ways to tell you the things which are most essential to me in the marriage state. As a whole they are attitudes not things. Being in good part an extrovert I react to these attitudes. Every now and then you do some little, almost insignificant thing that makes me so happy that were the world mine I would gladly give it to you and sink the price cheap. I remember with such pleasure the first time you thought of getting some ginger ale and cake for some guests who came to 250 W 150. It was months after we were married and the first genuinely kind move you had

made in that direction. I felt as proud of you as though you had just won a Nobel Prize. I still feel a pleasant afterglow from it though I have forgotten who the guests were or whether they enjoyed the cake or not. I can stand many slights to my own vanity much easier than I can think of my home being an inhospitable one.

Somehow or other you feel that I'm looking for unusual things all of the time. In truth most of the time the small ones make a much greater impression. If I should come home tired after a hard day work and a long train ride and you should offer to take my coat and hat and ask me to be seated—just the things most people would do for a stranger—I should probably just ooze with affection but it never has happened.

You say that my coming thrills you yet when I take the pains to wire you ahead of time then call you on the phone, eager to bask in your femininity, unless I specifically ask, you will not even take off those most unattractive always dirty looking house dresses. I look ahead for weeks at a time to seeing you, to letting down from affairs of the mind and 50% of the time I run into an argument on purely a masculine basis. I cannot come back here and write eulogies about the powers of pure reason that my wife is gifted with. I may not be a great flatterer but I am not a liar. Affection which is not spontaneous is unworthy of the name. Well over half of the letters you have written have been in the form of complaints—the things I don't do, or do do which you ought to be allowed to do, the letters I don't write or the lack of fire in those I do write, the standards of my family and the amount of money they make you spend, the money I don't save and the small amount I give you when my salary is considered etcetera etc., etc. I won't answer this stuff with poetry.

I'm trying to do certain things now which can be done now or never in the future. I am trying to get a foundation in which we can build a real structure in the future. I think that I am right in attempting to do it this way. All I ask in the way of help at the moment is an encouraging attitude on your part. I don't need your masculine brain, the need to feel that the things I do, I do for you, that should I do well it will make you proud, that should I not quite make the grade you will try to make it easier by gentle understanding, gracious womanly arts and not by snappy wisecracks. If I told you a thousand times I couldn't love you anymore than I do and in the best way I know I'm trying to be worthy of your love.

Charlie[47]

Apologies and amends doubtless followed all this, but the only satisfactory resolution to the Drews' marital conflict was going to be their physical reuniting. Realization of this may have played a part in a surprising decision he would announce just three weeks later.

Although the new program was for the benefit of Americans, rather than foreigners, the number of donors that came forward was, at first, less than for the Blood for Britain drive. It was true that the level of urgency was not as great: after all, the United States was not actually at war, whereas Londoners had been literally under the gun—or the bomb, to be precise—during the former effort. There might have been other reasons, too. As Drew noted in a symposium of the American Human Serum Association in June 1941, "The collection of blood is not only a scientific problem but also a complicated social matter, too."[48] Unfounded rumors about the collected blood not really going to England had caused temporary but noticeable drops in the number of donors presenting themselves the previous autumn. Later, another piece of harmful scuttlebutt claimed that the Red Cross was selling their collected plasma.

The social consideration of the most profound significance by far was the race of the blood donors. In the Blood for Britain program, as noted above, the decision was made early on to accept blood from black donors but to segregate the final pooled plasma product to avoid offending what were perceived to be the British sensibilities. However, in the exacting records and reports of the program, there is no evidence of this actually having been done. The technical considerations alone, not to mention the expense of running separate, parallel projects for whites and blacks, were likely prohibitive factors. In the new program, the Red Cross had no specific policy regarding black donors. Drew, at the same plasma symposium in June, said of blood donations, "there is no distinction made concerning race."[49]

That was true at the time Drew said it, but a change was coming.

In the effort to maximize outreach and increase the donor pool, one consideration that held appeal was a "move the mountain to Mohammed" concept of mobile blood drawing laboratories. Drew had admired (and recounted in his thesis) the extraordinary work of Frederic Durán-Jordà in the Spanish Civil War in transporting blood from population centers to the front lines. That program, though, involved drawing blood at fixed sites, then moving it to the front-line wounded. The British had taken things a step further with their Expeditionary Force in France in early 1940, incorporating mobile units that could both collect blood and distribute it (their fleet was essentially wiped out in the German advance). Distribution was not an issue for the Red Cross program, but the slow trickle of donors was. After all, it was reasoned, expecting significant numbers of the population to interrupt their daily lives and concerns to travel to the Red Cross site to have their blood drawn was asking a lot, particularly in peacetime. What if, instead, the "bloodletting" team were sent to them—that is, to their workplaces, schools, public events, and so on? The old bugaboo of contamination would be the biggest obstacle to "taking the show on the road," but, hopefully, upgrades in the closed system of blood drawing had eliminated that as a major issue for good. Once the concept had met with approval from the higher-ups the actual unit came together quickly. On March 10 Drew traveled with the new mobile blood bank, essentially a refrigerated trailer, on its maiden voyage. He reported the experience in a letter home:

> Hello my Sweet,
>
> Just had a most interesting day. Tested out one of the "Transfusion Trailers" . . . by attaching it to a Red Cross ambulance and, with the whole crew of nurses, traveled out to the State Agricultural School in Farmingdale, L.I. (about 35 miles) to take blood from the student body. We set up in the gymnasium and everything went extremely well. In spite of the heavy snow we did not get stuck. The refrigerator, which is run by a single motored gasoline engine attached to the compressor, just chugged along like a pop-pop motor boat all day. Worked swell.[50]

Only a few days after the Long Island blood trailer journey, Drew was scheduled to sit for the second part of the American Board of Surgery examination—the daunting oral certifying test. As with the qualifying exam, these tests were administered in selected sites across the country, usually in academic medical centers located as close as possible to the candidate's home. Drew was assigned to the Johns Hopkins Medical Center in Baltimore. As the date approached, he began to feel ill, having likely caught a virus on the maiden voyage of the bloodmobile, and drove to Maryland with a fever and waxing upper respiratory infection.

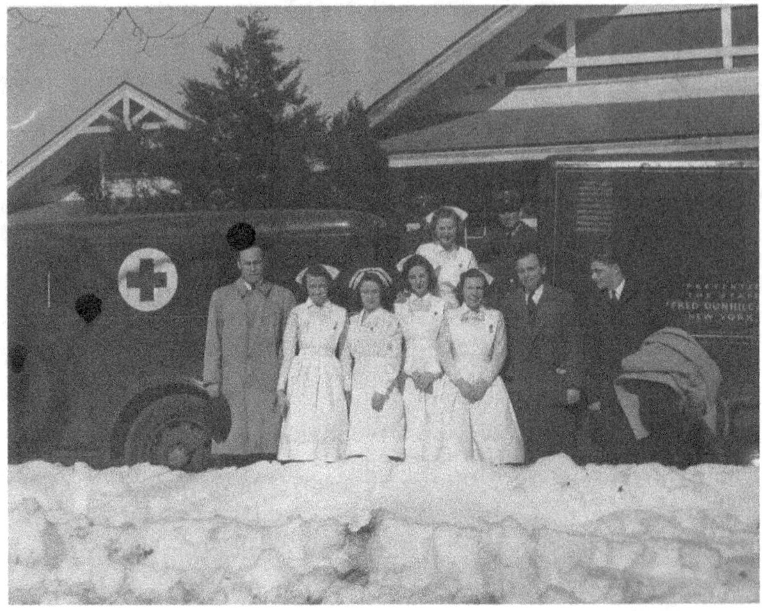

Figure 8.2 Drew and the "Transfusion Trailer" team on its test mission, March 10, 1941. Personal collection, Charlene Drew Jarvis.

When Drew appeared for the test on the surgical ward at Johns Hopkins on Friday morning, March 14, he was, as he might have put it, in pretty bad shape: "I took so many aspirin and sulfanilamide tablets trying to break up the cold and sniffed so much benzedrine my head was like a boiler factory and my mouth and nose so dry that breathing was difficult."[51]

The exam consisted of presentations of actual patients to the candidate. Physical examination and a limited perusal of the chart were permitted, along with inspection of X-rays and other objective test results. Then the candidate was expected to reveal what he believed to be the diagnosis and best plan of care. The examiner, typically a senior professor, would subsequently pepper the candidate with questions regarding this specific case, general queries about related anatomy and physiology, or, really, whatever came to mind. As the story goes, one of the patients Drew was presented elicited questions about, of all things, shock and its treatment with blood and plasma. One of his later trainees, Asa Yancey, recalled Drew telling him that he "replied with such detailed knowledge that the examiner went along the corridor, knocking on the doors of rooms where others were examining candidates, and urged several examiners to come and hear Drew's discussions of the use of blood in the severely ill and injured patient."[52]

A few days after the exam Drew described the experience for Lenore in the modestly low-key manner he typically employed in describing his own academic exploits: "Friday was a trying day. The morning exams went well, in the afternoon I began to falter. My nose began to run, my eyes ran and my brain slowed up. I don't know how the final results will be. I think I probably sneaked by. I was sorry not to have been in perfect shape for the exam because I really wanted to lay it on."[53]

When the marks came in the next month, Drew had made an outstanding score of 91 percent, which was "laying it on" by any standard.[54] He was now officially "board certified," a diplomate of the American Board of Surgery.

By the time he passed the board exam, Drew had already decided to resign his position with the Red Cross in New York and return to Howard and home. His extended leave of absence did not expire until the end of April, but Drew opted to resign a full month earlier than planned. He had hinted at this to Lenore back in February, reporting that "I am grooming Earl Taylor (to take over) as fast as I can."[55] Four weeks later he revealed more of his thinking while still leaving unspoken any specific reasons for cutting the mission short, "There are some things that I will leave unfinished here which I naturally would like to finish but I feel that the moment is propitious for pulling out and hence my decision to report for work at Howard a month before my leave is up."[56] His letter of resignation was dated March 17, 1941. On receiving it, the executive director of the New York Chapter of the Red Cross, Robert C. Davis, responded to Drew thus:

> I received your letter of March 17, 1941 telling me of the necessity for you to return to your work at Howard University and tendering your resignation as Medical Director of the Blood Bank on March 31, 1941.
>
> It is unnecessary for me to tell you how greatly I regret your leaving us and on behalf of the Red Cross and myself, personally, I want to thank you most sincerely for all that has been done, not only in the recent project for National Defense, but also in the prior one of Blood for Britain.
>
> Thanks to you the technical organization for the present project is splendidly established, and we will, of course, follow your suggestions."[57]

If any event or circumstance arose that directly motivated Drew to depart from New York and the nascent national plasma drive, it has not come down to us. In later years, some imaginative writers—and others with agendas to advance—conjured tales about Drew resigning in anger and protest because of Red Cross policy excluding African Americans from the donor pool. Although that execrable policy was coming, it did not exist until Drew had already returned to Howard. As noted above, at the Serum symposium in June 1941, months after his resignation, Drew went on record with the observation that no distinction was made in the Red Cross program regarding donor race.

Back at home in Washington, DC, Drew was ready to move on after focusing nearly three years of his professional life on researching and processing blood and plasma. His efforts in these areas had won great acclaim, and elevated his name in the medical profession far beyond where it would otherwise have been at this early stage in his career. Now, though, there were others to take up these torches. Drew's career in medicine, as well as his course in life, were about to undergo a significant change. From this time on, he would no longer devote most of his professional time either to pure science or his own ambitions, but nearly exclusively to helping others—his patients, medical students, surgery residents, and the African American community at large.

At age thirty-six, the accomplishments that would immortalize the name of Charles Drew were already behind him. The ones that would mean the most to the man and the legacy to which he aspired were yet to come.

9

Big Red

Howard University, 1941–45

When Edward Howes took over the Department of Surgery at Howard in 1936 it was with the understanding that under Dean Numa Adams's plan (as well as the GEB underwriting) the position was guaranteed for five years, after which a qualified Black surgeon would succeed him in the position. On June 30, 1941, the five years was up. After six months guiding sprawling academic- and government-sponsored programs at the highest level, on top of two years at the prestigious Columbia University and Presbyterian Hospital—engaged in intensive learning in both the research and clinical surgical arenas—Charles Drew was as prepared as any African American candidate could possibly be to take the next step and assume the leadership positions in surgery at Howard University and Freedmen's Hospital.

Howes had seemed an ill fit when he arrived on the Howard campus, but over the ensuing years he had come to understand and appreciate the place and its denizens. In turn, his colleagues and staff had grown fond of Howes and his gruffly amiable persona. Drew himself wrote about the man, "His own brusque manner and clipt speech added to his difficulties and to the difficulties of his assistants, but at the end of his five year term of office, he not only had overcome these obstacles but had won for himself the friendship of the vast majority of the people with whom he had to work and had laid a foundation for a truly modern and effective Department of Surgery."[1]

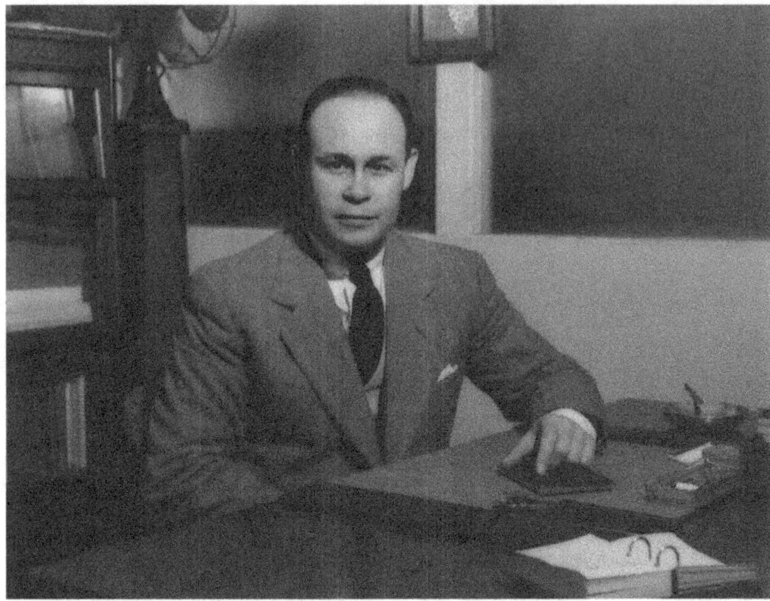

Figure 9.1 Drew in his office at Howard University. Personal collection, Charlene Drew Jarvis.

On the official recommendation of Joseph L. Johnson, acting dean of the medical school after the death of Adams, Drew assumed the twin crowns of chair of the Department of Surgery at Howard and chief of surgery at Freedmen's Hospital in October 1941.[2] That same month he was named as an examiner for the American Board of Surgery, donning the mantle of those questioners who had prodded him in Baltimore just seven months earlier. He was the first African American to be given this distinction.

It was around this time that Drew rewarded himself for his extraordinary efforts with the purchase of one item of minor luxury that was also eminently practical: a 1941 Ford 11A Super Deluxe four-door sedan, complete with leather seats and wood-grain dashboard. It would be his car for the rest of his life.

One of the many sayings of Charles Drew that were remembered and broadcast by his trainees in the years to come was, "The greatness of any institution depends upon the quality of the men it has turned out—likewise the greatness of any part of any institution is measured in the quality of its products."[3] As he embarked on his new journey as leader of the Howard University Department of Surgery, this statement, alongside the manifesto he had outlined to E. B. Henderson just before graduating from Columbia ("In American surgery there are no Negro representatives. . . . This attitude I should like to help change") defined the philosophy that would guide him. He added a more earthy version, too: "We're going to turn out surgeons here who will not have to apologize to anyone, anywhere."[4]

In continuing the policy of expansion and modernization that Howes had instituted, early in his tenure Drew initiated residency programs in the surgical specialties of orthopedics and urology, appointing Julius Nviaser and R. Frank Jones to lead those respective divisions. Drew's old co-resident J. Richard Laurey also finished his GEB fellowship training at the University of Michigan in 1941 and returned to Howard. Laurey was newly certified by the American Board of Surgery, too, and brought with him the skills to establish a program in thoracic surgery. Drew expanded efforts in otolaryngology and the growing field of anesthesiology, bringing in nurse anesthetists to improve efficiency.[5] He also, naturally, instituted the university's first blood bank and expanded the laboratory facilities and functions.

The academic program expanded in other ways, too. Drew initiated an annual lecture, named after the department's first African American chairman, Austin M. Curtis, as a vehicle to host visiting professors from other institutions. In the years to come, some of the biggest names in American surgery became Curtis lecturers. To raise interest among the medical students in surgery—and to recruit the best of them into his own training program—Drew initiated an annual grand prize for the graduating student with the highest rank in the subject. The honor was accompanied by $100—no mean sum in the early 1940s. The prize was named for Jesse Greene, a New York surgeon friend of Drew's who donated the money.[6]

Adding personnel and improving or installing new services and infrastructure were tangible means of advancing the agenda of academic modernization and horizon-stretching, with the underlying goal of producing the finest African American surgeons possible. No less important to Drew was inculcating, together with these improvements, the sometimes-conflicting spirits of uncompromising excellence and human charity. Leadership by example was his primary mode of communicating such values to the students and residents. It came in the lecture hall, in the clinics, and, most memorably, in the ORs and wards.

One example was often related by one of Drew's residents, Jack White, to his own trainees:

> A patient came in that he thought had a blockage of the intestinal tract. We call it intestinal obstruction. They were waiting to get some x-rays. At that time, we would get what we call a flat and an erect film of the abdomen. The patient would be lying down, and we would have the patient sit up. We would get a flat film lying down and one erect, an erect of the abdomen. They were making the afternoon rounds. A patient came in some three or four hours before that. They were making rounds, and Dr. Drew said, "Well, what about the x-rays?" Someone said, "Well, we're waiting for them to come and get him to take him around to x-ray." The man was dirty, he had a hospital gown on, but unkempt and unshaven. Dr. Drew immediately picked him up in his arms, put him on the gurney, and rolled him around to the x-ray department. "The residents and students," Dr. White said, "were so dumbfounded, we didn't know what to do. Dr. Drew was rolling the patient around to x-ray. He got the x-ray. He never said a word, but the lesson he taught us that day was so powerful it can never be forgotten." In other words, you waited for them to come and get him, he is an ill patient, they don't come, you take him around yourself. "Well, we're waiting for transportation to come and get him." "*You* are transportation."[7]

At home, two years after their wedding, Charles and Lenore finally settled down to some semblance of typical married life, at least the sort that could be expected among the never-ending responsibilities of a chief surgeon. Even before leaving New York City, in March, Drew reflected on the long-delayed joys to come:

> Now we shall have a chance to see for the first time really, just what married life is like. Up til now we have been more like sweethearts with special privileges than man and wife. Do you think that you can take it? Having a man around the house in the way all of the time. No more sleeping in, meals to get on time, though the culprit may not always show up, visitors to entertain, telephones ringing at weird hours of the night, tales of my atrocities in the hospital to put up with etc. etc. I think perhaps there may be a few things that I may add to your happiness to make up for these disrupting influences in your life, for instance I can bring the baby

> carriage up the steps at night, I can wax the floors (if I think it will not hurt my hands) I can take you to the movies (when I'm not on call) and I can help you get the back room straight. Perhaps I can put in some flowers in the back yard. More important perhaps, I can share more closely with you the day by day movie of Bebe's growth and trials and when the long days are through I can lie close (that is relatively close) to you and hear the story of your heart as it adds new verses to the poem of your life it is writing with the gold of each night's sunset and the silver of the soft moon's glow. And I too will weave a story, in prose no doubt and in harsher hues but even it will have much of loveliness in it for its central theme will be you. As the years go by the poetry of your heart and the prose of my song should blend until there is no line between them and with the increasing voices of our choir a real symphony could be created into which all the trials, tribulations, joys and aspirations that are common to man would be found but in a pattern all our own and harmonious beyond compare.[8]

Drew's remark about lying "relatively close" to Lenore was an allusion to her second pregnancy. On July 31, 1941, another daughter arrived. They named her after her father: Charlene Rosella Drew.[9]

One day around this time, Eva Drew was summoned from her classes at Miner to her brother's office at Howard. She found him there in a state of pleasant excitement. He had a task for her: to take a check he had written for $700 to the Rosslyn bank. There she was to apply it to the ancient mortgage on the Arlington home, which had been re-upped seemingly countless times to pay for urgent expenses, mostly his own education. Now it was payback time, in the brightest sense. This $700 represented the balance owed, and Eva was to take the bank receipt marked "paid in full" to her mother as a surprise. Decades later, Eva summarized the reaction of the elder Nora and the entire family in a brief and smiling phrase, "Oh, happy day!"[10]

In April of 1943 Drew returned to Tuskegee for the annual John A. Andrew free clinic and symposium (the same gathering en route to which he had met Lenore in 1939). As a leader in African American medicine, Drew felt an obligation to attend, but there was also great value in the opportunity to teach and learn, and certainly to provide care to the indigent patients who came from all over that part of the country. He made the long trek to Alabama every year he could.

At this 1943 meeting he received the first E. S. Jones Prize for Meritorious Research in the Medical Sciences, which carried with it a $50 award, for his work in blood research.[11]

There is, perhaps, no field of human endeavor in which the old maxim that "experience is the best teacher" is more accurate than surgery. Certainly, few involve such high stakes as the deliberate infliction of trauma to the human body in an attempt to improve or restore health.

The clinical experience of trainees at Freedmen's Hospital in the years before Numa Adams's reforms had been lionized by the house staff members themselves in what W. Montague Cobb called "defensive delusions."[12] The idea was that the indisputable inadequacies of their preclinical curriculum and physical plant were balanced by the "extensive bedside experience of the clinical years."[13] In truth, the surgical patient population was probably similar to that of any comparably sized urban hospital in the country, both in terms of numbers and the spectrum of encountered pathologies.

Now, though, in this emerging new era he hoped to define, Drew realized that expansion in both those axes was essential to accomplish his goals. He had already begun to move the Department of Surgery into new specialty areas and expand the clinics, reaching previously untapped cohorts of patients whose needs would provide the substrate for the surgical trainees' clinical requirements. It took a few years for the results to show up on the Freedmen's ledgers; in the academic year from July 1, 1944, to June 30, 1945, these were the clinic attendance figures:

Surgical Clinics

Clinic	Individual Visits
Emergency	24322
Surgical Dressing Clinic	3284
Surgical Diagnostic and Follow up	1793
Orthopedic	1285
Fracture	1656
Plaster Room	1094
Physical Therapy	7037
Podiatry	634

Urology (Male)	2371
Urology (Female)	600
Proctology	264
Thoracic Surgery (Approx.)	125
Eye	2614
Ear	278
Nose	179
Throat	1181
Oral Surgery	526
Blood Bank Donor Clinic	1964[14]

All these clinic visits were certainly a cause for optimism for the future of the medical school, the hospital, and the Department of Surgery. For Drew himself, the number of blood bank donors to come to Freedmen's Hospital must have been especially gratifying, particularly considering the chaos and controversy that had swirled around the Red Cross Blood Donor Service after his departure in April 1941.

Just weeks after Drew left the fledgling program, the NRC, acting on behalf of the US Army and Navy, established the Subcommittee on Blood Substitutes as the supervisory group for their Red Cross–administered national blood plasma drive. Two months later, the new Blood Donor Service was formally established (Earl Taylor, the Columbia-trained general surgeon mentioned by Drew as a possible successor in his February 14, 1941, letter to Lenore quoted above, did, in fact, become technical director).[15] It was subsequent to this, on November 5, that the blood donor policy excluding Blacks—which stemmed from the requirements of the rigidly segregated armed forces rather than the Red Cross per se—became active.[16]

Not much fuss was raised at first, but just weeks later, the attack on Pearl Harbor changed everything. With the country suddenly thrust into the Second World War, patriotic citizens across the country lined up to donate blood at the Red Cross centers in support. Many of them were African Americans, who were shocked and horrified to learn that their sacrifice was not only not needed but not even welcomed.

In short order, the Black newspapers got ahold of the story and emblazoned it on headlines from coast to coast: "Red Cross Bans Negro Blood" read the banner of the *Cleveland Call and Post* on December 27, and others of this ilk appeared far and wide. The entire Black community was aroused, and protests, both grassroots and organized in churches and civic groups (including the NAACP) followed. The howl rose so loudly and rapidly that an immediate official reply was necessary. After a flurry of impromptu meetings, on January 21, 1942, a new directive went into effect, generated by the Red Cross and the surgeons general of the Army and Navy—even approved by Secretary of War Henry Stimson.[17] This fresh mandate stifled few of the angry voices, though. Yes, blood would be collected from both whites and Blacks henceforth, but any plasma that it yielded was to be segregated and only administered to wounded who were members of the same race. The reason given was the wishes of the servicemen, although, as in the same considerations during the Blood for Britain project (or the white patients at Columbia and McGill, for that matter) if this was in good faith it was entirely assumption: no one bothered to ask the people in question.

The government considered the matter settled and would not deviate from this policy for the duration of the war. This did not, of course, mean that the people affected were satisfied or would not continue to clamber for a more reasoned course of action.

Inevitably Drew, as an African American with the highest profile and most unassailable of credentials in blood transfusion science, was approached for his thoughts. In fact, Howard University essentially invited this, composing a four-page press release in February 1942 under the headline: NEGRO SURGEON, OUTSTANDING AUTHORITY ON BLOOD TRANSFUSIONS AND BLOOD BANKS, WAS PERSON SELECTED AS MEDICAL SUPERVISOR OF NEW YORK RED CROSS MOVEMENT FOR PROCURING BLOOD PLASMA FOR BRITAIN AND NATIONAL DEFENSE.[18] This release, which included a brief biography of Drew, explicitly noted the irony of his contributions in light of the plasma segregation policy.[19]

By nature, buttressed by many years of education and training, Drew handled problems of every sort with a thoughtful, analytical approach. When journalists came calling, he maintained a measured, authoritative manner and suppressed any emotions he may naturally have been harboring. There were plenty of others to tackle the role of firebrand; he was a scientist who dealt in facts alone. Drew was quoted at length in the September 26, 1942, edition of the *Chicago Defender*, an African American paper:

> Is there a difference between the blood of different races? Is it possible to transmit the traits and characteristics of one race to a member of another race by means of blood transfusion? Is it possible to implant by blood transfusion potentialities in an individual of one race that will show up in succeeding generations? . . . these are not humorous questions to some people. They are important not only for white people who fear that they or their offspring will get Negro characteristics but by good people who fear they may get the blood of bad people and thereby lose some of their virtue. Or by healthy people who may have the blood of less healthy people infused in their veins . . . but one can say without any hesitation that no difficulties have been shown to exist between the bloods of different races which would in any way contraindicate the use of the blood from an individual of one race for the purpose of transfusion to an individual of another race providing bloods were of the same group.

Drew went on to discuss the larger issue of racial bigotry in America, its irrational basis, and, in a variation of a phrase and philosophy for which he would become especially well known, his theory of how to vanquish it:

> Like all other social problems where prejudice between races is concerned great difficulties face anyone who attempts to analyze the problems away. There are many white people who simply do not like Negroes and their reason for not liking them is that their fathers did not like Negroes nor their fathers before them. They have been taught since infancy that Negroes are an inferior race. . . .
>
> Only extensive education, continued wise government and an increasing unceasing fight on our part to disseminate the scientific facts and raise our levels of achievement can overcome this prejudice which to a large extent is founded on ignorance.[20]

These remarks were wise, but they circumvented the source of the controversy. In another setting that year, Drew addressed the blood donor policy directly: "I feel that the recent ruling of the United States Army and Navy regarding the refusal of colored blood donors is an indefensible one from any point of view . . . there is no scientific basis for the separation of the bloods of different races except on the basis of the individual blood types or groups."[21]

Drew's circumspect approach to the plasma segregation controversy was perfectly characteristic of the professorial mien that he wore after emerging from the crucible of formal medical education—or even before. Others, including some long-term friends and colleagues, hoped for a more aggressive posture. Mercer Cook, a friend since Dunbar who was instrumental in Drew's introduction to Lenore, had this to say in later years, "The whole issue of blood segregation was a difficult thing. Emotions were high. . . . There were blacks with Drew on it and there were blacks opposed to him. Some felt he didn't raise enough hell."[22]

Whether he was inspired by the passion of others or moved by an ongoing exposure to the harsh realities of the inadequate resources for medical care—and, indeed, all aspects of everyday life—among his fellow African Americans, as time passed Drew did grow more vocal in his criticisms of the government's policy. As W. Montague Cobb remarked, "He was not wholly indifferent to his value as a public hero."[23]

On April 27, 1943, Drew gave a talk on radio station KSD in St. Louis titled "The Negro Physician in the Present War Effort."[24] Here he provided a detailed analysis of the numbers of soldiers under arms as well as physicians who were Black, both in and out of the service, pointing out the wholly inadequate number of the latter, especially after accounting for those who had enlisted. At the close, though, Drew's speech shifted from the cold calculus of facts and figures to assert the fundamental patriotism of the Black serviceman, calling to mind the famous words of Frederick Douglass regarding the decision to permit African Americans to fight in the Union Army during the Civil War: "Once let the black man get upon his person the brass letter, U.S., let him get an eagle on his button, and a musket on his shoulder and bullets in his pocket, there is no power on earth that can deny he has earned the right to citizenship."[25]

> What do Negro physicians now in the Armed Services and those about to join up feel about their enlistment? With hardly a dissenting voice they feel that the important thing for all Americans at this time, whether black or white, is to get on with the winning of the war. They know costs will run high. Some will die.
>
> As a teacher of many of the younger officers now serving, I know that all their loyalty will never waver. Each will give a good account of himself in spite of the fact that the vast majority of Negro physicians enter the military service bitterly

> opposed to the Army's policy of segregation, unified in their distaste and dissatisfaction with the Navy's policy of exclusion and deeply conscious of the fact that while they serve those who go forth to rid the world of terror in far places, emancipation is not yet complete at home. They fight the sincere fight of men who know disenfranchisement and who long for freedom for themselves and all mankind. Freedom from want, freedom from fear, freedom from constant humiliation, freedom to rise by merit according to ability and freedom from the tyranny of small minds in high places. The Negro physician in this time of war serves at home and abroad in the armed forces and out of it, with devotion, ever hopeful that by service in a common cause in these times of great trial for the nation, he may prove himself worthy of sharing more completely in the common life of the nation when peace shall have been restored.
>
> He has never asked for more—after the war he is certain not to accept less.[26]

While issues of national public policy were too pervasive to be ignored, Drew's first responsibility was to his position at Howard: teaching the students, training the residents, and providing the best care possible to the patients. Of these tasks, sculpting the trainees into competent surgeons was undoubtedly the most challenging, a special charge he embraced with vigor.

The procedures Drew and the rest of the Howard surgical faculty were obligated to impart to their residents had not changed meaningfully from those outlined in the 1939 *Atlas of Surgical Operations* cited above. One particularly difficult challenge was obtaining enough cases over a sufficiently broad clinical range to accomplish the greatest goal: surgical competence in a variety of settings, and sufficient experience not only to engender confidence in the graduating surgeon but the opportunity to sit for the American Board of Surgery exam.

The volume of general surgical cases at Freedmen's Hospital in the academic year from July 1, 1944, to June 30, 1945, was reported as follows: appendicitis—166 cases, of which 15 were reported as "complex;" hernia—116, 94 inguinal, 14 umbilical, 1 femoral, 4 incisional (which could be interpreted as indicative of good closure technique) and 3 designated "other;" rectal—138, mostly hemorrhoids or fistulas; intestinal obstruction—36; thyroid—15; gall bladder—12, an oddly small number; infections—154, fairly evenly spread anatomically; benign neoplasms—35; malignant neoplasms—72, 17 gastric, 13 colon, 13 breast, the rest "other;" peptic ulcer—23, peripheral vascular disease—66,

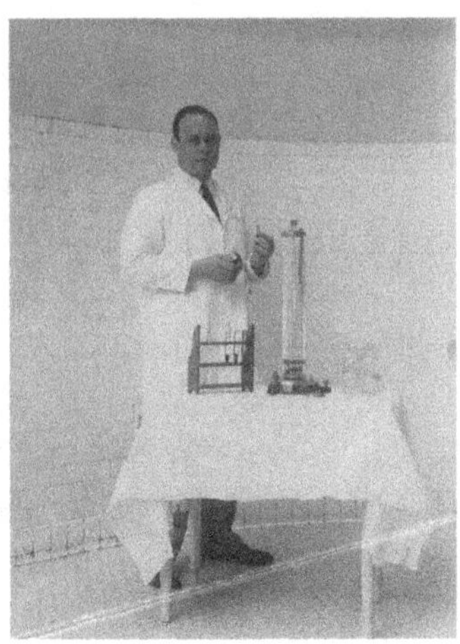

Figure 9.2 Drew posing with laboratory apparatus. Personal collection, Charlene Drew Jarvis.

diabetes—19, mostly gangrene cases treated presumably with amputation; varicose veins—27; skin lesions—104, these included burns and lacerations; other unreported trauma—81, mostly head injuries; and miscellaneous operative cases—140. With some overlap, the grand total was 1158 general surgical operations.[27]

This would not have been sufficient volume or variety to satisfy Drew that his men were getting exposure to enough cases, but the trend was positive. As the services grew, he filled in the gaps by continuing to provide the best example he could for "his boys."

Samuel Bullock, a fellow faculty member in the department and friend since the Dunbar High School years, later recalled, "That man was a perfectionist from the first day that I met him. . . . He thrived on doing things—and having others do them—that he could take pride in."[28]

"It's a delicate craft, an art." Drew said of his profession. "Each case marks the beginning or end of a life drama."[29]

Jack White, a surgery resident, remembered that "the precision and orderliness of his surgical technique matched elegantly his superbness as an athlete. His surgical talent was especially well seen in emergency situations, on which occasions his skill and judgment were matchless . . . His intuition and his instincts were so keen that he was said to have, above the head of his bed, a red light that went on the moment any of us, working under him at the hospital, made an erring step."[30]

Drew's temper, in something of a departure for leading academic surgeons of his era, had a long fuse. When one reached the end of it, though, there was usually hell to pay. The warning of an impending onslaught was evident to all, as his "buttermilk" face turned scarlet: "Suddenly you would know that he was angry about something," recalled one trainee. "Really angry, I mean. It didn't happen all the time but brother, when it did, there was just no hiding it. His eyes would flash. And he would flush beet-red. And you would know that he had had it."[31]

Like his father, Drew had an auburn tinge to his hair that became more distinct as he grew older. Between this and the crimson flush he displayed when angered, the nickname he earned after joining the Howard faculty, "Big Red," was no surprise.

"He was a strapping fellow—over six feet tall—and when he gave you that look it could curl your toes," a resident noted, recalling an embarrassing episode of mischief. "A group of us guys used to play a little poker. Oh, stakes were never high. But Drew had established this iron-clad rule: no gambling among interns. Well, along he comes in the midst of a game and the guys just panicked. Cards were hurriedly stuffed into desk drawers. All the money disappeared. Everything's fine except for one damned poker chip, which rolled down the aisle, finally stopping at his feet. He just stood there and stared."[32]

Lenore, who described her husband as "slow to anger but mighty in wrath," remembered an example in which he returned home from the hospital in a state of anger and wordlessly rifled through the kitchen sink closet, then announced that a law should exist making it a crime to store dangerous chemicals in ordinary containers. He had been involved that day in a case in which a toddler drank bleach that had been placed in a Coke bottle with fatal results. "What things made him angry?" she later wrote "Stupidity, meanness, pettiness, ugliness, criminal negligence (as in the case of the bleach bottle causing death)."[33]

Drew insisted on impeccable dress from his team, whether on the wards or in clinic—a standard to which he, of course, adhered (Lenore later remembered that he was "a plain but immaculate dresser," who owned just two suits but kept them spotless). One day on rounds, a medical student appeared in a particularly unkempt state. Drew chastised him for it: a physician's appearance was not only a reflection of their professionalism but a sign of respect for the patient and other caregivers. The student defended himself: he did not have enough time, was too busy with the work, and so on, to which Drew replied, "Well, *I'll* wash your clothes, *I'll* darn your socks, *I'll* clean your shoes."[34] Clearly, if the chief of surgery, far busier than anyone else on the team, could prioritize his appearance, so could they. That particular student's dress and demeanor were never an issue again, but the example demonstrated another aspect of Drew's perfectionism—one he applied to himself no less than others. "He was also angry with himself when he, too, came up short," said Lenore. "He was his own rigid taskmaster."[35]

In his wife's eyes, in later recollections at any rate, Drew was "a simple and uncomplicated person" who "didn't care much for complicated people." He enjoyed Western movies, but his favorite hobby was gardening: "The first thing he would do when he came home was go out and look at the flowers." Above all else, though, was an innate impulse to teach: "It was an education just to live with him . . . even when he would sit down with the children, he wanted them in possession of something when he got through with them."[36]

In June 1943 Drew was appointed a member of the American-Soviet Medical Society, an organization founded early that same year during the historically brief interlude when the United States and Union of Soviet Socialist Republics were allies.* Drew's membership was a natural outgrowth of his investigations into the origins of blood preservation technology, some of which had impressive (if somewhat dubious) origin in the Soviet Union, during his thesis research at Columbia. He wrote an article summarizing this information, entitled "The Role of Soviet Investigators in the Development of the Blood Bank," which appeared in the April 1944 issue of the organization's periodical, *American Review of Soviet Medicine.*

The Drews' third child—also a daughter, whom they named Rhea Sylvia, for the mother of Romulus and Remus, the legendary founders of Rome—was born on February 15, 1944. Around this time, the family moved from the apartment on Sherman Avenue to a university-owned house at 328 College Avenue NW. This three-story "comfortable old, big" home was much closer to the Howard campus and Freedmen's Hospital.[37]

Although his plate was more than full with his duties leading the Howard Department of Surgery—so much so, in fact, that against his wishes it turned out to be impractical for him to conduct any kind of basic science research of the sort that had propelled his career to great heights—other responsibilities

* This association kept a library of Soviet medical and science journals, and even motion pictures, in its New York offices. The famed McGill neurosurgeon Wilder Penfield and University of Pennsylvania surgical doyen I. S. Ravdin were members. The organization only lasted a few years, however, as membership dropped precipitously with the advent of the Cold War.

came to Drew as a matter of course. In January 1944 he was appointed chief of staff at Freedmen's Hospital, a position he held for two years, at which time he became, for another year, medical director. These were largely thankless administrative spots with unrelenting paperwork, minimal remuneration, and ill-defined authority, on top of which they conjured distressingly frequent opportunities to cause offense. Drew told his old friend W. Montague Cobb that "although the jobs did not particularly appeal to him, he might as well take them for a spell to fill out the record."[38] But Cobb also noted that "sometimes his intensity was such that in conference he could lose objectivity. And there were occasions when from too great an emphasis on the Department of Surgery . . . enthusiasm would make him fail to keep in perspective the contributory efforts of others . . . working toward the same goals in the broad field of medicine."[39] And another colleague wrote, "Charles R. Drew was a human being and as such had his faults. There were many who at times violently disagreed with him and temporarily were angered by him."[40]

In the years to come Drew would serve in leadership positions across a host of organizations, local and otherwise. He was a member of the Board of Trustees of the National Society for Crippled Children; the Board of Trustees of the District of Columbia Branch of the National Poliomyelitis Foundation; the Board of Directors of the District of Columbia Chapter of the American Cancer Society and the Deans' Committee of the Tuskegee Veterans Administration Hospital. Not least, Drew also served on the Executive Board of the Twelfth Street Branch of the YMCA, where he had first dominated swim races decades before.[41]

Perhaps the crowning achievement of these years, and even of Drew's life and career *in toto*, came in the summer of 1944. At a huge ceremony in Chicago, he was awarded the Spingarn Medal of the NAACP.

In 1914 J. E. Spingarn, then chair of the Board of Directors of the NAACP, established an annual award "for highest achievement of an American Negro."[42] In addition to the distinction, the recipient would receive a gold medal emblazoned with the figure of Lady Justice, sword and scales in hand alongside the words "For Merit." In the three decades since its inception, a "who's who" of African Americans of all walks of life—educators, writers, social activists, scientists—had won the award, among them W. E. B. DuBois, George Washington Carver, and Marian Anderson, the singer Drew had seen perform at the Lincoln Memorial in 1939. Two individuals personally familiar to Drew had already won the award, as well: Mordecai Johnson, the president of Howard University, and his old Dunbar and Amherst classmate, William H. Hastie, who was by now a noted jurist. Drew was notified that he had won in March 1944. The medal award ceremony was scheduled for July, during the four-day national NAACP conference in the Windy City.

On the morning of June 6, 1944, the momentous news of D-Day reached the country, and Americans from coast to coast were electrified by the reports. After listening to President Roosevelt's prayerful address to the nation an agitated Drew, unable to remain in the house amid the excitement, gathered the family—including little Sylvia, only four months old—and poured them into the Ford for a drive without specific destination: "We got in line and moved slowly through town down 14th Street," remembered Lenore. "Bells rang, whistles whistled, 'crankers' cranked. People yelled out of their car windows."[43]

As the date of the Spingarn Medal ceremony neared it came time to make travel arrangements. Drew decided to take the train to Chicago. He invited his mother, Lenore, and his kid sister Eva, who at twenty-three had never ridden in an "overnight" train before.[44]

The actual event was a gala affair on Sunday, July 16, 1944, a "mass meeting" in the open air at Washington Park lagoon on Chicago's South Side. The 2:30 P.M. festivities were preceded by a parade of civilian and military organizations that was led by the commander of the 8th Infantry, Illinois Reserve Militia. After this, the attendees sang the Star-Spangled Banner and "Lift Ev'ry Voice and Sing," then the NAACP Chorus followed with spirituals and Handel's "Hallelujah," which must have seemed a tough act to follow. After a speech by the publisher and department store magnate Marshall Field, Drew was introduced as the 29th Spingarn Medal winner (technically this was the 1943 award).[45]

Drew's speech at this ceremony touched on several points, but the central themes were the roles of blood and race in American culture in the context of

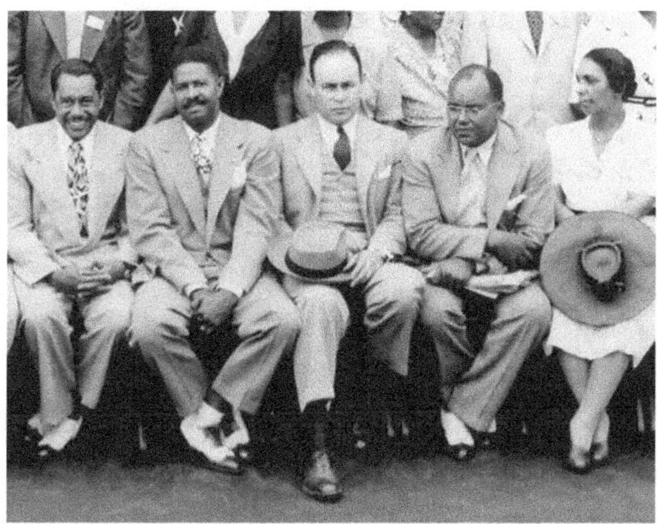

Figure 9.3 Drew in Chicago for the NAACP conference and Spingarn Medal award ceremony, June, 1944. Personal collection, Charlene Drew Jarvis.

the Second World War. After recounting some of the "bitter" correspondence he had received, including (as he mentioned in the *Chicago Defender* interview in 1942) inquiries into "whether it is possible to transmit characteristics of race by blood transfusions to another race," Drew pulled no punches in describing the unscientific thinking behind both the original decision to turn away Black blood donors and the subsequent one to segregate the acquired plasma. He also reflected on the entirely avoidable, dreadful consequences for the morale of African Americans:

> It is fundamentally wrong for any great nation to willfully discriminate against such a large group of its people. To the everlasting credit of the NAACP and many individuals, this first order (the Red Cross decision to exclude black blood donors) was fought bitterly. It finally was rescinded so that any citizen can give his blood if he so desires.
>
> Then came the next step. It is with something of sorrow today that I cannot give any hope that the separation of the blood will be discontinued . . . the same men who fight for this particular bit of discrimination are the gentleman who fight

all liberal policies. I recently was the subject for discussion by Bilbo in the senate for daring to say that all blood is alike.*

It is the unwillingness of the men now in charge of this program that they will not act to break up the segregation of the blood. One can say quite truthfully that on the battlefields nobody is very interested in where the plasma comes from when they are hurt. They get the first bottle they get their hands on.

The blood is being sent from all parts of the world. Is it is unfortunate that such a worthwhile and scientific bit of work should have been hampered by such stupidity.

The Spingarn Medal presentation has caused me to answer hundreds of people all over the world, asking about differences in race, color and blood. Many answers I do not know but I feel duty bound under such honors to become more aware of the great needs we have in all fields of activity when leadership is forced upon one in a manner quite comparable to this. As a task it has many good points and many which are trying. I am sure that people like Mr. Walter White are extraordinary.** I think that is why the NAACP is so important, because they have given leadership and I pledge you that in the future as I have tried in less degree in the past, I shall try to be worthy of this great honor. A great mass of people have been hurt sorely and unnecessarily by a form of discrimination which should never have come about. It is imperative therefore that we meet this new form and smash it as we must smash all the others.[46]

The Spingarn Medal speech was a departure for Drew, albeit one that had been brewing for some time. His manner—cool, unflappable, cerebral—never changed; that was his nature and it could not be altered. But a new passion had arisen in him and, along with it, a conviction to lead, visibly and vocally, sometimes in arenas far removed from academic medicine (he gave a similar speech the next month at a CIO labor rally in Washington). Drew believed that the reason he had received *this* honor from *this* organization at *this* time was a

*Theodore G. Bilbo was a US senator and dedicated segregationist from Mississippi. He quoted Drew on the equality of blood in transfusion during an attempt to halt legislation for the funding of Howard University.

**White was the long-time leader of the NAACP and a major figure in the Civil Rights Movement of the first half of the twentieth century.

righteous anger on the part of Black America toward the stinging injustice of the Red Cross program and their view that he, an African American scientist whose work contributed immensely to the program's realization, was the ideal knight to slay, or at least skewer, this dragon.

When Drew followed through on this unspoken accolade, he defined his public persona to those otherwise unfamiliar with him, for long beyond the end of his life.

10

This High-Walled Prison

Washington, 1946–50

When Drew delivered his inspiring speech at the presentation of the Spingarn Medal in July 1944, the invasion of Europe that began at the Normandy beaches on D-Day was already into its seventh week. There were many battles yet to be fought, lives to be lost, and units of plasma to be given, but the outcome of the conflict was inevitable and soon the war would be winding down.

It was certainly true that when World War II did conclude a year later the growing Civil Rights Movement in America had, from a practical perspective, barely begun, but the rallying cry about segregated blood was over (in fact, the Red Cross quietly stopped the practice in the peaceful days of 1948).

Charles Drew's role as a leader in the larger struggle would shift from protagonist against the injustice of a bigoted blood policy to advocate for racial equality in health care. This was a fight with many strategic fronts, and Drew developed a four-pronged plan, which he elucidated in a letter to one of his recently graduated residents, Asa Yancey, in 1947:

1. *Training of more undergraduate medical students*
2. *Training of more interns and residents*
3. *Better care for Negro patients and the right for Negro patients to be treated by their own physicians.*

4. *More opportunities for Negro physicians who are adequately trained to take part in the larger medical life of the community.*[1]

For Drew, as a surgeon and teacher of surgeons, the most effective means to the desired end was—and always would be—the education of ever more outstanding Black surgeons.

The question was how to accomplish this since the territory was uncharted. His education and experiences gave some clues, but the nature of the professional terrain Drew would have to negotiate for himself and his trainees in this setting was drastically different from anything he had encountered at McGill or Columbia. There would be political battles to fight in his own backyard at Howard as well as obstacles of racial bigotry and segregation not only in Washington, DC, but in medical training centers across the nation, and even in the professional associations that largely ran organized American medicine. He had no illusions about the difficulty of the task.

At many university medical centers, students and postgraduate trainees "rotate" at local institutions not directly affiliated with the home hospital in order to have a broader clinical experience than might otherwise be available. Surgery students in a suburban academic setting may spend time in an urban hospital to learn more about trauma, for example, or those in a rigidly scholastic facility may be afforded the opportunity to experience a private practice setting. At Howard University, though, such local opportunities did not exist.

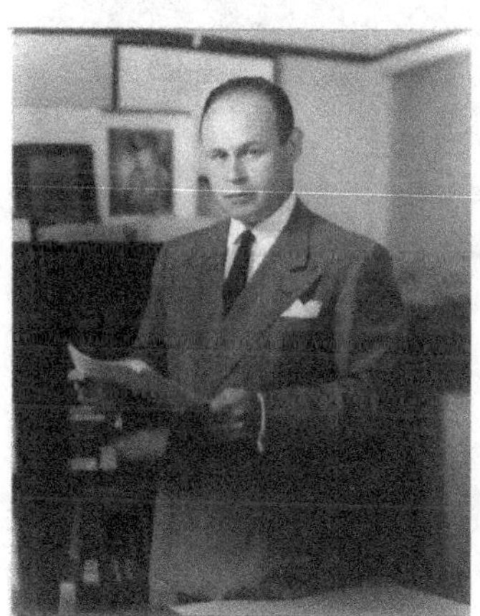

Figure 10.1 Charles Drew, Professor and Chair of Surgery at Howard University. Personal collection, Charlene Drew Jarvis.

Washington, DC, in the mid twentieth century retained many of the Southern characteristics that had defined the city since its founding. Sadly, strict segregation was among these: Jim Crow was alive and well in the nation's capital in the postwar years. Thus, even though there were a dozen other hospitals in the area, only Freedmen's was dedicated to caring for Blacks (three excluded African

Americans entirely). Segregation did not only apply to patients; African American doctors were denied privileges at the predominantly white hospitals, too. While a certain amount of wagon-circling pride developed in the Black community for "their" Freedmen's, the negative factors far outweighed any community loyalty.

Drew's trainees, and all the other Howard medical students, interns, and residents, were severely restricted in their clinical experiences, being confined, as they were, to a solitary facility which, with only about four hundred beds, was not on a par in terms of capacity with other urban general hospitals in the nation (for an extreme example, New Orleans' Charity Hospital, in a city with 5/8 the population of Washington, had over two thousand beds[2]). There were other inherent problems at Freedmen's, too. Although it was federally funded and thus in little danger of frankly failing, the nature of the financial support was so unpredictable (it depended on annual appropriations that waxed and waned according to the capricious whims of Congress) that administrators were paralyzed regarding capital expenses for expansion, improvements, or even

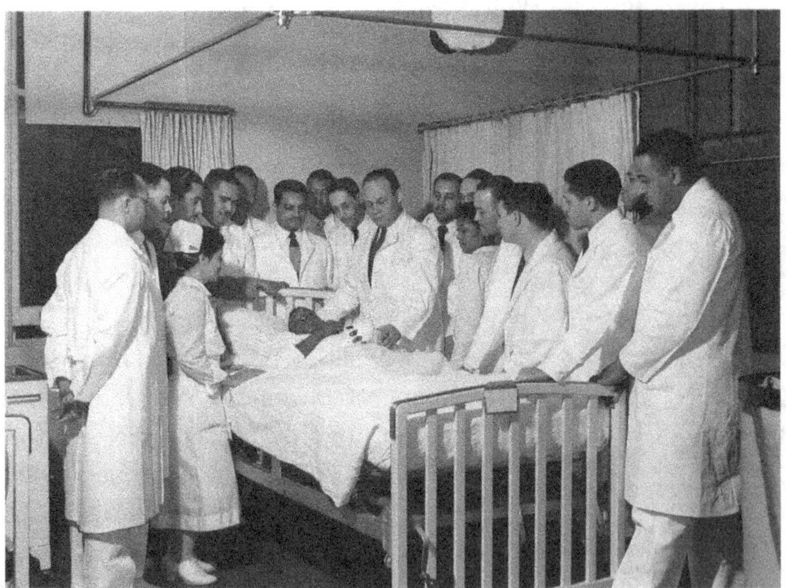

Figure 10.2 Drew teaching at the bedside. Personal collection, Charlene Drew Jarvis.

maintenance. As noted above, the single building dated to 1862 and was not only severely outdated but in dire disrepair, with crumbling open wards laid out in the Civil War–era pavilion design.

Faced with these realities, Drew endeavored to arrange opportunities for his men at the other area hospitals, an uphill battle with many forces arrayed in opposition. The most promising possibility was Gallinger Municipal Hospital, a large city-funded facility originally built in the 1920s to care for the indigent. A high percentage of inpatients at Gallinger were Black, which meant that, unlike the private facilities, resistance to African American doctors promised to be less deeply rooted, certainly among the clientele. The faculties of the medical schools of George Washington and Georgetown Universities provided the lion's share of the staff at Gallinger. Drew, following up on some progress that had already been made by the Howard administration in regard to placing the school's students and graduates, engaged his counterparts in the departments of surgery at Georgetown, Robert J. Coffey, and George Washington, Brian Blades. Letters to these two men were nearly identical:

> Our Administration, as you might know, has been anxious to extend our teaching opportunities and our local medical society has for years carried on a fight designed to eventually create openings for our fellows on the staff at Gallinger Hospital. When the proposition was placed before us in Surgery, we thought that our staff did not have the depth or strength to take on any new undertakings. We have been attempting to strengthen it and give it more depth. At the same time, several of our students were appointed on the staff as interns. I have had no unfavorable reports of their activities in the hospital, so I take this to mean that their work has been at least satisfactory and their presence has caused no unusual problems.
>
> The next area, it seems to me, which needs to be explored is that in which a group of assistant residents might he tried out—one under the supervision of the George Washington Staff and one under supervision of Georgetown. It would give us and you, I believe, an opportunity to observe whatever problems would arise with men at this level. I do not think that we can much longer dodge the responsibility of assisting in the care of the indigents at Gallinger since, as I understand it, nearly ninety per cent (90%) of the patients are Negroes; nor will the powers that be, be free from criticism as long as there are no Negro staff members.[3]

Both Blades and Coffey sent replies that were reservedly supportive. Coffey's indicated that Drew's effort had been ongoing:

> I read with a great deal of interest your comments about the set-up at Gallinger and, as I told you a year or two ago, I will support in every way your participation when you feel sufficiently manned in your department to handle it. If you would like to start out with one man, that will meet with my complete satisfaction. However, I would like to sit down and talk with you about it sometime at some length. Will you call me at some convenient time and we will arrange a meeting.[4]

If it was difficult to find positions for Howard graduates within the university's home city, the prospects further afield were even less promising. In effect, this was the same problem Drew had faced when he completed his time at McGill: residency and fellowship positions were simply not offered to Blacks (the exceptions for Howard's talented surgical trio of Drew, Laurey, and Manly from the previous decade had been due to General Education Board funding). Drew's strategy for his men, the same approach he had articulated in his 1942 *Chicago Defender* interview at the height of the blood segregation controversy, was to raise their levels of achievement to overcome the prejudice born of ignorance. But there was the catch: How could they prove their worth if they could not even get in the door?

One means of changing the minds of residency program directors, Drew recognized, was to bring Black surgeons into the mainstream—that is, into the national organizations that, in many ways, ran American medicine. These groups—the American Medical Association and the American College of Surgeons, to name two of the most important, especially in Drew's eyes—combined scholarly machinations with a heavy dose of socializing. It was in the "smoke-filled rooms" of the AMA, ACS, and other organizations that deals were done and careers were made. If Black surgeons could find entrée here, acceptance throughout the system was inevitable: fear of the unknown would be defeated by making the mysterious commonplace and the threatening familiar. In addition, the knowledge, and—to use a term from a later era—networking that might be acquired by members of the Black medical community would be invaluable.

It was probably for these very reasons, in addition to garden variety bigotry, that Drew and other African American physicians encountered steadfast resistance in attempting to join the associations.

The AMA traced its origins to 1847, when a determined cadre of well-meaning physicians banded together to raise the profession's poor educational and licensing standards, in a burst of ambitious idealism akin to that which drove the Flexner report many years later. After the Civil War the issue of admitting Black physicians to the association, then still relatively small and not the policy-influencing behemoth it would become in the twentieth century, inevitably arose. After some political maneuvering, the AMA absolved itself of responsibility for the issue in the 1870s by falling back on its status as a federation of constituent organizations. The national association per se would take no action; any decisions about admitting African Americans was left to the state and county medical associations that comprised it. If Blacks were admitted to the local groups, then they were allowed in the AMA. This was, of course, a de facto exclusion of African American physicians in the South from joining. In frustrated response, in 1895 African American physicians founded their own organization, the National Medical Association (NMA).[5]

In 1939, some six decades after the national governance of the AMA relinquished responsibility on the race question, a resolution was raised to abolish any denial of membership on the basis of "race, color, or creed," but it was defeated on the basis of interfering in local societies' "right of selection of (their) own members" (never mind that the AMA had interfered in issues of local constituent politics on other occasions).[6]

So it was that Drew faced a major challenge in attempting to get his trainees, and other Black physicians in the South, including the District of Columbia (where the local medical association refused to admit them), into the AMA. The import of this was not purely academic—in many hospitals throughout the country, membership in the AMA was a prerequisite for admitting privileges, and thus Black physicians were at a major disadvantage, economically and otherwise, if they could not join.[7] This gave the lie to the oft-cited trope at the time that there was no need for Blacks to join the AMA since they had their own group, a variation on the derelict "separate but equal" premise.

In early January 1947, ostensibly stirred by a historical article in the *Journal of the American Medical Association*, Drew fired a salvo directly at the head of the target: the editor, Morris Fishbein:

> January 13, 1947
>
> Dear Sir:
>
> In the January 11, 1947 Journal on page 101 under the general title, "History of the American Medical Association," there is a chapter, "Admission of Negro Delegates," which is worthy of comment.
>
> The material of this chapter is taken from the minutes of the Twenty-First Annual Session of the American Medical Association held in Washington, DC in 1870.
>
> The essence of the chapter is that by a vote of 115 to 90 men from the Department of Medicine of Howard University and Freedmen's Hospital were barred from membership.
>
> Today, seventy-seven years later, this ruling still stands. I shall not argue the case for admission as it stood in 1870, but I do feel that this age-long policy of discrimination under what guise or pretext is one of the dark pages in the history of an organization which otherwise has many bright ones.
>
> In 1870 Howard University was but three years old. Its professors, to a large degree, were large-souled physicians of the northern army who, while administering to the sick who came under their care through the Freedmen's Bureau, gave their time, often at great personal sacrifice and with rare devotion, in helping men who were but recently slaves to learn to assist the sick and afflicted of their race. Rejected by the District Medical Society, they helped form the National Medical Society so that there would be some medium for expression of their common problems and aims. Your pages now recite the story of their rejection by the American Medical Association.
>
> The men in Washington, the nation's capital, are still rejected although there can be no doubt of their qualifications by any standards, and so likewise are all of the Negro physicians who happen to live in the South.[8]

The preamble over, a passionate Drew then leveled volley after withering volley of fact to support the admission of African Americans to the AMA, revealing the gross injustice that it had not yet come to pass:

At Howard University for many years no physician has been considered for a position of professorial or associate professor rank in the preclinical area who has not earned a Ph. D. in his special field. In Freedmen's Hospital, the teaching hospital for the clinical years, a man must have successfully passed his specialty board to be considered for the position of assistant professor. The chief of every department and subdivision in the departments is a certified specialist in name and practice. Match these standards with those of the great hospitals of the land and they will be found good, but it will not grant them the privilege of discussing common problems with fellow physicians in the learned councils of the American Medical Association and celebrating its one hundredth birthday. One hundred years of racial bigotry and fatuous pretense; one hundred years of gross disinterest in a large section of the American people whose medical voice it purports to be—as regards the problem of Negroes which it raised in 1870; one hundred years of no progress to report. A sorry record.

The American Specialty Boards accept a man on the basis of merit; the American College of Surgeons has recently erased the infamous policy of discrimination and has made a man's ethical and surgical standards the sole measuring rod. The International Colleges open their doors to men of like training and interests regardless of race or nationality; but not the great American Medical Association.[9] If a small minority of county or state chapters persist in wagging the whole body, and the body as a whole makes no move to direct its own destiny, then it must be considered a body without true strength and purpose or one which likes the way it is going. The American Medical Association should not start its second century with unfinished business of this kind making mockery of its continuous protestations of leadership in medicine under the great and free American way of life.[10]

In his reply, dated January 22, 1947, Fishbein toed the ancient, if barely defensible, point-of-order company line:

Dear Doctor Drew: I have read with great interest your letter of January 13. . . . I will refer your letter to Dr. George F. Lull, Secretary of the American Medical

Association, so that it may be brought officially to the attention of the Board of Trustees. You realize, of course, that Negro physicians may now attain membership in the American Medical Association but that, according to our by-laws, it is necessary that membership be secured through entrance into a county medical society. It has always been the province of every county medical society to determine its own membership. There is no other way in which membership in the American Medical Association can be secured by anyone. Many Negro physicians are now members. As you are of course aware, representations have appeared before the House of Delegates of the American Medical Association. If a state medical society were to elect a Negro delegate, I am quite sure he would be received in the House of Delegates.[11]

Nothing in Fishbein's response was new to Charles Drew, of course, and his patience with the "that's the way it has always been" argument, or its "we can't control the local chapters" corollary had been worn to the breaking point:

January 30, 1947

Dear Dr. Fishbein:

You know and I know that it is utterly impossible for a Negro physician to become a member of a county medical society in the South. The American Medical Association has stood behind the bylaws which make this so as though God himself had written the bylaws and that they were immutable through the ages. These bylaws can and, I think, should be changed.

As I pointed out in my previous letter, the basic laws of the American College of Surgeons, the International College of Surgeons, and all of the specialty boards have been changed to allow the admission of qualified Negro physicians without reference to the place in which they practice.

I believe it would be a very simple thing, even with our segregated set-up, for the Board of Trustees of the American Medical Association to initiate changes which would grant membership to qualified men in the American Medical Association without going through county societies. Your letter is a most unrealistic document. The American Medical Association is made up of many men who honestly believe that they are members of a truly representative group of American physicians. They, I believe, would be surprised to know that a large segment of the physicians of this country who need, perhaps more than any other segment, the continuing contacts, the continuous postgraduate development, and the continuous stimulation of attendance at meetings where the learned men of the country discuss common problems, are denied such privileges on the basis of race alone.

I know that in the past it has been suggested to the American Medical Association that in those territories where Negroes are not eligible for membership in the county societies that their ethical and moral qualities be vouched for by the various state Negro societies. I have had the pleasure of taking part in the annual meetings of such societies in Maryland, Virginia, West Virginia, North and South Carolina, Alabama, Georgia, Mississippi, and Louisiana. They are all well organized. Several of these groups have had annual meetings in which as high as 94% of their total membership has taken part. They are a real and vital part of American medicine and should no longer have to explain on every application blank why they are not eligible for membership in the AMA. It is an unwarranted stigma. It is a cause of repeated humiliation. It is a constant indictment of the principles on which the American Medical Association is supposedly founded.

You know the answer, and I know the answer. I cannot understand why something is not done about it. If there are suggestions which you can make out of your greater intimacy with the problem I should appreciate hearing about them. We would be able, I am sure, to rally the Negro physicians of the country around any program which would promise emancipation. I think you could help this situation. I wish very sincerely that you would decide to do so.[12]

A clearly flustered Fishbein had no recourse at this juncture except to punt. He passed the buck to the association's secretary:

February 3, 1947

Dear Dr. Drew:

I have read with great interest your letter of January 30.

The question that you raise is quite outside my purview. I am, however, referring your letter to Dr. George F. Lull, Secretary of the Association, so that he may bring it to the attention of the Board of Trustees at their next meeting here in Chicago.[13]

Drew had already anticipated this and collected the correspondence between himself and Fishbein for forwarding to Lull:

> January 31, 1947
>
> Dear Dr. Lull:
>
> The enclosed copies of letters to Dr. Fishbein are self-explanatory. For years all such communications have stopped at the level of the Secretary of the American Medical Association. I hope that you will see fit to allow the matter to be brought before the House of Delegates, for I believe they as a group will feel that the present position as regards Negro physicians is an unjustifiable one.[14]

Lull's reply had nothing more to offer than Fishbein's, except to add that even if the rank-and-file of the association's national membership voted for a policy to end exclusion based on race the local chapters could simply ignore it:

> February 5, 1947
>
> Dear Doctor Drew:
>
> I received your letter of January 31, together with copies of the letters sent to Doctor Fishbein. The only way that this matter can be brought up in the House of Delegates is for a delegate to introduce it. I realize that this question is a troublesome one and I do not have the answer. It is entirely controlled by county and state associations. As you know the American Medical Association cannot dictate any policies to such organizations as we are organized as a federacy of constituent associations, so that even if a resolution was passed by the House of Delegates the state and local societies could still refuse to comply with it. It will have to be decided at each county and state level.[15]

As far as the American Medical Association was concerned, that was that. Charles Drew—or anyone else for that matter—might as well rage against a thunderstorm; in 1947 there was no power on Earth that would force the organization to change.[16]

The matter of the American College of Surgeons was different. As Drew had mentioned in his initial letter to Fishbein, that group had recently ceased refusing access to Blacks (in 1945). The history of discrimination in this, the largest and most powerful surgeons' organization in North America, was even more bizarre than that of the AMA. In fact, one of the founders of the ACS in 1913, Daniel Hale Williams of Chicago, was an African American surgeon.[17] After Williams, though, no Blacks were admitted until 1934, and then only one, Louis T. Wright of Harlem. Wright's admission was not without contention, though, and over the next years, entrenched, mostly Southern elements of the College fought against any further integration, using the same sort of quasi-legal legerdemain the AMA had employed, including deferment to local chapters and similar gambits. The tide of public as well as private sentiment was turning, however, and when some two hundred senior fellows of the College were directly asked the question in June 1945, a large majority favored admitting qualified African Americans.[18] The College's board of regents subsequently removed all official impediments to the admission of Blacks. That fall, four joined the organization.

Drew had not remained silent on this issue. Since his return to Howard as chief of surgery, he had waged a sometimes-rancorous campaign for the admission of Black surgeons to the college. He evidently applied for fellowship himself sometime around 1945, possibly before the exclusionary policy was rescinded, only to be rejected. Since he had two medical degrees from prestigious institutions, was the chair of an academic surgery department, and not just a diplomate of the American Board of Surgery but an examiner, this rejection rankled Drew beyond nearly all others. The ACS was not merely an organization of physicians of all stripes, as the AMA was, but an association of surgeons—his peers.

In the late summer of 1945 Drew sent a letter to John Scudder who had, as a surgeon and fellow of the college, written in support of Drew's candidacy. While thanking his old mentor for the help, Drew mentioned that he had approached the organization's leadership about being a kind of "test case" on admitting Blacks. He then touched on what he perceived to be the many failings of the college, which extended beyond obvious prejudice. The criticisms clearly reflect the knowledge that his own accomplishments far eclipsed those of accepted fellows who happened not to share his skin color:

> September 10, 1945
>
> Dear John:
>
> I got your note concerning the American College. Many thanks for your letter of recommendation. . . . Last year in a conference with Dr. Coller, Chairman of the recently revamped Committee on Admissions, I offered my services as a guinea pig when and if a test of the College was to be made.
>
> My first complaint against the College, of course, is, and has been, its bigotry; but probably a larger complaint would be that its admission requirements are too ill-defined and its standards too low for any institution which pretends to be representative of the best of American surgery. My contact with both the Canadians and the British has made it manifestly clear that they consider the American College of Surgeons to some degree a social organization whose scholastic and professional requirements, therefore, are purely secondary.
>
> In my discussions with Dr. Coller I suggested that there should be some sort of examination; as a matter of fact, my own feeling is that the American College would enhance its own status by accepting only candidates who have successfully passed Specialty Certifying Boards in Surgery and then have practiced that specialty with distinction, or at least satisfactorily, for a period of from three to five years.
>
> There are . . . dozens of very capable, well-trained Negro surgeons who can easily meet all requirements and who would be an honor to any organization. I hope that they will apply and are accepted.[19]

Five years later, the sting of rejection eased by much water under the bridge, Drew again applied. By this time more than thirty Black surgeons had become fellows of the college, and Frederick Coller of the University of Michigan, the chair of the ACS Admissions Committee mentioned by Drew, had been a visiting professor at Howard, where he gave the 1947 Austin Curtis lecture. Among those Drew approached for letters of recommendation were the other local surgery department chairmen Brian Blades of George Washington University and Robert Coffey of Georgetown, both of whom expressed enthusiastic support:

January 18, 1950

Dear Dr. Coffey

I am applying for Fellowship in the American College of Surgeons. I should like the privilege of using your name as one of the surgeons in my area who could vouch for my present surgical activities. I do not know the present attitude of the local Board of Regents. For five years before the acceptance of a Negro surgeon in 1945, I had waged a rather bitter battle with the American College of Surgeons, concerning the exclusion of qualified Negroes. I have purposefully waited for a period of time before making a personal application in this area, principally because I felt a little time was needed for some of the bitterness of our earlier discussions to have died down. I do not believe that there will be difficulty at this time since a number of men have been admitted from many sections of the country. I do feel it only fair, however, to mention this aspect to you. Our fellows have grown rapidly and well in Surgery out here at Howard University, and I feel that the further broadening influence of contact with the American College would be of tremendous help to them.[20]

January 25, 1950

Dear Dr. Drew:

You may be assured that I shall be delighted if you use my name in support of your application for Fellowship in the American College of Surgeons. Without reservation I don't believe that I have to tell you that I cannot think of a more deserving individual and one who would be more desirable in the American College of Surgeons.[21]

Robert Coffey, MD

As the winter of 1950 gave way to spring, Drew awaited the decision of the membership committee in far-off Chicago as to his fitness to join the American College of Surgeons.

In another wintertime four years before, Drew had found himself in most unusual company for an academic surgeon: among a "brilliant array of national and military leaders and outstanding stars of stage, radio, and screen" to celebrate National Negro Newspaper Week and the 119th anniversary of the Negro Press. This was a pair of radio programs, the first broadcast on CBS on Sunday, February 24, 1946, and the second on NBC the following week. Drew, who was doubtless selected because of his Spingarn Medal and newfound reputation as a public speaker, shared top billing with such luminaries as the actor Paul Robeson, vocalist Ella Fitzgerald, prize fighter Joe Louis, musician Lionel Hampton, old friend and judge William Hastie (who was now governor of the Virgin Islands), and an up-and-coming crooner named Frank Sinatra.[22]

Just three weeks later, Drew was in Boston to deliver a speech at the Temple Israel. If his head had been among the clouds in the company of the famous performers, he could be forgiven for harboring a different kind of pride on this occasion. The Temple Israel Brotherhood had established a scholarship fund in Drew's name to support a worthy Black student at one of the local medical schools: Tufts, Boston University, or Harvard.

Unquestionably deeply honored, Drew composed one of his most eloquent speeches for this event:

> Mr. Chairman:
>
> This scholarship which your group is creating is in the finest tradition of New England. It is fitting that such a program should be initiated here, for out of the heart and mind and blood of New England was forged the hammer which broke the chains of slavery. Out of its towns and hills and valleys went forth the fearless, Godlike, lonely men and women to teach these lowly and despised people so robbed and bound and ignorantly weak that God himself concealed their destiny. In those days you gave them hope. Into your schools and colleges came the first groups of those who had caught the dream of growing in knowledge and understanding and in service. From your schools have gone out the men and women who, in the past and today, play so large a role in attempting to complete the emancipation begun at an earlier day at such high cost to your spiritual ancestors.
>
> The Temple Israel Brotherhood, by its actions in the past and its action today, carries on in the great New England tradition. We of a younger generation of Negroes know well the significance of the names Garrison, Phillips, Stevens. We know how Shaw fell.[23] We humbly acknowledge a debt of gratitude.

Your present mode of action in establishing a scholarship in medicine for a Negro student is extraordinarily timely because there is a great need for just such aid. In the United States at the present time there are approximately 160,000 physicians. Only 2.3% of these physicians are Negroes—a total of 3,618—according to statistics released by the War Manpower Commission in 1944. For the population as a whole there is one physician for approximately every 750 people. When the ratio of Negro physicians to the 13,000,000 Negroes in the United States is considered, it is found that there is one Negro physician to every 4,000 individuals. In certain sections of the country this ratio reaches one Negro physician for every 5,000 colored persons; while in certain states the ratio is as great as one Negro physician to every 22,000 colored persons. This obviously is a woefully inadequate number. In certain sections of the country this great inadequacy is compensated for by the splendid care which our people can receive in large medical centers and clinics, but in other sections of the country no such services are available and the people die.

Of greater significance is the fact that the number of Negro physicians has gradually decreased during the ten-year period between 1932 and 1942. In 1932 there were 122 graduates. By 1938 this number had slipped to exactly half—61 graduates from all the medical schools in America. During this same period there was an 8% increase in the Negro population. At the present time statistics presented by Dr. Cornely of Howard University suggest that we may expect to lose by death 80 to 100 Negro physicians per year for the next ten years. These few facts represent the chief problem. What is the reason for this gradual decrease of trained men in a profession which all recognize to be so essential? There appear to be two chief causes: The first is the fact that medical education is extremely expensive, and the Negro is extremely poor. "How poor?" you ask. Richard Sterner, "The Negro Share" states that in the United States during the 1930–1940 period only 4% of Negroes made over $1,000 a year. It costs nearly a thousand dollars a year to attend a first-rate medical school. In 1935 he found that over 75% of Negro families of four made a total income of less than $900 a year—the sum established by the WPA as a minimum on which four people could live. (But they did live!) In the small villages of the South the average income for a family of four was found to be less than $330 a year. In the small cities the average was below $632 a year; and in New York City, the best income city in the country, the average for a family

> of four was below $980 a year. These facts, I believe, are sufficient to validate poverty as the first cause of lowered enrollment in the medical schools. The second great cause, and the one which is most active at the present time, is the widespread policy of exclusion which is so universal, even in New England, that the total number of graduates from all the 75 accredited white medical schools of the nation rarely exceeds eight or ten per year; and the opportunities for continued training in the various medical specialties in all of the clinical facilities associated with these great centers of medical teaching is rarely extended to more than a half dozen Negro postgraduate students in any given year although there are nearly 9,000 such places for such training. Even at Harvard, whose liberal attitude is well established, I can recall no instance of a Negro intern in any of the teaching hospitals associated with the college.
>
> This scholarship which you propose, therefore, answers the two dominant needs. It provides income sorely needed and creates an opportunity for the training of one more man in some institution other than Howard University College of Medicine in Washington, DC or Meharry Medical College in Nashville, Tennessee, both of which are overcrowded and overworked in attempting to work out a way of meeting this great need for thoroughly trained Negro physicians.
>
> That you have chosen to create this scholarship in my name is a great honor. I hope that the men who will be thus aided will prove themselves worthy of such aid, and that both they and I will repay you in the best way we can which is to be living up to the highest principles of good physicianship.[24]

Another significant distinction that came to Drew in 1947 was an honorary doctor of science degree from his old undergraduate institution, Amherst College (he had also received one from Virginia State College in 1945).

During the long decades when African Americans were not admitted to the American College of Surgeons, movements cropped up from time to time within the Black surgery community to create a separate organization for the excluded that would serve similar functions, as the National Medical Association had risen in response to the AMA. The closest thing to emerge was the Surgical Section of the NMA, which was formed in 1906.[25]

Drew became chairman of the Section in 1944 and held the position until his death. In August of 1947 he delivered the annual report of his group at the NMA meeting in Los Angeles. Although the fight was obviously far from over there was, in truth, much progress to trumpet. Drew noted that there were now Black surgical trainees in New York, Massachusetts, Illinois, Ohio, New Jersey, Kansas, Michigan, and California. Only two years before there had been just twelve Blacks in training above internship level in all branches of medicine in the entire United States. He went on to report that fourteen African Americans had successfully passed the American Board of Surgery examinations. Five were from Howard: Drew, Laurey, Clarence Green, Burke Syphax, and Hartford Burwell. Ten men had become fellows of the American College of Surgeons that year (though not, of course, Drew).[26]

At Los Angeles Drew also eulogized the Surgical Section's young but very accomplished secretary, Frederick Douglass Stubbs of Philadelphia, who had passed away from a heart attack at forty-one years of age. The annual surgical oration would be named in Stubbs's honor. In praising his deceased friend, Drew might have been describing himself:

> Frederick Douglass Stubbs had the background, the training, the brains, the heart, the understanding, the love of mankind and the will to serve which marked him as a natural leader. He knew our weaknesses and threw his great quiet strength into the struggle to better our poor lot. He saw the promise of our future and, stripped of all illusions, labored unceasingly to bring it to fruition . . . he might easily have basked without struggle on the income from an excellent practice of surgery. The amazing thing is that he did not choose to do so. I know of no problem which affected any of us in which he was not deeply interested. His method of doing something about these problems was not that of the propagandists whose loud mouthings at times do more harm than good, but that of a simple worker who by his own accomplishments and the inspiration he gave to all whom he touched created a record rarely equaled, seldom surpassed. He did not talk integration; he made himself so proficient that what were thought to have been insuperable barriers melted before his ability and tact.[27]

Drew closed with a poem by the Black writer and educator Leslie Pinckney Hill, which was intended to reflect honor on Stubbs but also revealed his own thoughts on leadership and the mighty price it exacts:

To be a leader! What is that to be?
To stand between a people- and their foes
And earn suspicion for a recompense;
To care for men more than they care themselves;
To keep a clear discriminating mind
Between the better counsel and the best;
To be a judge of men, that no one may rank
In estimation higher than his worth,
Nor fail of scope to prove his quality;
To search the motive that explains the act
Before it is accounted good or bad,
To trust a man, and yet not be dismayed
To find him faithless, going on again
To trust another; to build failure up
Into the tedious structure of success;
To meet the subtle enemy within
As well as him without, and vanquish both;
To see the cause betrayed by those who pledge
The strictest loyalty; to overmatch
The envious with magnanimity;
To labor through the day, and through the night
To watch and plan and exercise by prayer
The devil troop of doubts that tease the will;
To have a body that endures the strain
Of labor after labor, each in turn
Demanding more of nerve and hardihood;
To stand before your conscience offering
The utmost tithe of mortal sacrifice,
While selfish little critic parasites
Heckle and plot and spread malignant lies;
To walk through trouble with a heart that drips
The blood of agony, yet with a face
Of confidence and bright encouragement;
To do and do and die to raise a tribe
So robbed and bound and ignorantly weak

That God Himself conceals their destiny -
To be a leader! God, that is the cost ![28]

The issue of remuneration on which Drew praised Stubbs's selfless sacrifice was particularly applicable in his own case. His gross annual income as full professor and chair of surgery at Howard was $5,548 in 1943, $7,303 in 1945, and $8,199 in 1947.[29] If he had chosen, instead, to be a lab leader at a large pharmaceutical company—and he was known to all of them—Drew could have easily doubled or tripled those numbers, which would have been very welcome in a home with, now, four children (Charles, Jr., was born on October 30, 1945). Indeed, to give some sense of how much he might have earned in full-scale private practice, in the fiscal year 1944–45 Drew reported $1,380 in fees from a total of just *nine* private surgical patients at Freedmen's Hospital (the many others he operated on were house patients for whom he received no earmarked compensation beyond his standard salary). To add insult, the college of medicine took a 25 percent "surtax" of this private income—a practice Drew and his peers despised and fought against but one that was common in academic centers at that time.

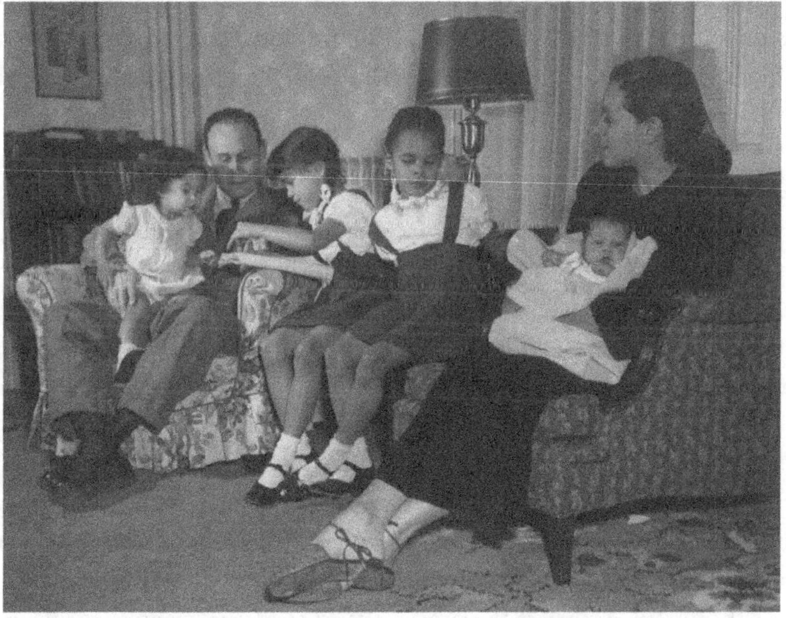

Figure 10.3 The Drew family, 1940. Personal collection, Charlene Drew Jarvis.

The following month Drew was back in his old stomping ground of New York City where he was asked to deliver an address of welcome at the opening of the Second General Assembly of the United Nations. The bulk of this speech was an appeal to the delegates to ratify the charter of the World Health Organization, which provided Drew the opportunity to deliver one of the memorable quotations for which he was becoming renowned: "The accidental boundaries of race, religion, nationality or language do not limit the spread of disease. No such boundaries must hinder the work of the men and women anywhere in the world who would fight this worldwide enemy, disease."[30]

Drew did not confine his public speaking to high-profile venues and events, nor his correspondence with the noted. Invitations came from churches and civic groups both near and far, and he would try to accommodate these whenever it was practicable among the heavy time burdens of his job and other responsibilities. Fan letters often crowded his mailbox, too. Early in 1947 Drew responded to a teacher in Fort Worth, Texas, who had written about a science program she had put together for her Black students in which he was featured prominently. After some modest deflections of credit, he moved into a brief but insightful consideration of the issue of race in American society and what her students might face in the future. With unforgettable imagery, the central thesis of Drew's overarching message to his students and all African Americans was nearing its classic form:

> Dear Mrs. Bates:
>
> I consider the program which you are sponsoring on January 29, 1947, as a great honor. One seldom merits such honor, for in the field of science wherever any advance is made the work of many people is involved and it always seems just a little bit unfair that one name should be chosen from the list for special commendation.
>
> To your students I would say this: There are so many things still unknown in almost every realm of knowledge, and the need for this knowledge is so great that in the very vast majority of instances any new addition not only is accepted but the individual who creates the work is accepted without very much regard to race, color, or creed. There are many difficulties to overcome it is true, but our greatest difficulty still remains in the fact that we do not have very much to offer which anyone wants. So much of our energy is spent in overcoming the constricting

> environment in which we live that little energy is left for creating new ideas or things. Whenever, however, one breaks out of this rather high-walled prison of the "Negro problem" by virtue of some worthwhile contribution, not only is he himself allowed more freedom, but a part of the wall crumbles.[31] And so it should be the aim of every student in science to knock down at least one or two bricks by virtue of his accomplishments.[32]

In the spring of 1949 Drew put the finishing administrative touches on the Department of Surgery's new Division of Neurosurgery, which was headed by his former general surgery resident, Clarence S. Greene. Greene had studied the subject in Montreal for two years under Drew's old professor from McGill University, Wilder Penfield.

That same season Drew was approached by James C. Evans, a civilian aide to the War Department who was familiar with his work, about joining a contingent of American physicians on a mission to Europe for the US Army.[33] The purpose of this mission, according to the orders that were eventually issued,

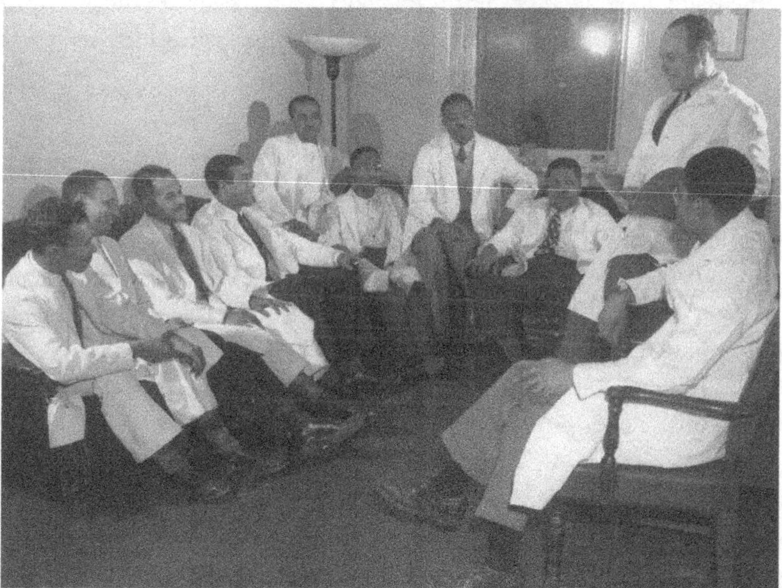

Figure 10.4 Drew in an informal moment with surgery trainees. Personal collection, Charlene Drew Jarvis.

was "promoting and improving further quality of medical care and instruction in Army Medical Installations in the American Occupied Zone of Europe."[34] Drew, who had never traveled outside of North America, was happy to accept the role of civilian surgical consultant.

Prior to departing, Drew was given the opportunity to familiarize himself with the military medical system by spending some time in the wards and laboratories at Walter Reed Hospital located in nearby Bethesda, Maryland.

Three other physicians would round out what was known as the Consulting Team: William Middleton, an internist from Madison, Wisconsin; Rudolph Reich, an orthopedic specialist out of Cleveland, Ohio; and an anesthesiologist from Hartford, Connecticut, named Ralph M. Tovell. Middleton, who had been on active duty in the Army in both world wars and thus knew not only the military medical routine but many individuals within it, became the de facto leader of the group. Drew got along well with the other consultants, finding them individually pleasant and very capable in their fields.

Orders were issued on June 15, and the trip commenced exactly two weeks later, the team arriving in Frankfurt by way of the Azores on the afternoon of June 30. Their itinerary was extensive and compact, with thirteen scheduled inspections in a little more than three weeks:

1. Heidelberg, Germany—130th Station Hospital—7-1-49
2. Stuttgart, Germany—387th Station Hospital—7-3-49
3. Munich, Germany—98th General Hospital—7-5-49
4. Vienna, Austria—110th Station Hospital—7-8-49
5. Linz, Austria—124th Station Hospital—7-10-49
6. Salzburg, Austria—57th Field Hospital, 2 H.U.—7-11-49
7. Regensburg, Germany—250th Station Hospital—7-14-49
8. Nurnberg, Germany—385th Station Hospital—7-15-49
9. Wurzberg, Germany—57th Field Hospital, 1 H.U.—7-18-49
10. Frankfurt, Germany—97th General Hospital—7-19-49
11. Giessen, Germany—388th Station Hospital—7-21-49
12. Bremerhaven, Germany—319th Station Hospital—7-22-49
13. Wiesbaden, Germany—317th Station Hospital—7-23-49

Drew sent a telegram to Lenore from Frankfurt informing her of his safe arrival. The first inspection was scheduled for the following day in Heidelberg, about an hour's drive to the south. Getting up early enough turned out not to be a problem, as Middleton insisted that the whole team get up at 6 A.M. and begin work, which Drew called an "apparent unbreakable habit" that was the group's lone, good-natured complaint.

Heidelberg was the site of the US Army Headquarters in Europe, including the medical corps. Although the physician general in charge was not present, Drew and the others were cordially welcomed by the other officers before they began their tasks.

The ranking officer at Heidelberg's 130th Station Hospital was a young lieutenant colonel for whom a civilian consultant team was something new. The visitors were initially unsure of themselves, as well, but they had devised a plan in their first few days together and put it into execution with immediate success.

On arrival at the installation in the morning, they would have a general conference with the commanding officer and the chiefs of the major divisions. Here, salient problems would be discussed and a program for the visit outlined. If operative procedures were scheduled, Drew would observe until the morning's work was completed, "being helpful if possible." If no operations were posted for that morning, he would make ward rounds with the chief of the service, as would occur in a university hospital. Each case would be presented in detail by the officer-in-charge and discussed in relationship to accepted principles of therapy in both Army and civilian hospitals.

In the afternoon, one of two procedures was followed. In the larger centers, if any morning rounds had not been completed, these were now finished; in the smaller centers, the surgical staff gathered for an informal discussion of surgical problems arising either in that installation or in the delivery of surgical care systemwide.

At some time during each visit, Drew sat down for a private conference with each member of the surgical staff, gauging that member's own personal attitude toward the assignment, interest in the Army as a career, and any personal difficulties.

In the late afternoon the consultants gave a formal presentation, complete with "lantern" slides if projecting apparatus was available (Drew brought about two hundred slides along). The surgical component of this covered what Drew considered the "five basic surgical problems": hemorrhage, shock, pain, infection, and wound healing.

Drew found the Army medical facilities at Heidelberg to be adequate; they suffered in comparison to those of the local university hospital, but that was understandable. The physicians and staff went about their business with admirable dedication and professionalism, although he had some criticism for the chief of the surgical service, a position with which he was intimately familiar in the civilian milieu: "One would like to see his routines better established and a somewhat more polished professional manner, especially in a center like Heidelberg where critical non-medical personnel abounds."[35] Drew was surprised to see that catgut sutures were still being used in most cases at Heidelberg (these had been largely superseded by alternative materials in the United States).

The Consultant Team stayed in Heidelberg for two days, then took the train on the morning of July 3 to their next stop, Stuttgart. Once there, Drew took up his pen to share his thoughts with Lenore on the first European city he had the opportunity to see and explore:

> The most striking thing in Heidelberg, the old 13th century university town which by common agreement was spared by the war, was the beauty of its two mountains, Konigstuhl on the north side of the Neckar river and Heiligenberg on the South with its ancient looking, sturdy red stone houses climbing each slope upwards from the banks of the river. There is quaintness and disrepair in the university buildings. Nothing matches the modern splendor of our schools. The clinic buildings are shabby.
>
> We have very little direct contact with the Germans. Americans have taken over the best hotels, the best hospitals, the best homes for their officers. We are a party of an invading army. They accept it rather stoically, we feel it.
>
> We use American scrip for money and have not yet been able to get German marks. We eat in prescribed areas, live with the army and travel in American cars on German trains. I should like to return to Heidelberg someday when the tension of war is gone. On the roads outside of town and the small villages one sees the women with their hoes working the fields as they did 100 years ago. The villages have narrow streets, the peasants look as though they are out of story

> books—plodding, hardworking, unemotional—only the kids are happy. There seem to be thousands of kids, hundreds of bicycles on every road and lane. Automobiles are seldom seen out of town. The farms are beautiful. Every inch of ground is used. The chief crops seem to be wheat, barley, potatoes, clover for fodder, poppies for poppy seed, oats, some mustard and a few beans. Have seen very few tractors. On these farms the world has not changed very fast.[36]

Along the train route to Stuttgart, Drew had seen firsthand the physical evidence of the war, now four years after its end:

> In the other towns I have seen so far the one overwhelming impression is that of staggering destruction. Mannheim, once a proud industrial center, has been leveled to the ground. Heilbronn, which resisted the 7th Army's advance, is not much more than a shell. Even now, four years later, very little rebuilding has taken place. The once great station here at Stuttgart still has no roof and there are scars on every hand. The Germans were not hurt like this during the first war. They have been whipped till it hurts this time. They don't like it but still are not too anxious to have all of the Americans go because there is real fear that the Russians will walk in. War is even in its aftermath an almost totally unhappy thing.[37]

Over the next three weeks, Drew completed the tour of the thirteen US Army installations and recorded his official thoughts, which were generally positive, for each of them. In his final report there were some recommendations for improvement, and unabashed observations regarding personnel: "Lt. Col . . . is a sound neurosurgeon and was popular with his Staff in spite of the monocle and Prussian crew haircut. . . ." "Capt . . . highlighted for us some of the major psychological problems of a young Jewish Officer in a land where antisemitism is still rampant and the ghosts of five million destroyed people haunt the land. He is a well-trained, capable physician." "I got the feeling that Lt . . . on the Obstetrical Service felt his inadequacy at times but made up for the lack of training with great conscientiousness to duty. It might be fairer to put one with a little more experience in an area as busy and as isolated." There were also things to be said about the organizations, coming from the perspective of a seasoned leader: "The Service is well covered. Routines for handling suddenly increased numbers are well worked out. They work well with the Medical Staff on all difficult cases. This was not a happy 'family', however, for there was universal disaffection with the Hospital administration. The area is worth looking into, for such a situation eventually leads to a lower level of patient care even where the letter-of-the-law is rigidly enforced."[38]

Drew's next letter to Lenore was from Munich, from which he also sent colorful postcards for the children: "We rode through the courtyard of the palace of the Bavarian kings. Even in ruins there is splendor which staggers. No wonder the people revolted." After a few days in the new role, he felt more comfortable with the challenges: "The days are full, almost crowded with new problems, new people, new situations. So far I think I have done alright." Americans were given military certificates to use as cash—Germans were not permitted to hold this "scrip." In reality, though, Drew found that "a carton of cigarettes still is the best money in the country. For instance we tip a waiter two cigarettes, the Porter who carried 10 bags for four of us got 10 . . . a carton will bring 20 to 25 marks—equivalent to from 7 to $8. I sold one of my $10 script notes for 50 German marks in order to buy German stamps to put on the children's postcards."[39]

From Munich it was on to Austria. Drew found Vienna, in Soviet-controlled territory and under four-power rule like Berlin, a somewhat uncomfortable mix of Old-World cosmopolitan opulence and bristling Cold War tension. He leapt at the chance to visit the famous Allgemeines Krankenhaus, the legendary hospital where Ignaz Semmelweiss made his observations on childbed fever and Karl Landsteiner (who was on the Columbia faculty when Drew was there) had discovered the blood types. To his surprise, Drew found the Krankenhaus to be well behind American institutions. Ever conscious of music, he basked in the city of Mozart, Beethoven, and Schubert: "It is a city of lost dreams and music. Every little cafe has music. I have not had a meal outside of the hospital where there is not music—all kinds—from Beethoven to very good American swing."[40]

On July 11 Drew wrote from Salzburg, a city he found beautiful:

My Sweet,

Outside of my window tonight the river runs by with the sound that is both beautiful and lonely. I miss you tonight, I've missed you all day as I drove about 190 kilometers from Linz to Salzburg. All the way down we hung close to a series of lakes nestling in the Austrian Alps.

It was lovely for the first time—there were no signs of the horrible destruction of war. The peasants were in the field cutting and sheathing wheat by hand as they have done for centuries. We passed a hundred pastoral scenes to delight the eye of an artist. Almost universally the men wear short leather pants (lederhosen) with or without their short gray or green coats and Alpine hats. The women wear simple dresses with built in aprons, kerchiefs around their heads and for the most part they are barefooted while working in the fields. Wheat is being harvested in this area and it makes a striking picture with blue water below the geometrical farms that stretch far up the mountain slides.

Salzburg, like most of the other cities passed in the last week, lies in the valley by a river with mountain peaks on all sides. It is an interesting town in the daytime, unbelievably striking and beautiful at night when floodlights from the heights of one of the mountain ranges light up the city. It looks like an Alpine scene on a great stage. It shines like a jewel in a great verdant crown of hills.

I miss you so much

with all my love goodnight[41]

A week later he was in Nurnberg, former home of the immense Nazi rallies, which provided a stark contrast. War damage was heavy in the city, and entrance was forbidden to all except US military personnel. Drew encountered a large detachment of Black troops here and was asked to speak at church services. He recorded his thoughts for Lenore:

This was my first contact with Negro troops on the trip. At Chapel there were about 25 German brides, many of whom had their brown skin offspring with them. This relationship there seemed quite alright; they looked like any other family groups in church. Afterwards I had lunch at the officers mess and picked up some rather interesting data. In the outfit I visited there are 900 men. During the last 19 months there have been approximately 176 marriages. Since January the authorities made the regulations stiffer and the rate has slowed up. Now marriages are not permitted until the man is within three months of his departure for the States. He must place $1000 in escrow with family welfare office and the girl

> must be okayed by the CIC (counterintelligence) and the Provost Marshall (to check morals status). What has simply happened is that the boys now live with girls out of wedlock. There have been 196 babies born to such couples during the last year. The chaplain estimates that 80 to 90% of the men have "homes" in the city. This of course infuriates many of the Germans but they dare not protest. The white soldiers do not like it and many fights ensue. Tonight, looking down on the main Plaza of the city from my hotel room, I should say that at least 2/3 of the troops were walking off arm and arm with some fraulein within the first 50 yards from the bus stop. It is not nice, as a matter of fact, makes me just a little sick in the stomach—but this is a victorious army, the Negroes are a part of it, there are few German men, the girls are still hungry and the Americans feed them, dress them and fill their wombs. More than the towns have been destroyed in Germany—the moral codes have been destroyed—values are not the same.[42]

By July 25 Drew and the rest of the Consulting Team were back in Heidelberg, where they reported to General Guy Denit, medical commanding officer of the European Theater, who was back in town. Denit spent three hours with the Consultants and "seemed extremely interested in every suggestion made which might improve the care of the patients in his Command and the morale of his Officers."[43]

The Consultants had several recommendations, some of which pertained to their own function, which they believed was of significant value but recognized could be disruptive to the units' routine. In a larger sense, though, their suggestions were intended to optimize the educational and practice environment for the military physicians—from practical considerations such as providing slide and movie projectors where they were lacking to organizing didactic sessions and conferences. They did not have much in the way of criticism regarding patient care—only that the military medical environment in the installations they encountered was potentially conducive to stagnation, which could lead to practices that lagged the state of the art.

After the command meeting in Heidelberg, the Consultant Team dissolved. Their report, which Drew composed, was dated September 15, 1949, and delivered to the surgeon general of the army, Major General Raymond Bliss.

Drew had a few weeks on his own in Europe before he was scheduled to fly back to the States from England on August 13. Like any good American tourist, he made plans to visit Paris and London. Before setting off for the City of Light he reflected on the good fortune of being asked to join the Consultants mission: "It has been a marvelous experience," he wrote Lenore. "Except under auspices such as those under which we did it such a tour would be impossible . . . I would enjoy it so much more if you were here to share it with me."[44]

Drew also summarized the trip in a letter to his sister Nora:

> So far I have been to Frankfurt, Heidelberg, Stuttgart, Munich, Nurnberg, Giesen, Weisbaden, Bremen, Bremerhaven, Kassef, Mainz, Heilbronn, Wurtzburg, Regensburg and several smaller towns in Germany; to Linz, Salzburg and Vienna in Austria and after 30 days of exciting work a great deal of traveling by all known means of locomotion—planes, 1st class trains, 3rd class trains, military trains, touring cars, jeeps, and trucks—I finished my assignment. I have visited every medical installation in the European Command. I travelled with rank equivalent to a general, and the so-called VIP (very important person) category. It has been an unusual experience.
>
> I have had an opportunity to see much more than medicine—the beautiful farms of the Neckar valley, the castles on the Rhine, Hitler's Eagle's Nest atop the Bavarian Alps near Berchtesgarden, Salzburg at night like a huge stage setting in some far off make believe land, the Schoenburg palace and the graves of the Hapsburgs, the mountain top land of the good king of Wurtenberg and his Russian Princess bride, the Haus der Kunst in Nuremberg where Hitler built dreams of a world capital . . . I'll tell you about it.
>
> Charlie[45]

Drew arrived in Paris on July 27, finding that his recent Consultant teammate, the anesthesiologist Ralph Tovell, was in town with his family. The Tovells had two rooms at the Ambassador Hotel and invited Drew to stay in one with their son, which saved him a great deal of money (what the son had to say about it was not recorded).

Drew was refreshed by the appearance of the French capital, untouched by the war's devastation. He could see no outward evidence of the German occupation aside from the absence of statues that had been melted down for their metal. For the most part, though, he found the French people less personally appealing than their German counterparts: "The men of Germany as a whole are manly brutes when compared to the average pasty, dapper, hand kissing little Frenchmen. The women of Germany are a buxom, healthy looking, unmade up, but totally females of the type built for carrying and not for speed when compared with the slim, chic, well dressed sleek models that roam this town. They are not prettier they are in better shape and made-up fancier."[46]

He studied the French language (two years of which he had taken back at Amherst twenty years before), went on bus tours of the Île de la Cité and Versailles, walked the Left Bank, and generally tried to get what he called "a bird's eye view" of Paris. He also visited the local US Army hospital, although it was not part of his official Consultant's tour. The contrasts Drew encountered left a particularly deep impression, although he tried to keep a generous spirit and realized that the brief time he had to observe was not nearly enough to grasp a foreign culture:

> Paris is a great city,—full of grandeur and squalor, great beauty in the midst of much ugliness—a deeply religious place nestled in the most universal debauchery I have seen. The moral code in Europe is a different thing from that at home and the attitude here in France requires a lot of understanding. In Germany there is an extreme surplus of women and they are hungry. Moreover they throughout the war were encouraged to have children, they still tacitly are encouraged to rebuild the nations manpower. Many things are overlooked. Here the naked female form is idolized, worshipped one might say, but woman's place is not a high one as a whole. There are so many of them, competition is so keen, and extramarital relationships from kings to commoner such a part of France's history and present thinking that a stranger has a difficult time establishing just where the values lie. Certainly it would be unwise to attempt it in a few days.[47]

On August 8 Drew took the afternoon train to Calais, then boarded a boat to Dover. From there another train took him to London where he checked into the Mt. Royal Hotel on Oxford Street in Marylebone.[48]

He took in Grosvenor and Berkeley Squares, Piccadilly Circus, Regent Street and Pall Mall, St. James Palace and Whitehall. Finally, Drew found himself at the Houses of Parliament "with Big Ben smiling down at the Thames River below and hiding, for a moment, the greatest building of them all, Westminster Abbey." He spent three hours among the interred luminaries and royalty in the magnificent architecture of the Abbey "and enjoyed every minute in a quiet contemplative way."[49]

Of the Europeans he encountered in the memorable journey Drew clearly held those he saw in London in highest regard: "Here the people are slim, bright eyed, clean looking. The gentlemen impeccable, and the women markedly different from Paris. One cannot but admire the British."[50]

A few days later he was back home in Washington.

Shortly before leaving for his European tour, Drew had heard that his old biology professor from Amherst, Otto Glaser, was retiring to emeritus status. He and other former students created a fund to help their old teacher negotiate the vicissitudes of retirement more securely. Drew also composed a heartfelt letter to Glaser, reporting his own accomplishments as one might to a proud parent and reflecting any praise he had received back on the instruction from which he had benefited, decades before:

> Throughout this entire period, my research efforts have been confined largely to the field of "Water Balance in Surgery", Shock, Blood Transfusions, Preservation of Blood, Blood Substitutes, etc. Much of this interest undoubtedly stems from your early teaching and interest in the relationships of fluid distribution in the developing embryo as a factor in its differentiation and definitive form. I still feel that my senior essay on "Growth" was one of the best things I have done; and certainly, the preparation of this paper opened up more new fields to me than any similar exercise I have carried out since leaving Amherst. . . . It is with a sense of real gratitude and deep affection that I wish you many years of care-free leisure to work at the things you like to do best.[51]

Not long after his return from the continent Drew received a reply from Glaser:

> Dear Charlie Drew:
>
> The treasurer of the College has told me about the fund you helped raise for my benefit. I can't tell you how much I appreciate this generous act—not only for what it means in concrete terms—but especially as it expresses so much good will and is evidence that the old days remain alive.

> You were and are one of those who make a teachers' life worthwhile. I have followed your career with great satisfaction and was proud and more than pleased when the College gave you the honorary DSc. I still wish we might at that time have had a chance to talk—perhaps our paths may cross again. . . .
>
> As my mind plays over the past, it is curious how vividly certain little things loom up—things you may not and perhaps could not recall. There was the time when as I was walking by, you came tripping lightly down the stairs of Tertsy's emporium. I don't think you saw me—but the grace and beauty of your young movements have left an indelible impression. Could you do it now? Another thing I cannot forget is the football game during which one of the opponents tried to get you out by trying to twist your ankle, I saw how that hurt and was glad to see its purpose fail. . . . There are happy memories and you are one of them.[52]

In October, Drew was asked to come to New York City to give a lecture to the annual meeting of the Association for the Study of Negro Life and History.[53] He chose to speak on the topic of "Negro Scholars in Scientific Research." Drew delivered a lengthy list of Black American scholars who had made contributions of significance to the scientific world, and took a special interest in four whom he had seen in a Hall of Fame at the New York World's Fair nine years before: Benjamin Banneker, a mathematician and surveyor who helped lay out the new city of Washington, DC, in the late eighteenth century; George Washington Carver, the agricultural chemist; Ernest Everett Just, a groundbreaking biologist who had won the first Spingarn Medal; and Daniel Hale Williams, the founding member of the American College of Surgeons noted above.

Drew reflected on the dreadful toll that racial prejudice exacted on these four men who were celebrated for their greatness after their time had passed. (Just could not secure an academic appointment at a large university despite the profound nature of his research, and Williams led a life of seclusion rather than face the indignities of bigotry.)

"Each was a gifted man," said Drew. "Each helped make the road easier for those who must come behind, but each had a problem added to the problems of his scientific endeavors, which he could not surmount."[54]

In years to come, others would give similar speeches about him.

From the Foggy Bottom years through the times in Arlington and the world beyond, Christmas had always been a special season for Charles Drew. Now, with his own family, he did the best he could to maintain the traditions that had defined the holiday throughout his youth—and add some new ones, as well.

On Christmas Eve, he and the children bundled into the venerable family Ford and chugged downtown to see the brightly decorated windows at Woodward and Lothrop's (Lenore remained at home to prepare the meal and wrap gifts). From there, it was off to the Ellipse to gawk at the fabulous, brilliantly illuminated White House Christmas tree. Next, suitably inspired by this sight, they drove to the tree lot markets to select their own spruce—a lengthy process, given Drew's tendency toward perfectionism. Back at home everyone chipped in to decorate the new tree, bathed in the fresh scent of pruned pine.[55]

Christmas meant rounds of a different kind from those he made at Freedmen's: joyous jaunts to the Gregory house in the Southeast district and across the river to see Grandmother Drew, along with Joseph and his family, in Arlington. Though the family income was modest, the children never wanted from a lack of presents and squabbled laughingly over who got the most. The Christmas of 1949 seemed to pass all too swiftly, but then they always did.

As the new year, and with it a new decade, rolled around, Drew had settled into the intermittently comfortable routine attendant to an eminent position at Howard University and in the African American community. Professionally, he continued to be embroiled in the struggle to be recognized as a fellow of the American College of Surgeons, in addition to all the other battles across the country in which he and his comrades and colleagues fought to improve the health care of Blacks by elevating the training and education of their physicians: "It must be held as a basic principle of our thinking and a continuing hope that in the not too distant future plans for the medical care of patients will not be made on the basis of race or economic status but on the basis of best preserving and

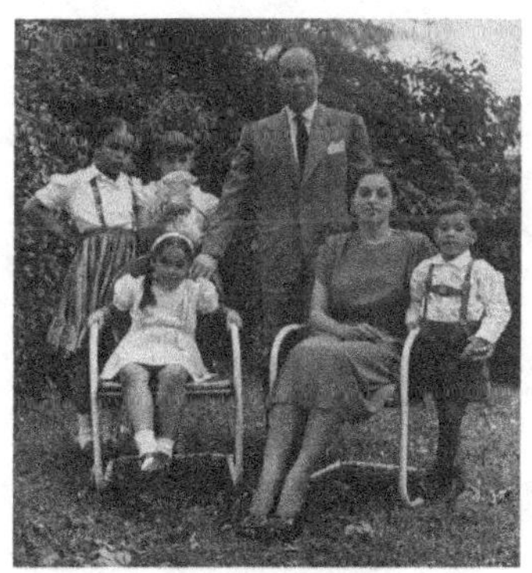

Figure 10.5 At home with the family, circa 1950. Personal collection, Charlene Drew Jarvis.

improving the health of the nation. Such a happy state does not at the present time exist, therefore it is necessary to plan for the health needs of Negroes and the training of Negro personnel as a special programme."[56]

Some of the efforts to nurture this consistent message had begun to bear fruit. In addition to the newfound success Black surgeons were enjoying among the credentialing organizations, Drew's trainees had begun to fill positions in other medical centers across the country, both in training scenarios and as attending physicians. One of these was Jack White, for whom Drew arranged a residency year with the US Public Health Service at the Marine Hospital in Brighton, Massachusetts. Drew recognized that such positions could serve more purposes than simply providing experience and training: they could spread the word about what was happening at Howard and, if the trainee happened to return or simply communicate his experiences, broaden the horizons of the home institution the way his own time at Columbia had. In a reply letter to White, Drew both expressed these convictions with eloquence and reminded White that he would always be a part of the Howard surgery community:

> I know you must feel that I have sent you off to the far, cold Northland and left you to work out your destiny as best you could without further interest on our part. This is not true. We still love you and are extremely interested in what you do, what you think, and what you plan for the future.
>
> I took the liberty of reading to the fellows that section of your last letter which presented a comparative analysis of procedures there with those here. This type of information, I feel, is of inestimable value. Each service has a character of its own, and only when one knows how many services are run will he have sufficient background to select those routines from each, which best suits his needs and skills. . . . Our horizons are being widened by the residents all the time, and the things they write back, sharing with us, as it were, their daily experiences, enriches us all and at the same time forges the bonds which unite us even more firmly, so that each man is inspired to do more and more on his own, in order to be worthy of the fine companionship of such a group. In the individual accomplishments of each man lies the success or failure of the group as a whole. The success of the group as a whole is the basis for any tradition which we may create. In such tradition lies the sense of discipleship and the inspiration which serves as a guide for

> those who come after, so that each man's job is not just his job alone, but a part of a greater job whose horizons we at present can only dimly imagine, for they are beyond our view.
>
> The thing which we have not had in the past is a group bound by similar training, aspirations and ideals to which we can feel that we belong. The sense of belonging is of extraordinary importance to man as individuals and as groups. The sense of continuously being an outsider requires the greatest type of moral courage to overcome before actual accomplishments can be begun. Our fellows are rapidly creating something which gives them a sense of "belonging to." Within the protection of this feeling, they should be able to accomplish more than the fellows who have gone before.[57]

When White finished this year of training in Boston, he proceeded to another arranged for him by Drew at Memorial Hospital in New York City, which was famous for its advanced cancer treatments. Drew had initiated a Tumor Clinic Program in 1948 and wanted White to lead it; the Memorial fellowship would give the young man a head start. Drew's efforts to secure the position for White were aided by the fact that the head of the Memorial program was Cornelius Rhoads, Drew's immediate superior in both the Blood for Britain and American Red Cross plasma programs (Rhoads had given one of the first Austin M. Curtis lectures in 1942). White went on to found the Howard University Cancer Center, which was thereafter known as "the house that Jack built."

Toward the end of March, Drew began to finalize arrangements for his near-annual trip to the John A. Andrew Society meeting and clinic. He was now on the Dean's Committee of the Veterans Administration hospital in Tuskegee where one of his former trainees, Asa Yancey, was chief of surgery. Drew had arranged for a current Howard resident, John R. Ford, to gain additional training under Yancey. As the travel date neared, Drew invited Ford to come along.

The original plan had been for Drew and Samuel Bullock, another staff surgeon at Howard who was a friend from the Dunbar days, to fly to Alabama. As a cash-strapped resident, though, Ford could not afford such luxuries. Instead, Drew, Bullock, Ford, and another surgery resident named Walter R. Johnson would make the trek by car—just as Drew had with his two friends on the 1938 trip that led to his meeting Lenore. Bullock offered the use of his nearly new 1949 Buick Roadmaster, much the superior long-distance touring car to Drew's well-worn Ford, and the question of transportation was set.

Lodging was the same issue it had always been for African Americans on the road in the South, but by now the routine of a stopover in Atlanta was well rehearsed for Drew: he had made reservations for the troupe at the Butler Street YMCA. The four men would leave Washington after their work week was complete, in the very early hours of Saturday, April 1. The Andrew Clinic did not start until Monday, so, although the journey was a long one, they would have plenty of time to get there.

Friday, March 31, 1950, began at the usual weekday time for Drew with resident rounds at Freedmen's at 6:30 A.M.[58] He had just one operative case that day, a radical mastectomy that was scheduled at 8 A.M. When this was completed, he headed to the medical school to give the Introduction to Surgery 203 lecture to the sophomore class. The topic was one he could probably have covered in his sleep, "Shock, Blood Plasma, and Water Balance." Following lunch, the entire afternoon was devoted to administrative business for the Department of Surgery. At around 5 P.M. Drew went home for dinner and some time with his family. He had a busy evening ahead.

At 7 P.M. Drew attended the Chi Eta Phi Nursing Society dinner, where he gave a speech. After this, he went to the student council banquet, which lasted until 10 p.m. Before going home for some last-minute packing, Drew made rounds at the hospital, checking with particular interest on his postoperative patient from the morning.

After midnight he bade goodbye to Lenore and went to meet the other three physicians at Freedmen's, where they packed into Bullock's Roadmaster and started off for Atlanta under a bright, full moon. The car was abuzz with pleasant conversation as the men recounted their busy days.

11

Alamance

April 1, 1950

From his front row seat in the lecture hall, nineteen-year-old Lasalle Leffall could hear every word and see each scribbled blackboard note of Professor Walter Booker's Saturday morning pharmacology lecture. Already a second-year student at Howard University Medical School, the precocious Leffall had a habit of placing himself as close to the teacher as possible so as not to miss a single morsel of information cast his way. From this vantage point he had a good view when lab technician Bill "Long Tall" Miller—all 6'4" of him—came into the class from the rear door and approached Professor Booker for a sidebar conversation. Leffall could not hear the whispered words, but he saw the professor's face grow ashen and contorted. Booker turned to Miller and said, "You shouldn't joke like *that* on April Fool's Day." Miller straightened and shook his head, "Oh, I would never make a joke like that."

With a stunned expression, the professor faced his class.

"I have some very bad news for you," he said, voice trembling. "Our chief of surgery was just killed in a tragic automobile accident on his way to a medical meeting in Tuskegee, Alabama."

The class absorbed this inconceivable report in shocked silence. Was it possible? Could the brilliant, famous, towering figure—who had just lectured to them on shock *the previous day*—really be gone? Booker looked at his startled pupils and realized any hope of meaningful teaching was gone for the day. He could only close his lecture book and murmur, "Class is dismissed."[1]

After Drew took the wheel of Bullock's car, conversation in the passenger compartment began to die down. Already exhausted by their full days and lengthy road trip, the men were overwhelmed by the sedative effect of the food, coffee notwithstanding, and began to drift off to sleep. Soon only Drew remained awake. Bullock was in the passenger seat, with Johnson in the seat behind him. Ford was behind Drew.[2]

The miles passed. They crossed the border into North Carolina on Route 49, keeping a steady, brisk pace of about 70 miles per hour. At around 7:50 A.M. Bullock was suddenly awakened by violent shaking. Opening his eyes he saw that the Buick had drifted onto the right shoulder of the road. With a voice of sudden alarm he shouted, "Hey Charlie!"[3]

Drew, who had evidently been dozing, jumped with a start, saw what was happening and wrenched the steering wheel to the left. The tires shrieked against the asphalt; he had overcorrected. Careening sharply to the left, the sedan barreled into the embankment, flew wildly in the air and, landing sideways, began to tumble through a plowed cornfield.

The Buick had no seat belts.* Ford was catapulted clear of the rolling vehicle. Bullock was tossed to the floor of the passenger side like a ragdoll. The sedan rolled three times. As it finally came to a shuddering halt about thirty yards from the road, right side up, Johnson found himself still in the back seat on the passenger side.

After the sudden and violent awakening Johnson was confused and disoriented, but uninjured. At first, sitting in an unnatural quiet with no one else visible, he thought he was alone. He noticed that the left side doors of the Buick were both open. With gathering awareness, Johnson saw that Bullock was wedged under the dashboard. He helped his professor, who was also unhurt—apart from bumps and bruises—out of the car. The two men circled the wreck, trying to take in the damage and their surroundings. There were two farmhouses visible; otherwise, only cultivated fields and the state route.

* Only one US automobile manufacturer, Nash, offered seat belts as an option at this time.

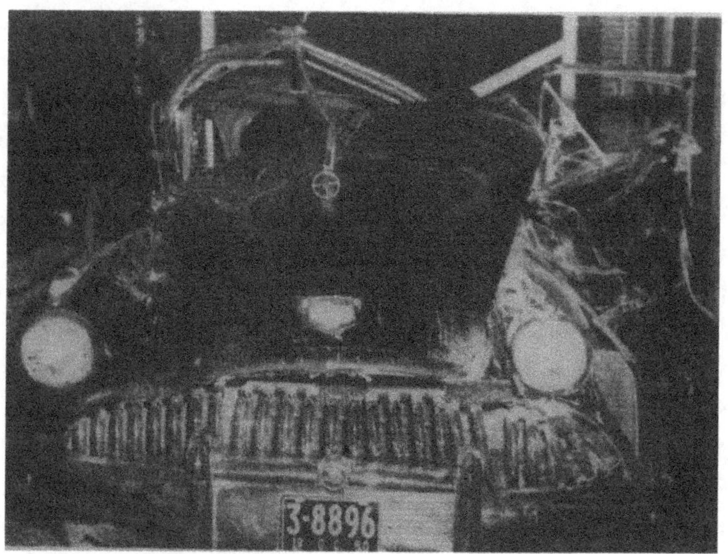

Figure 11.1 Samuel Bullock's Buick Roadmaster photographed shortly after the accident, April, 1950. *Carolina Times* April 8, 1950, p.1.

The roof of the Buick was caved in, the windshield shattered, and the left side of the car crushed like a tin can. They came upon Drew, lying on his back, half-in and half-out of the car at the driver's side door. His foot had been caught under the brake pedal and this prevented him from being launched out of the passenger compartment. Instead, the big sedan had rolled over him: "He was alive, his breathing was irregular, and his face was pale and contorted as if in pain. Dr. Bullock examined the upper extremities while I examined the lower. There was an avulsion of the quadriceps muscle of the left leg; there was no frank hemorrhage, not even from the avulsed injury. There was no bleeding from the mouth, nose, or ears. He was obviously in shock."[4]

At this point they saw Ford, who was about ten yards away, holding his left arm. He had been thrown from the rolling car. Johnson went to him and, making a quick examination, confirmed that his left humerus was fractured. He told Ford to put his hand between the buttons of his shirt to act as a sling. Ford could see that Drew was seriously injured and told Johnson he had an overcoat in the car that they could use to cover him.

Soon, passing motorists realized what had happened and stopped to help; one went into town and telephoned an ambulance, which arrived in about fifteen minutes along with a state highway patrol car. Drew was carefully lifted onto a stretcher and placed in the rear of the ambulance. Johnson accompanied him on the trip to the hospital. Ford, with his fractured arm, was brought in by a motorist. Bullock collected as many of the group's belongings as he could from the wreck and was transported by a policeman.

Their destination was Alamance County General Hospital in Burlington, North Carolina. This forty-eight-bed private facility, the only one in the county, was about five miles from where the accident occurred, which was just north of the town of Haw River.

The ambulance came to a stop on the north side of the hospital, a red brick neoclassical building with a white colonnade portico, at 8:30 A.M. Johnson helped the ambulance attendants wheel Drew on a gurney down the entrance ramp into the emergency room, which was on the ground floor under the elevated portico. Hospital personnel began to collect vital signs and perform a survey physical exam of Drew. Like all hospitals in the South, Alamance Hospital was segregated, but it had a small Black ward with five beds, located in the basement. There was just one emergency room, though, which served patients of all races.

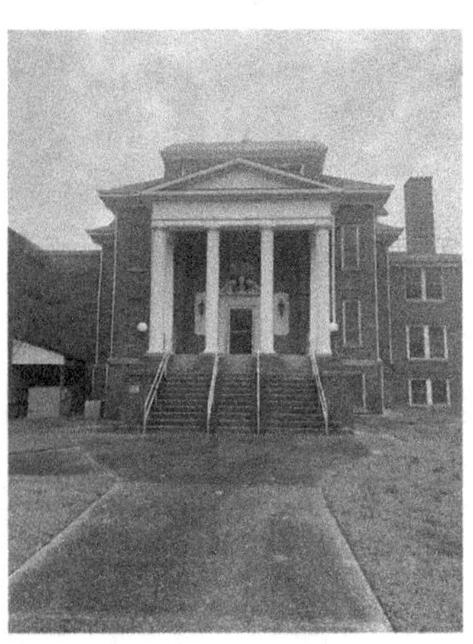

Figure 11.2 The former Alamance County General Hospital. Photo by author April 2024.

Johnson saw that Drew "was still alive, periodically gasping." A "tall, ruddy, brown-haired man in a long, white coat" came into the room and assessed the situation. It was George Carrington, a surgeon and one of the hospital's two physician owners. He began issuing orders in "a commanding voice," calling for intravenous fluids and a tourniquet* to be placed around Drew's right arm.[5] He then relinquished care to the physicians on call, the brothers Harold and Charles Kernodle, al-

* This was likely to facilitate placement of an IV.

though he and the hospital's other surgeon-owner, Ralph Brooks, continued to look in as the case unfolded.

At this point Johnson was ushered out of the emergency room into a waiting area. Before leaving, he told the Kernodle brothers who their patient was. Soon Bullock arrived and asked about Drew. Johnson said that their chief was still alive, the last he knew. Bullock was having back pain and so he and Ford were

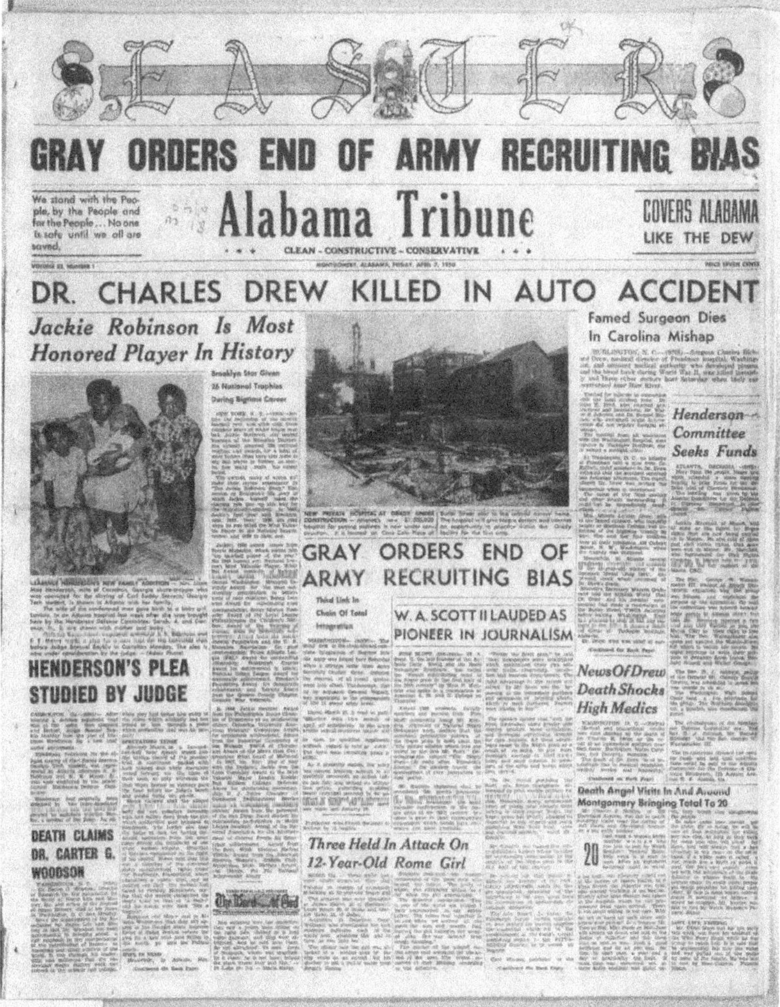

EASTER

GRAY ORDERS END OF ARMY RECRUITING BIAS

We stand with the People, by the People and for the People ... No one is safe until we all are saved.

Alabama Tribune

COVERS ALABAMA LIKE THE DEW

CLEAN - CONSTRUCTIVE - CONSERVATIVE

DR. CHARLES DREW KILLED IN AUTO ACCIDENT

Jackie Robinson Is Most Honored Player In History

Famed Surgeon Dies In Carolina Mishap

Henderson Committee Seeks Funds

GRAY ORDERS END OF ARMY RECRUITING BIAS

W. A. SCOTT II LAUDED AS PIONEER IN JOURNALISM

HENDERSON'S PLEA STUDIED BY JUDGE

News Of Drew Death Shocks High Medics

Death Angel Visits In And Around Montgomery Bringing Total To 20

DEATH CLAIMS DR. CARTER G. WOODSON

Three Held In Attack On 12-Year-Old Rome Girl

Figure 11.3 Drew's death was headline news in black papers nationwide.

taken for X-rays. Ford was admitted to the Black inpatient basement ward because of his fracture.[6]

The Kernodle brothers did not recognize Drew by his appearance, but both knew the name that Ford gave them. Harold, who was an orthopedic surgeon, had served in the war and knew Drew from his role in the plasma field. Charles, a general surgeon, had once worked in the blood bank as a resident at Duke, where he had heard the name. "We knew what we were dealing with," Harold later remembered.[7]

The Duke University Medical Center, as well as the University of North Carolina hospitals, were thirty miles away. Both offered far superior trauma resources to what Alamance County could provide, but, in such a desperate case, the forty-five-minute time for transport was out of the question.[8]

On another floor of the hospital an operation was about to begin when the nurse anesthetist, Lucille Crabtree, was summoned *stat* to the emergency room. Eschewing the elevator, she swept down the stairs to find the urgent chaos of the scene spread before her. To Crabtree, the identity of the patient and his companions was both unknown and inconsequential: "We just knew they were victims. I didn't know they were doctors until later in the day. . . . Dr. Drew was on the main operating table. Right away I tried to get an open airway. Another attendant tried to get an IV going."[9]

The emergency team initiated standard resuscitation measures, which had not yet been distilled into the streamlined protocols of today. Crabtree placed an endotracheal tube and administered oxygen, the team gave IV fluids, supplemented by plasma. Accounts differ as to whether whole blood was administered; Charles Kernodle remembered that there was insufficient time for a proper type and crossmatch.[10] From the start, all the physicians involved in the emergency room care recognized that Drew's case was, if not hopeless, at least desperate. Charles Kernodle noted on his first examination that Drew's pupils were fixed and dilated as well as unresponsive to light; grave signs of catastrophic neurologic injury. Crabtree remembered, "His chest was crushed, his head was crushed and broken. There was nothing anyone could do—not even Duke, he was torn up too bad."[11]

In the waiting area, Bullock and Johnson kept up their grim vigil. After more than an hour had passed, one of the treating physicians came out to talk with them. "We tried," he said. "We did the best we could." It was 10:10 A.M.[12]

Two months shy of his forty-sixth birthday, Dr. Charles Richard Drew was gone.

12

Epilogue

The Life and Legacy of Dr. Charles Drew

Lenore Drew was at home on Saturday morning, April 1, when a physician from Howard named Lillian Wiggins came to the door. As she heard the nightmarish news "everything went cold," she remembered. "But there was no real recognition of what had happened." Other Howard colleagues of her husband began to arrive to comfort and grieve with one another. Bebe, who was nine years old, later remembered her mother sitting on the couch between two men who stared silently and sorrowfully at their shoes.[1]

Joseph Drew received the news in a call from a friend. Dubious, he telephoned the Howard University Department of Surgery, where the sad fact was confirmed. Indeed, the whole medical school was in shock. "Medical students, residents, young attending staff members, colleagues, and employees at all levels and in all categories wept unabashedly and unashamedly," recalled Paul Cornely, a Howard physician who had succeeded Drew as medical director at Freedmen's Hospital.[2]

When Nora found out, she told her husband Francis, "Go to Mama"—to the Arlington house where her mother and namesake would surely be devastated at the dreadful news.[3]

Back in North Carolina, C. Mason Quick, a physician friend of Drew's who was interning at Kate Bitting Reynolds Hospital in nearby Winston-Salem, had received a call from Bullock shortly after the victims arrived at Alamance

General. He made the hour-long drive to Burlington as quickly as he safely could and stepped into the hospital just as Drew was being pronounced dead. Grief-stricken, Quick took the still-stunned Bullock and Johnson back to the crash site, where they all looked over the sad scene once more and collected what belongings of their own, as well as their late friend, remained.

Drew's body was taken from the emergency room beneath the columns of the Alamance County Hospital portico to the Sharpe Memorial Chapel, a black funeral home in Burlington. Quick, Bullock, and Johnson came by to be sure everything was in order for transport of the body back to Washington, then left for Winston-Salem, where the two Howard University physicians caught a flight home. As word got out, scores of African Americans descended on the Sharpe chapel, hoping in vain for a look at the great Charles Drew in repose. Late in the day, a hearse from Washington's McGuire funeral home arrived for Drew's body.[4]

At Tuskegee, those gathered for the Andrew Clinic were shocked and distraught at the news. There was talk of canceling the event, but, before long, all agreed that that would not be Drew's wish. The conference went on, though covered in an inescapable, somber pall.[5]

A day or two later, Joseph Drew and his sister Nora, accompanied by Burke Syphax, went to Lincoln Cemetery just across the border of the southeastern District of Columbia in Suitland, Maryland, to look for a grave site. Joe wandered the grounds for a seemingly interminable time, looking around and murmuring over and over, as much to himself as his companions, that his brother's grave had to be on "the highest spot."[6]

Telegrams and notes of mourning and sympathy came into Howard and the Drew home from across the world. A message from President Roosevelt's widow, Eleanor, was among them, as were notes from the author Pearl S. Buck; Major General Raymond Bliss, surgeon general of the army; Mary McLeod Bethune, founder of Bethune-Cookman College; the eminent historian John Hope Franklin; DeWitt Stetten, president of the Blood Transfusion Betterment Association; and Coach Tuss McLaughry, who wrote, "Charlie's untimely passing is a loss not only to his many friends, but to all humanity. He was one of the finest individuals I have ever known. My close friendship with him at Amherst and afterward is something that I will always cherish."[7]

The funeral was set for Wednesday, April 5, at 1 p.m. at the Nineteenth Street Baptist Church. Drew's body lay in state at Rankin Chapel on the Howard University campus all day Tuesday and Wednesday morning. Thousands came to pass by the casket and pay their respects. Florists in the city could not keep up with the demand. W. Montague Cobb described the scene: "The endless procession which passed through Rankin Chapel from noon to midnight as he lay in-state in an atmosphere of moving beauty and dignity were a token of the extent to which his character and achievements had gripped the public imagination."[8]

One of the mourners approached the bier in a wheelchair. She sat beside the casket for a moment and murmured quietly to the body of the fallen doctor then, turning, asked to meet Drew's mother. Nora was nearby, clothed in black. The woman was rolled beside her and spoke gently.

"Do you see this?" She pointed at the stump of her leg. "This is my baby. I was dying and some other doctors had given up on me. Your beautiful son told me he thought he could save me, but he'd have to amputate my leg. I told him to go ahead. I believed him. You see this stump? It's my baby. God bless you for having my savior."[9]

Fifteen hundred people crowded into and around the church Wednesday afternoon. Reverend Jerry Moore officiated. The eulogy was given by Mordecai Johnson, the venerable and revered President of Howard University, who spoke for over an hour. "In my 24 years at Howard University," he declared, "I don't recall such a staggering loss. Dr. Drew's death has been felt by students and graduates all over the world." Johnson went on to laud Drew's accomplishments in breaking through all barriers of prejudice to accomplish great things, "If he had died at 37, he would have been listed among the great benefactors of the human race." Rather than rest on those laurels, however, Drew had gone on to ignore the temptations of a career with greater reward to devote himself to the education of Black surgeons. "Here we have what rarely happens in history . . . a life which crowds into a handful of years significance so great men will never be able to forget it."[10]

The pall bearers were Drew's three old friends from Dunbar High School and Amherst College, William H. Hastie, Mercer Cook, and W. Montague Cobb, as well as R. Frank Jones and Burke Syphax from the department of surgery and Leonard Hall. Allen Whipple and John Scudder came down from New York to serve as honorary pallbearers.

In Tuskegee, at exactly one o'clock, as the funeral began in Washington, the entire Andrew Clinic stopped for a minute of silence.[11]

Thousands of people and vehicles comprised the miles-long funeral procession to Lincoln Cemetery; more than one onlooker compared it to that of President Franklin D. Roosevelt, five years before.

Drew's friend and counterpart at Meharry Medical College, chair of surgery Matthew Walker, composed a thoughtful and moving tribute:

> Not often in the life of an institution has such a valuable man as Dr. Charles Drew met such an untimely death in the height of his career. The Surgical Department here at Meharry is deeply grieved over the passing of this outstanding surgeon, scientist, and educator. And we can well understand how deeply you, his family and others feel at this loss. As another evidence of his farsightedness and greatness of his work he has trained a group of efficient men around him which will assure Howard University the same high caliber of surgery to which it has been accustomed, although I must admit that nobody can take the place of Charlie Drew. He was loyal to the administration, interested in the development of men and interested in all problems regarding our race; however, his greatness was not limited to our race. It so happens that he was my personal friend and I am most deeply grieved. For the rest of my life I will be urged on by the great spirit of Charlie Drew who died enroute to give service as he lived giving service.[12]

On Monday, April 10, 1950, the Honorable Hubert Humphrey of Minnesota rose to address his colleagues of the 81st Congress in the chamber of the United States Senate:

> Mr. President, on April 1 Dr. Charles Drew, an outstanding Negro physician and a member of our District of Columbia community, was killed in an automobile accident. Dr. Drew was a pioneer in the field of blood plasma and as a result of his brilliant research in that field saved thousands of British and American lives during the war. In 1943 he won the Spingarn medal for 'the highest and noblest achievement by an American Negro.' In 1940 he was

> awarded a doctorate in medical science by Columbia University and was most recently professor of surgery at Howard University and chief surgeon at Freedmen's Hospital.
>
> Dr. Drew's tragic accident is a profound loss to the whole American community. It is fitting that we in the Senate of the United States give his achievements due recognition and express to his family, to his friends and to the members of the Negro race our sorrow at the loss of this great American.
>
> I ask unanimous consent to have printed in the Appendix of the Congressional Record an editorial paying tribute to Dr. Drew which appeared in the *Washington Post* for April 6, 1950, as well as the obituary notice of his death, which appeared in the April 2, 1950, issue of the *New York Times*.[13]

After noting that Drew was one of "the most gifted of American surgeons," Humphrey went on to say that he "chose to devote his gifts to the advancement of medicine rather than to the advancement of personal career or to winning the monetary rewards that were easily within reach. He will be missed, however, not alone by his own race but by his whole profession and by men everywhere who value scientific devotion and integrity."[14]

Drew's friends and colleagues recognized that he had not amassed a great deal of money on which his family could now live, with not only their beloved father and husband but their sole source of income gone.[15] Almost immediately these benefactors set up the Charles R. Drew Memorial Foundation, chaired by R. Frank Jones, to help Lenore, widowed at age thirty six, and the four children: Bebe, now nine years old; Charlene, eight; Sylvia, six; and Charles Jr., four. Contributions came from friends and admirers across the nation.

The house at 328 College Avenue was owned by Howard University, and with that affiliation now officially severed, the Drews could not stay. In February 1952 they moved into a home at 4409 Eighteenth St. NW. The foundation provided $18,000 of the $32,500 purchase price; the rest would be paid by the family. The lion's share of this, and the means of support for the Drews in the years to come, was a pension that Lenore received from the university amounting to three-quarters of her husband's salary. She was entitled to this because her husband had died in the course of his work.[16]

In November 1951 Drew's name finally came up for election to fellowship in the American College of Surgeons. The assistant director of the organization later wrote, "When the application was presented to the Credentials Committee . . . we were informed of Drew's death in April of 1950, but the committee stated that they would have granted him full fellowship if he had been living." The Board of Regents then took the extraordinary step of conferring on Drew Fellowship of the College posthumously, the only time in the history of the organization that such a gesture was made.[17]

An unfortunate coda to the life of Charles Drew began to play out within weeks of his death. From sources that have never been elucidated, the rumor rose that Drew could have survived the injuries from his automobile accident but that he had been refused or received negligent care because he was Black. Variations on this unsupported theme proliferated, perhaps the most insidious incorporating the infuriating element of irony: that Drew could have survived but he, the surgeon-scientist famous for helping to elucidate the principles of blood banking, had been specifically denied a lifesaving transfusion because of his race.

There were certainly instances in the Jim Crow era when African Americans were denied treatment at white hospitals, or otherwise suffered from absent or suboptimal care for no other reason than their race, but even the very earliest news stories about the Drew accident, in both the Black and mainstream press, carried quotes from the survivors—Bullock, Ford, and Johnson, physicians all—that Drew had been given the best care available at little Alamance County Hospital. Those survivors continued to refute the false narrative throughout their lives, buttressed by the recollections of the Kernodle brothers, C. Mason Quick, Lucille Crabtree, and many others—including Lenore Drew herself, who, shortly after the funeral, penned a note to Ralph Brooks, co-owner of Alamance General Hospital, thanking him for the care her late husband had received.[18] Nevertheless, the myth of Drew's unnecessary death grew deep and strong roots, a veritable industry of misplaced rage that endured for decades before finally succumbing to the overwhelming weight of the evidence.

In April 1985 the son of Drew's sister Nora, Colonel Frederick Drew Gregory, took the Spingarn Medal his uncle had won onboard the space shuttle *Challenger*, where it orbited the Earth for a week.

A year later, on April 5, 1986, a memorial marker to Drew was unveiled along state route 49 in Alamance County, North Carolina, near the site of the automobile accident. The public event was heavily attended and featured choral music and speeches by many of Drew's admirers and colleagues, as well as his brother Joseph and daughter Charlene. The rectangular gray granite was engraved, "In Memory of Charles Richard Drew 1904–1950" and a bronze plaque beneath was emblazoned with these words:

CHARLES RICHARD DREW
1904–1950
BLACK SCIENTIST AND SURGEON
PIONEER IN THE PRESERVATION OF BLOOD PLASMA
MEDICAL DIRECTOR FOR THE BLOOD-FOR-BRITAIN PROJECT, 1940
DIRECTOR OF THE FIRST AMERICAN RED CROSS BLOOD BANK, 1941
TEACHER TO A GENERATION OF AMERICAN DOCTORS,
FREEDMEN'S HOSPITAL, HOWARD UNIVERSITY, WASHINGTON, DC
OUTSTANDING ATHLETE, AMHERST COLLEGE AND MCGILL UNIVERSITY
MEMBER OF OMEGA PSI PHI FRATERNITY
STEADFAST FOE OF RACIAL INJUSTICE
DIED IN ALAMANCE GENERAL HOSPITAL, 1 APRIL, 1950,
AFTER AN AUTOMOBILE ACCIDENT AT THIS SITE
"THERE MUST ALWAYS BE THE CONTINUING STRUGGLE TO MAKE THE INCREASING KNOWLEDGE OF THE WORLD / BEAR SOME FRUIT IN INCREASED UNDERSTANDING AND IN THE PRODUCTION OF HUMAN HAPPINESS."
CHARLES R. DREW

Four years later, a ten-mile stretch of route 49, including the monument at the accident site, was renamed the Charles Richard Drew Memorial Highway.

After the death of her son, Nora Burrell Drew remained active in the Nineteenth Street Baptist Church in Washington, DC, receiving numerous awards there for her exceptional service, particularly in the Jennie Dean Society. She passed away in 1962 at the age of eighty-one.

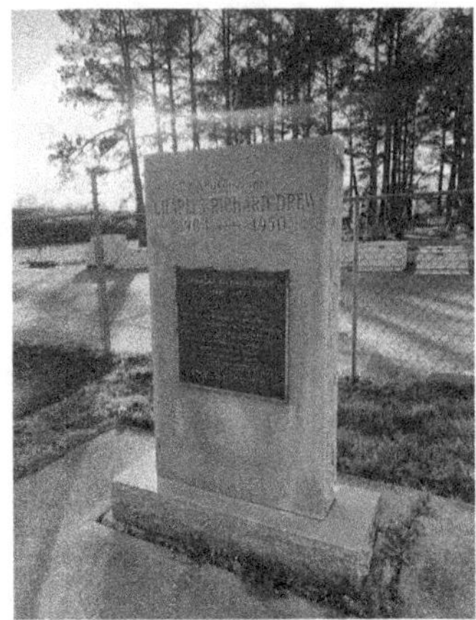

Figure 12.1 The Memorial to Charles Drew on N.C. route 49 in Alamance County, North Carolina.

Joseph Drew was a teacher in the Washington, DC, school system throughout his working life. He obtained a master's degree from Columbia University in 1963. He and Grace, who had a long career with the National Labor Relations Board and was considered the family historian, had three sons. Richard, their first son, died of a brain tumor while at the US Naval Academy; Jay (for Joseph) was a combat pilot in Vietnam; and Eric was successful in business. Joseph Sr. passed away in 1991, Grace in 2009.

Nora Drew Gregory remained a teacher in the public schools and, after retiring, became a leader in the District of Columbia Library system. Her husband Francis was also a teacher and leading administrator in the schools and DC libraries. A neighborhood library is named for him. The Gregorys had one son, Frederick Drew Gregory, who became an astronaut with NASA, flying on three space shuttle missions—as pilot of *Challenger* (where he carried his uncle's Spingarn Medal) and commander of missions aboard *Discovery* and *Atlantis*. He was the first African American to command a space mission. Nora passed away in 2011.

Eva, the youngest of Drew's siblings, also became a teacher after graduating from Miner Teacher's College. She married Phillip Johnson who, unfortunately, suffered from multiple sclerosis. After his death Eva remarried, this time to a New Yorker named John Pennington. The pair moved to St. Albans, New York, where they lived for thirty-five years. After her second husband's death, Eva returned to Arlington, Virginia, where she passed away a few months after Nora in 2011.

Minnie Lenore Robbins Drew successfully reared her four children, Bebe, Charlene, Sylvia, and Charlie, through college, then returned to the career she had set aside on meeting Charles Drew in 1939. She became a teacher at Burdick Vocational School, the United Planning Organization, and Morgan State College, where she was associate professor of home economics education and head of the Department of Home Economics. Spare hours found Lenore at the National Gallery of Art or listening to her beloved Wagner, Puccini, Gilbert and Sullivan, and Debussy. She passed away on January 25, 1992, and was buried alongside her husband in Lincoln Cemetery.

Bebe Drew Price earned a degree in French from Trinity College in Washington, DC, and taught that language in the District of Columbia Public Schools. She subsequently married Dr. Kline A. Price Jr. and managed his office while raising four children. The call to medicine was great. Bebe enrolled in the Howard University Medical School, loved her courses, especially in biochemistry, and then found that the two-year practicum had to give way to her duties at home. She has four very accomplished children. Kelly Price Noble, PhD, is an executive with a national veteran's group and clinical researcher in Parkinsonism in San Diego; Kline Armand Price III is an avid skier and bicyclist in Colorado; Kendall Drew Price, MD, is a pathologist in St Paul, Minnesota; and Reverend Kathryn Charlene Price Bronson, is in the final stages of her doctor of ministry studies at the Duke University Divinity School.

Charlene Drew Jarvis, PhD, graduated from Oberlin College with a degree in psychology, then earned a master's in psychology from Howard University and a doctorate in neuropsychology from the University of Maryland. After a decade of neurological research at the National Institute of Mental Health at NIH, she won political office after the assassination of Martin Luther King Jr. and became a political force in Washington, DC. She was later president of YMCA-founded Southeastern University. Among the honorary degrees she received were two from her father's *alma matri*, Amherst College and McGill University. From her first marriage came Ernest Drew Jarvis, an accomplished leader in the commercial real estate sector in Washington, DC, and the late Peter David Jarvis. She has two grandchildren, Ernest Drew (EJ) and Jacob Drew Jarvis. Her second marriage to Dr. DeMaurice (Bucky) Moses, an award-winning physician, occurred in 2013.

Sylvia Drew, JD, graduated from Vassar College and the Howard University School of Law. She spent many years as an attorney at the NAACP Fund in New York, challenging health disparities among African Americans and Native Americans. Moving to California with her husband, the late Ardie Ivie, Sylvia worked with the California Endowment on health access issues, led the T.H.E. Clinic in Los Angeles, was director of the Office of Civil Rights at the HHS, and was chief of staff to a powerful Los Angeles politician. She is now the special assistant to the president of the Charles R. Drew University of Medicine and Science in Los Angeles. Sylvia's children, Leslie Ivie, an attorney in private practice, and Drew Ardie Ivie, an avid bicyclist, still live in Los Angeles.

Charles R. Drew Jr. earned a degree in sociology from Howard University and became a teacher in the District of Columbia public school system. He also counseled families in poverty at the Washington Hospital Center. Ever the raconteur, Charlie could regale his listeners with stories, delivered standing up with his hands in his pockets, or using his hands especially at the punch line. He passed away in 2008.

Richard Laurey, Drew's fellow resident under E. L. Howes in the 1930s, succeeded his fallen colleague as chairman of the Howard University Department of Surgery. Laurey held the position for five years, then was succeeded by former Drew resident Clarence S. Green. Burke Syphax, another Drew trainee, took over in 1957. These men led the Department of Surgery on a continuing uphill trajectory. In 1970 Lasalle Leffall, the young medical student whose class was interrupted by the dreadful news of the chief's death, became head of the department, and carried the torch still further. Leffall was awarded the first Charles R. Drew Endowed Chair of Surgery in 1992. As one of Drew's trainees, Charles D. Watts observed, "What (Drew) did at Howard didn't collapse when he died. It was continued, very ably, by later chief surgeons. . . . Black surgical training has never been the same."[19]

Freedmen's Hospital finally closed its doors as a health care facility in 1975, replaced by the modern Howard University Hospital. The old building still stands, though, repurposed to house the university's John H. Johnson School of Communications. The new hospital is located on the former site of Griffith Stadium, where many years ago a young Charles Drew led Company E of the Dunbar High School cadets in review.

The name of Charles R. Drew lives on in a hundred places today: from the Charles R. Drew University of Medicine and Science in Los Angeles, California, to dozens of clinics, schools, libraries, and laboratories across the continent. At his undergraduate alma mater, Amherst College, there is a Charles Drew Memorial Cultural House residence; in Montreal, where he attended medical school, a Parc Charles-Drew; and at Columbia University, where his greatest scientific accomplishments occurred, a Charles Drew Premedical Society. In June 1981 the United States Postal Service issued a stamp in his honor, and in 2010 the 690-foot navy cargo ship *USNS Charles Drew* was launched. In his hometown of Washington, DC, the Charles Drew Memorial Bridge spans the neighborhoods of Edgewood and Brookland. The list goes on.

There can be little doubt, however, that the greatest legacy left by Charles Richard Drew was his indomitable spirit. His achievements in science, specifically the consolidation and furthering of knowledge in the field of blood preservation and the harnessing of technology and logistics to lead the way in wide-scale blood collection and processing, place Drew in the top ranks of physician-scientists produced by the United States in the twentieth century. This is to say nothing of the fact that this work contributed enormously to saving countless thousands of lives on the battlefields of World War II and beyond. Yet, despite that spectacular and profound contribution, it is his example, especially to the ranks of African American physicians he trained and inspired, but, more widely, to all who strive against mindless prejudice or devote something of their existence to the betterment of others, that lives on—immortal and unbroken.

"Excellence of performance will transcend artificial barriers created by man."

Notes

Chapter 2

1. Interview with Joseph L. Drew and Grace Ridgeley Drew, December 7, 1983. DC Public Library Oral History Project, 32.

2. Drew and Drew, interview, 11. Grace Ridgeley Drew: "[Never having the opportunity to teach] was a big disappointment to her." In that period married women were prohibited from teaching in the District of Columbia.

3. None of the Drew or Burrell homes in Foggy Bottom are still standing. The Burrell house, 1806 E Street NW, was located at the current site of the Department of the Interior Museum. By family tradition, when President Theodore Roosevelt passed the house riding through Foggy Bottom on the way to the White House, he would tip his hat at the matriarch and say "Morning, Emma." She would reply, "Morning, Teddy." 821 Twenty-First Street NW was near that thoroughfare's intersection with I Street. A period building, likely of similar appearance, still stands at 825 Twenty First Street NW.

4. Eva Drew Pennington, unpublished memoirs. Personal collection of Charlene Drew Jarvis. Some sources state that Drew was named after his paternal uncle, but his youngest sister, Eva, asserted that it was in honor of Dr. Marshall. Emma Burrell worked with the physician for many years in her capacity as a midwife.

5. Ulysses S. Wharton, notes for speech, undated. Personal collection of Charlene Drew Jarvis.

6. Pennington, unpublished memoirs.

7. W. Montague Cobb, speech at opening ceremony of Black History Week, Walter Reed Army Medical Center, Bethesda, MD, February 10, 1974. W. Montague

Cobb Collection, Stuart A. Rose Manuscript, Archives, and Rare Book Library, Emory University. Cobb/MSS 1413, Doctor Charles Drew.

8. M. M. Greenlee, *A Foggy Bottom Family: An Early Twentieth Century Account. An Oral History Interview with Nora Drew Gregory* (Washington, DC: The District of Columbia Public Library, 1995), 7.

9. Pennington, unpublished memoirs.

10. Interview with Joseph L. Drew and Grace Ridgeley Drew, 52.

11. Pennington, unpublished memoirs.

12. Pennington, unpublished memoirs.

13. Rawlins Park, which still exists, was named for John Rawlins, a Union general and confidant of Ulysses S. Grant who, after the Civil War, became an outspoken advocate of civil rights for Blacks.

14. Greenlee, *A Foggy Bottom Family*, 43.

15. Greenlee, *A Foggy Bottom Family*, 7.

16. Greenlee, *A Foggy Bottom Family*, 17.

17. Spencie Love, *One Blood: The Death and Resurrection of Charles R. Drew* (Chapel Hill: The University of North Carolina Press, 1996), 99.

18. R. A. Davis, G. J. Horton, D. V. Robinson et al., "Hidden in Plain Sight: The Culture of Excellent Black High Schools in the Era of Jim Crow," *Gifted Child Today* 47 (2024): 14–39.

19. *Saturae*, Paul Laurence Dunbar High School Yearbook, 1922. Charles R. Drew Papers, Moorland-Spingarn Research Center, Howard University, 134: 5–15.

20. "Dunbar High School (May 28, 1922)." *Sunday Star*, Washington, DC, 26.

21. Love, *One Blood*, 105.

22. *Saturae*, 1922.

23. Love, *One Blood*, 104.

24. Love, *One Blood*, 104.

25. Love, *One Blood*, 104.

26. Greenlee, *A Foggy Bottom Family*, 44.

27. Love, *One Blood*, 104.

28. Love, *One Blood*, 104. According to Drew's friend W. Montague Cobb, he began playing the saxophone while at Morgan College in 1926–28.

29. Pennington, unpublished memoirs.

30. Charles R. Drew Papers, Moorland-Spingarn Research Center, Howard University, 135: 5–15.

31. Pennington, unpublished memoirs.

32. Charles R. Drew application for Rosenwald Fellowship. May 1, 1931. Personal collection of Charlene Drew Jarvis.

33. Another factor that cannot have fostered a desire to stay in Washington, DC, was the infamous race riots that affected the city for several days in July 1919. Although the violence did not extend to Foggy Bottom, the entire community was undeniably shaken.

34. *The Drew Family Home, Arlington, Virginia, 1920 to 1992*. Personal collection of Charlene Drew Jarvis.

35. *Drew Family Home*.

36. Pennington, unpublished memoirs.

37. Interview with Joseph L. Drew and Grace Ridgeley Drew, 9.

38. "Dunbar Athletes Lead in School Track Meet," *Evening Star*, May 27, 1922, Washington, DC, 12.

39. In addition to Charles Drew, Dunbar boasted a constellation of alumni and faculty of the highest achievement in the arts, academia, science, and government, a listing of which is beyond the scope of this text. Ironically, the elimination of segregation in the District of Columbia school system in the 1950s had a deleterious effect on Dunbar High School. In earlier years the school achieved high academic standards by selectively admitting students from outside the Truxton Circle neighborhood; after the ruling the constraint to accept students only from the immediate locale eliminated this advantage.

40. H. Wade, *Black Men of Amherst* (Amherst, MA: Amherst College, 1976), 24. The Dunbar-Amherst connection was largely established by William Tecumseh Sherman Jackson, an outstanding scholar and athlete who was a member of Amherst's Class of 1892. After college he became an educator and was principal of the M Street School from 1906 to 1909.

41. Letter A. Meiklejohn to C. R. Drew, May 20, 1922. Charles R. Drew Papers, Moorland-Spingarn Research Center, Howard University, 135: 5–22. Biographical materials on Drew over the years have almost universally referred to his being awarded an athletic scholarship to Amherst, but a source for this assertion has proven to be elusive. President Meiklejohn's offer letter contains no such language, and Drew himself referred to his scholarship as being "scholastic." Charles R. Drew application for Rosenwald Fellowship (May 1, 1931). Personal collection of Charlene Drew Jarvis.

42. Amherst College Course Catalog, 1922–23.

43. *Saturae*, 1922.

44. Charles R. Drew Papers, Moorland-Spingarn Research Center, Howard University, 135:5–15. Among the many mentions of Charlie Drew in this edition of the *Saturae* was his classmate Francis Syphax's fanciful narrative of a future reunion in which Drew, having successfully pursued his goal of becoming an electrical engineer, attends the reception as vice president of the Chicago-Milwaukee Electric

Railroad, alongside "his pretty Boston bride." Charles R. Drew Papers, Moorland-Spingarn Research Center, Howard University, 135: 5–14.

Chapter 3

1. *The Class of 1926 Freshman Bible*, in Amherst College Administrative Publications Collection (Box 14), Amherst College Archives and Special Collections, Amherst College Library.

2. *The Class of 1926 Freshman Bible.*

3. A. Meiklejohn, *The Liberal College* (Boston: Marshal Jones, 1920), 38.

4. Wade, *Black Men of Amherst*, 5.

5. *The Class of 1926 Freshman Bible.*

6. *The Class of 1926 Freshman Bible.* The freshman regulations ceased on February 1, which was, as noted earlier, the due date for the final installment of tuition.

7. *The Class of 1926 Freshman Bible.* The statue depicts the nymph Sabrina being summoned in Milton's masque, Comus. As of this writing, the sculpture's whereabouts are unknown. College Hall, which is still standing, was a church in the town of Amherst before being purchased by the school. Among the luminaries to speak there before its repurposing was the noted Black abolitionist Frederick Douglass.

8. Amherst College Course Catalog, 1922–1923.

9. Transcript of Charles R. Drew, Amherst College Registrar's Office.

10. Transcript of Charles R. Drew.

11. *The Class of 1926 Freshman Bible.*

12. S. King, *The Consecrated Eminence: The Story of the Campus and Buildings of Amherst College* (Amherst, MA: Amherst College, 1951), 5. Scatchard later moved to MIT where, during World War II, he worked on the Manhattan Project as well as the government's blood plasma fractionation program.

13. "Dunbar High School," *The Sunday Star*, Washington, DC, October 29, 1922, 16.

14. "Pine Tree State Athletes, with Tootell Scoring 13 Points, End Engineers' Run of Track Victories," *The Boston Globe*, May 20, 1923, 20.

15. *Olio* Amherst College Yearbook, 1924.

16. Transcript of Charles R. Drew.

17. Transcript of Charles R. Drew.

18. Eva Drew Pennington, unpublished memoirs.

19. Transcript of Charles R. Drew.

20. The East-West Shrine Game pitted teams of collegiate all-stars against one another.

21. Letter D. O. McLaughry to R. Hardwick, August 17, 1966, Howard University, Moorland-Spingarn Research Center, Charles R. Drew Papers 136: 1–6.

22. Sport comment, *The New York Age* (New York: October 23, 1923), 6.

23. *Olio* Amherst College Yearbook, 1924.

24. Love, *One Blood*, 107.

25. W. Taylor, *A Glance at Amherst Athletics*, accessed July 21, 2023, https://www.amherst.edu/library/archives/sources-on-college-history-/virtual-history-bookshelf/etext-tower. Among Drew's extant papers is an envelope from the Boston section of the American Olympic Committee postmarked June 9, 1924. Unfortunately, it is empty.

26. *The Class of 1926 Freshman Bible.* Drew's mother displayed his trophies at home, where young Eva made it her job to keep them well polished. From time to time the young girl also convinced Mrs. Drew to put flowers in the cup-shaped awards.

27. Transcript of Charles R. Drew.

28. Transcript of Charles R. Drew.

29. "Amherst Tuning Up for Battle with Bowdoin," *Portland Evening Express and Daily Advertiser*, October 8, 1924, 6.

30. Letter D. O. McLaughry to R. Hardwick, August 17, 1966, Howard University, Moorland-Spingarn Research Center, Charles R. Drew Papers 136: 1–6.

31. *Olio*, 1924.

32. "Williams Team Holds Last Strenuous Drill," *The North Adams Transcript*, November 13, 1924, 14.

33. *Olio*, 1926, 152.

34. The origins of this trophy were described in the *Freshman Bible* for the Class of 1926: "The Tom Ashley Memorial Football trophy was given by Homans Robinson, '16, in memory of T. W. Ashley, who was killed in action in Belleau Wood in 1918 and is presented annually to the retiring member of the team who in the opinion of a committee consisting of Dr. Phillips, the coach and the Captain-elect, has best 'played the game.'"

35. *Olio*, 1926, 154.

36. O. Pilat, "A New Plateau of Life," in *Amherst Alumni News* (undated), Howard University, Moorland-Spingarn Research Center, Charles R. Drew Papers 135, 7–2. See also "Amherst Trainer, Peerless 'Builder of Men,' Praised by Grad," *The Pittsburgh Courier*, July 16, 1927, 1. F. Dwight "Doc" Newport was a local product of the Amherst area who became an assistant manager for the College's football and baseball teams shortly after finishing public school. At this point in time, he had been affiliated with Amherst for thirty-eight years, twenty-two as athletic trainer. Newport was universally loved and respected by his student-athletes.

37. "Drew Permanently Lost to Amherst," *Greenfield Daily Recorder*, January 16, 1925, 8.

38. "The Medical Context of Calvin, Jr.'s Untimely Death," accessed December 23, 2023, https://coolidgefoundation.org/blog/the-medical-context-of-calvin-jr-s-untimely-death/.

39. Letter D. O. McLaughry to R. Hardwick, August 17, 1966, Howard University, Moorland-Spingarn Research Center, Charles R. Drew Papers 136: 1–6. It is likely that Drew avulsed a ligament or tendon, resulting in the periosteal lesion, a tearing of the membrane that overlies bone. On a form he filled out in 1931, Drew recorded these as injuries he sustained in football: "broken ankles, rib and right wrist." Charles R. Drew application for Rosenwald Fellowship (May 1, 1931). Personal collection of Charlene Drew Jarvis.

40. *Olio* Amherst College Yearbook, 1926.

41. W. M. Cobb, "Charles Richard Drew, M.D., 1904–1950," *Journal of the National Medical Association* 42 (1950): 241.

42. *Olio*, 1926.

43. Howard University, Moorland-Spingarn Research Center, Charles R. Drew Papers 134: 5–21.

44. Charles R. Drew Papers 134: 5–21.

45. Transcript of Charles R. Drew.

46. Pennington, unpublished memoirs.

47. Letter E. H. Bensley to N. E. Edelen, May 11, 1966, McGill University Archives, P130-Drew_DrCharlesRichard-Folder1.

48. D. Hepburn, "The Life of Dr. Charles R. Drew," *Our World*, 1950, 25.

49. Transcript of Charles R. Drew.

50. Drew may well have noticed a recommendation in the Amherst College Course Catalog that "students intending to enter a medical school should elect (Biology) course 1 and 4." He had, of course, already finished Biology 1. A reported story that Dean Esty encouraged Drew's increased attention to scholarship with the admonition "Negro athletes are a dime a dozen" lacks attribution and appears to be apocryphal. John C. Esty was dean of admissions at Amherst in the 1950s and 1960s, long after Drew's years of attendance.

51. Cobb, "Charles Richard Drew," 241.

52. Cobb, "Charles Richard Drew," 241.

53. *The Class of 1926 Freshman Bible.*

54. *Olio*, 1926.

55. D. O. McLaughry, "The Best Player I Ever Coached," *Saturday Evening Post*, December 1952. In addition to playing collegiate and professional football, Tuss McLaughry served in the military in both world wars. After leaving Amherst he coached football for many years at Brown and Dartmouth Universities and was a major figure in the American Football Coaches Association. That

organization's highest honor, awarded annually to an American (or Americans) for distinction in service to others, is named for McLaughry. Recipients have included US presidents, astronauts, and distinguished figures from the worlds of the arts, military, and entertainment. National Football Foundation, "Tuss McLaughry," accessed December 29, 2023, https://footballfoundation.org/hof-search.aspx?hof=1597.

56. Cobb, "Charles Richard Drew," 240.

57. Cobb, "Charles Richard Drew," 240.

58. C. R. Drew, "Growth," Howard University. Moorland-Spingarn Research Center. Charles R. Drew Papers 134: 5–18.

59. "Williams Track Team Faces Amherst Rival," *The North Adams Transcript*, May 4, 1926, 11.

60. *Olio* Amherst College Yearbook, 1927.

61. Transcript of Charles R. Drew.

62. *Olio*, 1927.

63. Pennington, unpublished memoirs.

64. "Alumni Day at Amherst," *The Holyoke Daily Transcript*, June 21, 1926, 9.

65. *The Holyoke Daily Transcript*.

66. *The Class of 1926 Freshman Bible*.

Chapter 4

1. Howard University, Moorland-Spingarn Research Center, "Charles R. Drew Papers," 199: 1–6.

2. Morgan State University, "Our History," accessed December 23, 2023, https://www.morgan.edu/about/our-history. Morgan State became a university in 1975.

3. Newark, A. C., "Athletes Win Junior A. A. U. Meet," *Evening Star*, July 4, 1926, 49. Flippin later set national hurdling and pentathlon records. He became a distinguished physician at the University of Pennsylvania and the head doctor for the National Football League.

4. "College Football Results," accessed August 19, 2023, https://college-football-results.com/.

5. *The Morganite* (undated); Howard University, "Charles R. Drew Papers," 199: 2–9.

6. "College Football Results." Many of the early records of smaller college sports teams are incomplete or conflicting. The information provided here derives from the College Football Data Warehouse, a website that contains the most comprehensive compendium of such records.

7. *The Morganite* (undated); Howard University, "Charles R. Drew Papers," 199: 2–9. In later years Hill became assistant football and head basketball coach, as well as a professor, at Morgan.

8. *The Morganite* (undated).

9. *The Morganite* (undated).

10. "'Lanky' Jones and His Morgan College Quint Topples Howard, 24–19," *The Pittsburgh Courier*, January 15, 1927, 13.

11. "Morgan Halts Hampton, 20–10," *The Pittsburgh Courier*, March 19, 1927, 17.

12. W. M. Cobb, "Charles Richard Drew, M.D., 1904–1950," *Journal of the National Medical Association* 42 (1950): 241.

13. Both of Cook's parents were accomplished musicians; his father was a mentor of the legendary jazz artist Duke Ellington. During the time when Drew was at Morgan College, Cook was assistant professor of Romance languages at Howard University.

14. "Dear Omega," by Charles Drew and Mercer Cook, Gamma Xi Chapter of the Omega Psi Phi Fraternity, Inc., accessed August 21, 2023, https://www.gammaxiques.org/omega-dear.html.

15. Howard University, "Charles R. Drew Papers," 199: 1–19, 22.

16. Obituary for Lee Waller Smith, *The Boston Globe*, February 5, 2012, B10. Lelia went on to marry John Caswell Smith, a writer and sociologist who had a lengthy career at Bennington College in Vermont. She died in Cambridge, Massachusetts, in 2012 at the age of 103.

17. "Banquet Will Feature Father and Son Week," *Evening Star*, December 7, 1927, 17.

18. "Morgan College Downs Cheyney 57–0," *The Black Dispatch*, October 20, 1927, 8.

19. "Institute Held to 0–0 Tie by Morgan College," *The Pittsburgh Courier*, November 5, 1927, 18.

20. "Storer College Holds Morgan to 13-13- Tie," *The New York Age*, November 12, 1927, 6.

21. "Morgan Coach Gives up Job to Study Medicine," *The Baltimore Afro-American*, n.d., 12. Personal collection of Charlene Drew Jarvis.

22. C. E. Wynes, *Charles Richard Drew: The Man and the Myth* (Champaign: University of Illinois Press, 1988), 16.

23. Wynes, *Charles Richard Drew*, 16.

24. Howard University, "Charles R. Drew Papers," 199: 1–15.

25. Howard University, "Charles R. Drew Papers," 199: 1–6.

26. Love, *One Blood*, 113.

27. McGill Bicentennial, "West Indian Medical Students Protest Admission Quotas," accessed July 27, 2023, https://200.mcgill.ca/history/gamma-medical

-league-students-protest-and-petition-the-board-of-governors-over-quotas-put-in-place-by-mcgill-medicine/.

28. Letter J. C. Simpson to L. W. Douglas, January 14, 1938, McGill University Archives RG2 c46 file 442.

29. Letter J. C. Mackenzie to V. W. Lippard, October 17, 1939, Charles Drew Administrative Records, Archives & Special Collections, Health Sciences Library, Columbia University.

Chapter 5

1. "1926–1932 Annual Announcement of the Medical Faculty of McGill College," 1930, 107, https://archive.org/details/McGillLibrary-osl_robe_journal_1930-1935_99-103-session-17634/page/n107/mode/2up?q=1829.

2. W. Osler, "Books and Men," *Boston Medical and Surgical Journal* 1901 (144): 60–61.

3. "1926–1932 Annual Announcement."

4. To illustrate some of the flexibility involved with the medical school class schedule, there are existing class notes that indicate Drew attended lectures in internal medicine—a Third Division subject—in March 1930, his second year and fifth term. Howard University, Moorland-Spingarn Research Center, "Charles R. Drew Papers" 134:8–13.

5. "1926–1932 Annual Announcement."

6. "1926–1932 Annual Announcement."

7. Letter from C. R. Drew to R. Drew, undated. Personal collection of Charlene Drew Jarvis.

8. "1926–1932 Annual Announcement."

9. Letter from C. R. Drew to R. Drew, undated. Personal collection of Charlene Drew Jarvis.

10. "Two Records Go at McGill Track Meet," *The Montreal Gazette*, October 13, 1928, 24.

11. "One Record Falls as McGill Beats Varsity at Track," *The Montreal Gazette*, October 20, 1928, 22.

12. "Drew, McGill Track Ace, May Turn out for Senior Rugby," *The Montreal Gazette*, October 23, 1928, 16.

13. "Medicine Winners in Wood Cup Final," *The Montreal Gazette*, November 15, 1928, 19.

14. Letter from C. R. Drew to N. Drew (undated). Personal collection of Charlene Drew Jarvis.

15. Eva Drew Pennington, unpublished memoirs.

16. McGill University, "Calendar for the Session 1928–1929," 1928, https://archive.org/details/McGillLibrary-rbsc_calendar_mcgill_college_1928-1929_octavo13936-20947/page/356/.

17. University Notes: McGill University. *Canadian Medical Association Journal* (1934): 96.

18. The Royal Victoria Hospital, Montreal, Canada: "Forty-first Annual Report," 157, https://digital.library.mcgill.ca/images/penfieldfonds/large/penrvhannual_report1934.pdf. Some previous Drew biographical materials have confused John Beattie with William Walter Beattie, an unrelated Canadian bacteriologist at McGill who led a briefly contemporaneous career. Drew may have encountered W. W. Beattie in the classroom, as well. Ironically, W. W. Beattie was killed in an accident while on a research leave of absence in London, England, in 1934.

19. W. Montague Cobb collection, Stuart A. Rose Manuscript, Archives, and Rare Book Library, Emory University. Cobb MSS 1413, "Dr. Charles Drew." The Francis Pool and adjacent junior high school were named for Dr. John R. Francis, a distinguished African American obstetrician in the Washington, DC, community.

20. "Francis Swimmers Take Easy Victory," *Evening Star*, September 1, 1929, 42.

21. McGill University, "Calendar for the Session 1928–1929." Two of Drew's biochemistry exams have survived, one from November 1929 and one from January 1930. He scored, respectively, a 79 and a 74. In the absence of a class distribution, little can be imputed from these numbers, but based on his aggregate class standing they must have been at least satisfactory. Howard University, "Charles R. Drew Papers," 134: 7–2.

22. "Medicine Gains Honors on Track, *The Montreal Gazette*, October 12, 1929, 21.

23. "Varsity Obtains Stranglehold on Track Meet Title," *The Montreal Gazette*, October 19, 1929, 21.

24. Howard University, "Charles R. Drew Papers." Also found at https://profiles.nlm.nih.gov/spotlight/bg/catalog/nlm:nlmuid-101584649X49-doc.

25. Howard University, "Charles R. Drew Papers." Also found at https://profiles.nlm.nih.gov/spotlight/bg/catalog/nlm:nlmuid-101584649X49-doc.

26. Howard University, "Charles R. Drew Papers." Also found at https://profiles.nlm.nih.gov/spotlight/bg/catalog/nlm:nlmuid-101584649X49-doc.

27. Howard University, "Charles R. Drew Papers." Also found at https://profiles.nlm.nih.gov/spotlight/bg/catalog/nlm:nlmuid-101584649X49-doc.

28. Some sources have reported that Drew waited tables while at Amherst as well, but no primary evidence of this has surfaced.

29. Letter from D. O. McLaughry to Richard Hardwick, August 17, 1966. Howard University, "Charles R. Drew Papers." Also found at https://profiles.nlm.nih.gov/spotlight/bg/catalog/nlm:nlmuid-101584649X137-doc.

30. McGill University Calendar for the Session 1928–1929. https://archive.org/details/McGillLibrary-rbsc_calendar_mcgill_college_1928-1929_octavo13936-20947/page/362/mode/2up.

31. Pennington, unpublished memoirs.

32. Pennington, unpublished memoirs.

33. Interview with Joseph L. Drew and Grace Ridgeley Drew, December 7, 1983, DC Public Library Oral History Project, 72.

34. Pennington, unpublished memoirs.

35. Ernest R. Ball and J. Keirn Brennan, "Let the Rest of the World Go By" *Historic Sheet Music Collection,* (1919): 832. https://digitalcommons.conncoll.edu/sheetmusic/832.

36. Howard University, "Charles R. Drew Papers," 134: 6–17.

37. McGill University, "Calendar for the Session 1928–1929."

38. "McGill Athletes Gain Track Title in Kingston Meet" (October 18, 1930), *The Montreal Gazette*, 18.

39. McGill athletes gain track title in Kingston meet (October 25, 1930), *The Montreal Gazette*, 21.

40. Pennington, unpublished memoirs.

41. Charles R. Drew application for Rosenwald Fellowship (May 1, 1931). Personal collection of Charlene Drew Jarvis.

42. "The Four Principles of Philanthropy," *Social Service Review* 36 (1962): 452.

43. E. R. Embree and J. Waxman, *Investment in People: The Story of the Julius Rosenwald Fund* (New York, Harper and Bros., 1949).

44. Charles R. Drew application for Rosenwald Fellowship (May 1, 1931). Personal collection of Charlene Drew Jarvis.

45. Embree and Waxman, *Investment in People.*

46. M. Maxwell, *Charlie Drew's Book of Thoughts about God and Love and Beauty.* Personal collection of Charlene Drew Jarvis.

47. Maxwell, *Charlie Drew's Book.*

48. Pennington, unpublished memoirs.

49. Letter May Maxwell to C. R. Drew, February 1, 1934. Howard University, "Charles R. Drew Papers," 134: 1–17.

50. Pennington, unpublished memoirs.

51. V. Nakhjavani, *The Maxwells of Montreal*, vol. 2 (George Ronald Publishing, 2016). In 1937 Mary Maxwell wed Shoghi Effendi, the grandson of 'Abdu'l-Bahá, who was Guardian of the Bahá'í Faith, the highest authority in the religion. She became known as Amatu'l-Bahá Rúhíyyih Khánum and, after Effendi's death in 1957, took on the mantle of propagator and protector of Bahá'í. She wrote several books and traveled to 185 countries, meeting a litany of cultural and political leaders, including

heads of state, in a long life that ended in January of 2000, when the former Mary Maxwell was eighty-nine.

52. Personal collection of Charlene Drew Jarvis.

53. Technically, the McGill Faculty of Medicine regarded the second- and third-year classes bacteriology and pathology as clinical sciences although they did not involve actual patient contact.

54. "Four Records of Long Standing Go at McGill Meet," *The Montreal Gazette*, October 10, 1931, 17.

55. "McGill Athletes Keep Track Title by Large Margin," *The Montreal Gazette*, October 17, 1931, 18.

56. 1926–1932 Annual Announcement of the Medical Faculty of McGill College. https://archive.org/details/McGillLibrary-osl_robe_journal_1930-1935_99-103-session-17634/page/n155/mode/2up.

57. Howard University, "Charles R. Drew Papers," 134:8–13.

58. Pennington, unpublished memoirs. The former Vashti Smith was married to Drew's old friend, Mercer Cook.

59. Pennington, unpublished memoirs.

60. Pennington, unpublished memoirs.

61. *Old McGill*, 1933, 92. yearbooks.mcgill.ca/viewbook.php?campus=downtown&book_id=1933#page/1/mode/2up.

62. *Old McGill*, 253.

63. *Old McGill*, 256.

64. Letter C. R. Drew to E. R. Embree, April 9, 1948. Personal collection of Charlene Drew Jarvis.

65. The Dr. J. Francis Williams Scholarship. Annual Announcement of the Medical Faculty of McGill College 1926, 40, https://archive.org/details/McGillLibrary-osl_robe_journal_1930-1935_99-103-session-17634/page/n45/mode/2up.

66. Letter C. R. Drew to E. R. Embree, April 9, 1948. Personal collection of Charlene Drew Jarvis.

67. "Two Records Fall in McGill's 60th Interfaculty Meet," *The Montreal Gazette*, October 15, 1932, 17.

68. "McGill Scores 73 Points on Track to Retain Title," *The Montreal Gazette*, October 22, 1932, 14.

69. "Edwards Beaten, but McGill Scores," *The Montreal Gazette*, March 20, 1933, 17.

70. Howard University, "Charles R. Drew Papers," 134: 8–13.

71. The Wasserman test was the first blood test for syphilis. It has been superseded by superior methods.

72. Howard University, "Charles R. Drew Papers," 134: 8–13.

73. McGill University, "Calendar for the Session 1934–1935," 1934, https://archive.org/details/McGillLibrary-rbsc_calendar_mcgill_college_1934-1935_octavo13936-20923/page/310/mode/2up.

74. A 1939 letter of recommendation from the McGill surgeon Alfred Bazin states that Drew "obtained aggregate honours in his 1st and 5th years and Grade B plus in the other three years." Letter A Bazin to VW Lippard, October 12, 1939. Charles Drew Administrative Records. Archives & Special Collections, Health Sciences Library, Columbia University.

75. "Final Year Lists in All Faculties Posted at McGill," *The Montreal Gazette*, May 22, 1933, 11. The number of people in Drew's Faculty of Medicine graduation class is not clear. A contemporary newspaper article from the *Montreal Gazette* indicates that eighty-three MDCM degrees were awarded by McGill in May 1933. In December 1935, Drew noted on an evaluation form for the Rosenwald Fund that there were ninety-six students in his class. In 1948, in a letter to the Rosenwald Fund at the conclusion of that foundation's mission, he indicated that his class numbered 137 students. A woman named Ruth P. Dow placed first in Drew's class. She went on to join the faculty of McGill as a bacteriologist, primarily employed at the Alexandra Hospital, which specialized in childhood infectious diseases at the time.

76. McGill University, "Calendar for the Session 1934–1935, https://archive.org/details/McGillLibrary-rbsc_calendar_mcgill_college_1934-1935_octavo13936-20923/page/324/mode/2up.

77. "Blood Against the Blitz," *Ebony* 1 (1946): 31. The first appearance of this story is in an article about Drew from the January 1946 issue of *Ebony*. Although he is not quoted in the article, other items of Drew's personal history are reported accurately and he may have been the source. In other versions, Drew saved two men who suffered electrical burns with fluid infusion or a transfusion of his own blood. Later appearing variants include John Beattie alongside Drew, although Beattie was not a clinician and was likely either in England already or preparing to leave.

78. Letter C. R. Drew to W. M. Cobb, December 7, 1934. W. Montague Cobb collection, Stuart A. Rose Manuscript, Archives, and Rare Book Library, Emory University. Cobb/MSS 1413, "Doctor Charles Drew."

79. The letter of rejection from the Mayo Clinic does not survive, although there is an envelope addressed to Drew from the institution, dated December 8, 1934. The recollections of family and colleagues are, however, unequivocal. "Howard University, Charles R. Drew Papers," 135:1–17. There are notes on Buddhism in Drew's hand on the envelope: "Buddha Gautama 560 B.C. – the wis- white elephant dream, All existence involves suffering; suffering is roused by desire, especially the desire for continuance of existence; the suppression of desires will lead to extinction

of suffering Whatever is subject to origination is subject also to cessation or destruction."

80. R. S. Jason, "Charles Richard Drew." Speech at the dedication of Charles R. Drew Elementary School in Washington, D.C., April 1960. Howard University, "Charles R. Drew Papers," 136:1–2.

81. Letter C. R. Drew to W. M. Cobb, December 7, 1934. W. Montague Cobb collection, Stuart A. Rose Manuscript, Archives, and Rare Book Library, Emory University. Cobb/MSS 1413, "Doctor Charles Drew."

82. W. M. Cobb, "Charles Richard Drew, M.D., 1904-1950," *Journal of the National Medical Association* 42 (1950): 242.

83. Letter A. Bazin to V. W. Lippard, October 12, 1939. Charles Drew Administrative Records. Archives & Special Collections, Health Sciences Library, Columbia University.

84. R. Lambert R. Commentary on W. M. Cobb, "Numa P. G. Adams, M.D. 1885–1940," *Journal of the National Medical Association* 43 (1951): 54. Robert A. Lambert, an important figure on the Rockefeller Boards who had a lengthy professional relationship with Dean Adams, later noted that his diary from 1934 contained a reference to Adams being already interested in recruiting Drew in 1934, when he was an intern at Montreal General Hospital; Pennington, unpublished memoirs.

85. Pennington, unpublished memoirs.

Chapter 6

1. "1932–1933: Catalog of the Officers and Students of Howard University (1932)," *Howard University Catalogs*, 54. https://dh.howard.edu/hucatalogs/54.

2. Howard was wounded at the Battle of Fair Oaks in Virginia in 1862, an action for which he received the Medal of Honor. An imposing equestrian statue of Howard overlooks East Cemetery Hill at Gettysburg, where Howard was in overall command of the Federal forces for several hours on the first day of that epic battle. He later commanded the Army of the Tennessee in the western theater of the Civil War under Sherman.

3. W. Dyson, *Founding of the School of Medicine of Howard University* (Howard University General Publications, 1929), 5. https://dh.howard.edu/hupub/5. The initial classes were held on the second floor of a building in which one of the professors lived. Anatomic dissections took place here, too, until the family living on the first floor discovered the fact.

4. W. M. Cobb, "Numa P. G. Adams, M. D. 1885–1940," *Journal of the National Medical Association* 43, no. 1 (1951): 46.

5. Cobb, "Numa P. G. Adams," 49.

6. A. Flexner, *Medical Education in the United Sates and Canada* (Washington, DC: Science and Health Publications, 1910).

7. Although the origins of the NIH date to the nineteenth century, the organization only became a significant source of federal funding for medical education and research following World War II.

8. T. Bonner, "Searching for Abraham Flexner," *Academic Medicine* 73 (1998): 160–66. Flexner has received considerable negative attention from historians in recent years for what have been interpreted as derogatory remarks in his report regarding African Americans. It bears noting, however, that the evidence of his actions contradicts such characterization. As secretary of the GEB, Flexner was personally responsible for the distribution of large sums of money for Black education, particularly in the South. He was also reportedly the individual who persuaded Julius Rosenwald to establish the Fellowships for African American scholars, of which Charles Drew, as we have seen, was a notable recipient. After leaving the GEB, Flexner also became a member of the Board of Trustees of Howard University and its chairman in 1933.

9. C. E. Wynes, *Charles Richard Drew: The Man and the Myth* (University of Illinois Press, 1988), 36.

10. L. LeFall and B. Syphax, "The Howard University Department of Surgery and Freedmen's Hospital," in *A Century of Black Surgeons: The U.S.A. Experience*, ed. C. Organ and M. Kosiba (Transcript Press, 1987), 10; LeFall and Syphax, 9. To inaugurate a full-fledged clinical training program, Adams first had to obtain the approval of the Council on Medical Education and Hospitals of the American Medical Association (this organization continues today as the Accreditation Council for Graduate Medical Education). He succeeded in these efforts in February 1935, receiving permission to start such programs at Howard in obstetrics and gynecology, internal medicine, pediatrics, and surgery.

11. LeFall and Syphax, 9.

12. The Howard Department of Surgery had only one officially recognized position of surgery resident, which was held by Manly. When they moved into their clinical training years, Drew and Laurey were technically "assistants in surgery." Practically speaking, there was no difference. Laurey's first year was spent in a similar role to Drew but in the physiology department.

13. Howard University, Moorland-Spingarn Research Center, "Charles R. Drew Papers," 199–201: 4.

14. "1938–1939: Catalog of the Officers and Students of Howard University," *Howard University Catalogs*, 1938, 55. https://dh.howard.edu/hucatalogs/55.

15. Rudolph Virchow was a German physician, scientist, and polymath of the nineteenth century who is widely regarded as one of the founders of modern pathology. As noted earlier, McGill legend William Osler studied under Virchow in the 1870s.

16. C. R. Drew, "Pathology 170 Class Notes," January 7, 1935. https://profiles.nlm.nih.gov/spotlight/bg/catalog/nlm:nlmuid-101584649X89-doc.

17. "1938–1939: Catalog," 55.

18. Numa P. G. Adams, "Charles Drew's Faculty Evaluation from Howard University School of Medicine," National Library of Medicine, https://profiles.nlm.nih.gov/spotlight/bg/catalog/nlm:nlmuid-101584649X100-doc.

19. Howard University, "Charles R. Drew Papers," 134–39: 10.

20. Howard University, "Charles R. Drew Papers," 134–39: 21. As of July 1, 1937, Drew also owed Amherst $411 in student loans.

21. "The Drew Family Home, Arlington, Virginia, 1920 to 1992." Personal collection of Charlene Drew Jarvis.

22. "Drew Family Home."

23. L. LeFall and B. Syphax, "The Howard University Department of Surgery and Freedmen's Hospital," in *A Century of Black Surgeons: The U.S.A. Experience*, ed. C. Organ and M. Kosiba (Transcript Press, 1987), 11.

24. This text remains in print and is currently in its eleventh edition under the title, *Zollinger's Atlas of Surgical Operations*.

25. E. Cutler and R. Zollinger, *Atlas of Surgical Operations* (New York: MacMillan, 1939).

26. Eva Drew Pennington, unpublished memoirs.

27. "Drew Family Home."

28. Pennington, unpublished memoirs.

29. Pennington, unpublished memoirs.

30. Pennington, unpublished memoirs.

31. Pennington, unpublished memoirs.

32. Charles R. Drew, "Routines for Students on General Surgical Wards," National Library of Medicine, https://profiles.nlm.nih.gov/spotlight/bg/catalog/nlm:nlmuid-101584649X99-doc.

33. "Application for Admission to Graduate Studies in Clinical Medicine Leading to the Degree of Doctor of Medical Science," Charles Drew Administrative Records, Archives & Special Collections, Health Sciences Library, Columbia University, May 15, 1939. At this same time, Laurey began a fellowship in thoracic surgery at the University of Michigan. Manly continued as assistant in surgery for two more years at Howard but took a year-long GEB fellowship in orthopedics at the University of Iowa in 1940.

Chapter 7

1. As is often the case in the history of surgery, there are other valid claimants to the title of originator of the Whipple procedure; consideration of their merits is

beyond the scope of this book. Whipple also lent his name to the constellation of clinical signs of hyperinsulinemia known as Whipple's Triad.

2. J. Howard, *The Life and Times of Allen Oldfather Whipple: The Missionary and Surgeon* (Toledo: Communica, 2007).

3. Letter A. O. Whipple to V. W. Lippard, October 16, 1939. Charles Drew Administrative Records, Archives & Special Collections, Health Sciences Library, Columbia University.

4. "Our History," Columbia Medicine, accessed December 10, 2023, https://www.vagelos.columbia.edu/departments-centers/department-medicine/about-us/our-history.

5. Letter A. O. Whipple to V. W. Lippard, October 16, 1939. Charles Drew Administrative Records, Archives & Special Collections, Health Sciences Library, Columbia University.

6. "A Letter from a Distinguished Emeritus Member of BBANYS," *Newsletter* (Blood Bank Association of New York State, 1970–71); 5:3.

7. "Letter from a Distinguished Emeritus Member," 4.

8. Letter C. R. Drew to N. Drew, June 18, 1938. Personal collection of Charlene Drew Jarvis.

9. J. Scudder, C. R. Drew, and L. W. Sloan, "Anhydremia in Appendicitis," *Surgical Clinics of North America* 19 (1939): 295–306. J. Scudder, M. E. Smith, and C. R. Drew, "Plasma Potassium Content of Cardiac Blood at Death," *American Journal of Physiology* 126 (1939): 337–40.

10. Program of the John A. Andrew Clinical Society, April 1942, https://www.nlm.nih.gov/exhibition/forallthepeople/img/639.pdf.

11. Wormley was the grandson of a congressman from North Carolina and a hotelier in Washington, DC. He attended college at Dartmouth.

12. Schomburg Center for Research in Black Culture, Manuscripts, Archives and Rare Books Division, The New York Public Library, "The Negro Motorist Green Book: 1939" New York Public Library Digital Collections, accessed December 29, 2023, https://digitalcollections.nypl.org/items/911d3420-83da-0132-687a-58d385a7b928. This prejudice was not confined to lodging. Restaurants, gas stations, and other facilities were also frequently off-limits to African Americans, which greatly complicated any travel. Several guidebooks were published, most notably *The Negro Motorist Green Book*, to aid Black travelers in finding establishments that would serve them.

13. Biography of Minnie Lenore Robbins. Personal collection of Charlene Drew Jarvis. On her birth certificate the middle name is recorded as Lenora. Pennsylvania Historical and Museum Commission; Harrisburg, PA; *Pennsylvania (State). Birth Certificates, 1906–1913;* Box Number: *444*; Certificate Number Range: *Philadelphia (Jackewski)—Washington (Furlong).*

14. Telegram C. R. Drew to M. L. Robbins, April 5, 1939. Personal collection of Charlene Drew Jarvis. By family tradition, on arrival late in the night Drew brushed past a nonplussed house mother to get to Lenore.

15. Lenore Robbins Drew, "Unforgettable Charlie Drew," *Reader's Digest*, 1978, 112, 135.

16. Letter C. R. Drew to M. L. Robbins, April 13, 1939. Personal collection of Charlene Drew Jarvis.

17. Letter C. R. Drew to M. L. Robbins, April 13, 1939.

18. Letter C. R. Drew to M. L. Robbins, April 13, 1939. Anderson's legendary Lincoln Memorial concert, which drew an in-person audience of seventy-five thousand and was live broadcast across the nation to millions more, was organized after she was prohibited from singing at Constitution Hall by the Daughters of the American Revolution. NAACP President Walter White, Eleanor Roosevelt (who resigned from the DAR in protest), and Secretary of the Interior Harold Ickes were mainly responsible for the auspicious venue change. Ickes introduced Anderson after an impassioned speech denouncing ongoing racial prejudice in the United States. Cary O'Dell, "NBC Radio Coverage of Marian Anderson's Recital at the Lincoln Memorial," April 9, 1939. https://www.loc.gov/static/programs/national-recording-preservation-board/documents/MarianAndersonLincolnMem.pdf.

19. Letter C. R. Drew to M. L. Robbins, April 9, 1939. Personal collection of Charlene Drew Jarvis.

20. Letter C. R. Drew to M. L. Robbins, April 13, 1939.

21. Letter C. R. Drew to M. L. Robbins, April 16, 1939. Personal collection of Charlene Drew Jarvis.

22. Letter C. R. Drew to M. L. Robbins, April 16, 1939.

23. Letter C. R. Drew to M. L. Robbins, May 3, 1939. Personal collection of Charlene Drew Jarvis.

24. Letter C. R. Drew to M. L. Robbins, May 3, 1939.

25. Letter C. R. Drew to M. L. Robbins, May 3, 1939.

26. Letter C. R. Drew to M. L. Robbins, May 7, 1939. Personal collection of Charlene Drew Jarvis.

27. Helen Stoddard was a Canadian-born, Columbia-trained nurse who would serve as head nurse of the blood bank until 1945.

28. Memorandum, "Things to do," May 11, 1939. https://profiles.nlm.nih.gov/spotlight/bg/catalog/nlm:nlmuid-101584649X139-doc.

29. Letter C. R. Drew to M. L. Robbins, May 11, 1939.

30. Whipple AO, Department of Surgery, in Annual Report of the President and Treasurer to the Trustees with Accompanying Documents for the Year Ending June 30, 1939. New York, Morningside Heights, 1939, 134.

31. "Letter from a Distinguished Emeritus Member," 3.

32. Letter C. R. Drew to M. L. Robbins, May 17, 1939. Personal collection of Charlene Drew Jarvis.

33. In several of these early letters Drew mentions potential employment for Lenore at Howard University, in the departments of home economics, nursing, and even theater (at Spelman College Lenore was involved in theater productions). He arranged meetings for her with the leaders of these departments, but it is not known if they took place.

34. Letter C. R. Drew to M. L. Robbins, May 21, 1939. Personal collection of Charlene Drew Jarvis.

35. Robert A. Lambert, MD, noted earlier, was associate director of the Medical Sciences Program of the Rockefeller Foundation.

36. Letter C. R. Drew to M. L. Robbins, May 21, 1939.

37. Letter C. R. Drew to M. L. Robbins, May 21, 1939.

38. Letter C. R. Drew to M. L. Robbins, May 21, 1939.

39. Letter A. O. Whipple to V. W. Lippard, October 16, 1939, Charles Drew Administrative Records, Archives & Special Collections, Health Sciences Library, Columbia University.

40. Spencie Love, *One Blood: The Death and Resurrection of Charles R. Drew* (University of North Carolina Press, 1996), 121.

41. Letter M. L. Robbins to parents, June 10, 1939. Personal collection of Charlene Drew Jarvis.

42. Letter M. L. Robbins to parents, June 10, 1939.

43. Letter C. R. Drew to M. L. Robbins, June 9, 1939. Personal collection of Charlene Drew Jarvis.

44. Letter C. R. Drew to M. L. Robbins, July 3, 1939. Personal collection of Charlene Drew Jarvis.

45. Letter C. R. Drew to M. L. Robbins, July 3, 1939.

46. Letter V. W. Lippard to A. O. Whipple, October 10, 1939, Charles Drew Administrative Records, Archives & Special Collections, Health Sciences Library, Columbia University.

47. Letter N. P. G. Adams to V. W. Lippard, October 11, 1939, Charles Drew Administrative Records, Archives & Special Collections, Health Sciences Library, Columbia University.

48. Letter J. C. Mackenzie to V. W. Lippard, October 17, 1939, Charles Drew Administrative Records, Archives & Special Collections, Health Sciences Library, Columbia University.

49. Letter A. Bazin to V. W. Lippard, October 12, 1939, Charles Drew Administrative Records, Archives & Special Collections, Health Sciences Library, Columbia University.

50. Letter J. C. Mackenzie to V. W. Lippard, October 17, 1939, Charles Drew Administrative Records, Archives & Special Collections, Health Sciences Library, Columbia University; Letter A. Bazin to V. W. Lippard, October 12, 1939, Charles Drew Administrative Records, Archives & Special Collections, Health Sciences Library, Columbia University.

51. "Application for Admission to Graduate Studies in Clinical Medicine Leading to the Degree of Doctor of Medical Science," May 15, 1939, Charles Drew Administrative Records, Archives & Special Collections, Health Sciences Library, Columbia University.

52. Letter C. R. Drew to M. L. Robbins, July 12, 1939. Personal collection of Charlene Drew Jarvis.

53. Letter C. R. Drew to M. L. Robbins, July 19, 1939. Personal collection of Charlene Drew Jarvis.

54. Letter C. R. Drew to M. L. Robbins, July 19, 1939. Drew had used the expression "bright new steel" to describe the men tested by athletics in his widely reprinted *Morganite* article from thirteen years before.

55. C. R. Drew, *Banked Blood: A Study in Blood Preservation*. Submitted in partial fulfillment of the requirements for the degree of doctor of medical science in the Faculty of Medicine (Columbia University, 1940), 205–8.

56. Drew, *Banked Blood*, 208.

57. Drew, *Banked Blood*, 2.

58. Eva Drew Pennington, unpublished memoirs.

59. Pennington, unpublished memoirs.

60. F. D. Jordà, "El Servicio de Transfusión de Sangre de Barcelona," *Técnices y Utiliaje. Rev. Sanided de Guerra* 1 (1937): 621.

61. Beginning around this time, and extending even to the present day, was a protracted and energetic controversy—beyond the scope of the present text—centered around the infusion of colloid solutions (water with insoluble particles such as proteins, e.g., serum, plasma, or a solution of proteins such as albumin) or crystalloid ones (water with electrolytes) in shock and fluid resuscitation.

62. J. Scudder, R. L. Zwever, and A. O. Whipple, "Acute Intestinal Obstruction. Evaluation of Results in Twenty-one Hundred Fifty Cases; with Detailed Studies of Twenty-five Showing Potassium as a Toxic Factor," *Annals of Surgery* 107 (1938): 161–99.

63. Scudder filed a patent for this design on April 1, 1939. In October 1942 he had the patent assigned to Drew with the stipulation that any proceeds from the invention be applied to surgical research at Howard University. "Apparatus for Preserving Blood," US 2301710 A. Serial No. 265, 560.

64. Drew, *Banked Blood*, 203–4.

65. United States Census 1940, Census Place: *New York, New York, New York*; Roll: *m-t0627-02671*; Page: *5B*; Enumeration District: *31–1949A*.

66. Drew, *Banked Blood*, 212. In an article written for *Reader's Digest* in 1978, "Unforgettable Charle Drew," Lenore stated that she worked as a volunteer at the blood bank. The 1940 United States Census recorder who visited the Drew apartment on April 8, 1940, reported Lenore's income as $1,200 per annum. Drew's income was reported as "0," and no occupation was given for him. Although valuable, the dependability of census records is limited. Drew himself reported an income of $1,800 on his application for the Columbia graduate program.

67. Drew, *Banked Blood*.

68. "Memorandum from Charles R. Drew to John Bush (on the establishment of a permanent 'blood bank')," January 31, 1940, https://profiles.nlm.nih.gov/spotlight/bg/catalog/nlm:nlmuid-101584649X21-doc.

69. Letter A. O. Whipple to V. W. Lippard, April 16, 1940. Charles Drew Administrative Records. Archives & Special Collections, Health Sciences Library, Columbia University.

70. "Letter from a Distinguished Emeritus Member," 4.

71. "Letter from a Distinguished Emeritus Member," 4. Drew's doctoral thesis was never published, although from this work he did generate no less than nine papers that appeared in the literature. In chronological order of publication, these were Scudder J, Smith ME, and Drew CR, "Plasma Potassium Content of Cardiac Blood at Death," *American Journal of Physiology* 126 (1939); Scudder J, Drew CR, Corcoran DR, and Bull DC, "Studies in Blood Transfusion: Repartition of Potassium in Cells and Plasma," *Journal of the American Medical Association* 112, no. 22 (3 June 1939); Drew CR, Edsall K, and Edsall J, "Studies in Blood Preservation: Fate of Cellular Elements in Relation to Potassium Diffusion," *Journal of Laboratory and Clinical Medicine* 25, no. 3 (December 1939); Smith ME, Tuthill E, Drew CR, and Scudder J, "Studies in Blood Preservation: Some Effects of Carbon Dioxide," Journal of Biological Chemistry,133, no. 2 (1940); Drew CR, Scudder J, Papps J, "Controlled Fluid Therapy with Hematocrit, Specific Gravity, and Plasma Protein Determinations, *Surgery, Gynecology, and Obstetrics* 70 (May 1940); Scudder J, Drew CR, and Virgil G. Damon, "Studies on the Preservation of Placental Blood," *American Journal of Obstetrics and Gynecology* 40 (July 1940); Scudder J, Bishop K, and Drew CR, "Studies in Blood Preservation: The Shape of the Container," *Journal of the American Medical Association* 115 (27 July 1940); Bull DC and Drew CR, "The Preservation of Blood," *Annals of Surgery* 112, no. 4 (October 1940); and Drew CR, and Scudder J, "Studies in Blood Preservation: Fate of Cellular Elements and Prothrombin in Citrated Blood," *Journal of Laboratory and Clinical Medicine* 26, no. 9 (June 1941).

72. M. Ravitch, *A Century of Surgery: The History of the American Surgical Association* (Philadelphia: J. D. Lippincott, 1981), 820–22. Which author presented the Drew/Bull paper was not recorded.

73. E. B. Henderson, *The Negro in Sports* (Washington, DC: Associated Publishers, 1939).

74. Letter C. R. Drew to E. B. Henderson, May 31, 1940, https://profiles.nlm.nih.gov/spotlight/bg/catalog/nlm:nlmuid-101584649X87-doc.

75. Program for 196th Annual Commencement, Columbia University, June 4, 1940. Personal collection of Charlene Drew Jarvis.

76. Letter C. R. Drew to E. R. Embree, April 9, 1948. Personal collection of Charlene Drew Jarvis.

Chapter 8

1. "A Letter from a Distinguished Emeritus Member of BBANYS," *Newsletter* (Blood Bank Association of New York State, 1970–71), 5:4.

2. G. R. Ward, "Transfusion of Plasma," *British Medical Journal* 1 (1918): 301.

3. J. Watson, S. Pati, and M. Schreiber, "Plasma Transfusion: History, Current Realities, and Novel Improvements," *Shock* 46 (2016): 469. Both of these men provided Scudder with plasma for his electrophoresis experiments.

4. "Dans les champs de l'observation le hasard ne favorise que les esprits prepares." Pasteur made this remark in his inaugural speech as professor and dean of the Faculty of Science at the University of Lille on December 7, 1854.

5. "Letter from a Distinguished Emeritus Member," 4.

6. Executive Order 2859—National Research Council of the National Academy of Sciences, May 11, 1918, accessed December 12, 2023, http://www.presidency.ucsb.edu/ws/index.php?pid=58834. The National Research Council was created in 1916 under the overall charter of the National Academy of Sciences. Its existence was formalized under an executive order from President Woodrow Wilson that read, in part, that the mission of the council was "to stimulate research in the mathematical, physical, and biological sciences, and in the application of these sciences to engineering, agriculture, medicine, and other useful arts, with the object of increasing knowledge, of strengthening the national defense, and of contributing in other ways to the public welfare." Since it was created during the First World War, the main focus of the council at that time was research for military purposes. In 1940, with the threat of war looming, the work of the organization moved in that direction again.

7. D. Stetten, "The Blood Plasma for Great Britain Project," *Bulletin of the New York Academy of Medicine* 17 (1941): 27–28.

8. *Report of the Blood Transfusion Betterment Association Concerning the Project for Supplying Blood Plasma to England, Which Has Been Carried on Jointly with the American Red Cross from August, 1940 to January, 1941: Narrative Account of Work and Medical Report* (New York: Blood Transfusion Association, 1941), 4.

9. *Blood Transfusion Betterment Association*, 4.

10. *Blood Transfusion Betterment Association*, 5.

11. Letter C. R. Drew to N. Drew, October 25, 1940. Personal collection of Charlene Drew Jarvis. Lenore later indicated that the name "Bebe" originated with the Columbia nurses.

12. William Warrick Cardoza was a pediatrician at Howard University, noted for his work on sickle cell anemia.

13. Letter C. R. Drew to L. Drew, August 13, 1940. Personal collection of Charlene Drew Jarvis.

14. W. M. Cobb, "Numa P. G. Adams, M. D. 1885–1940," *Journal of the National Medical Association* 43 (1951): 46. Writing in eulogy a decade after Adams's death, W. Montague Cobb held that the former dean, who had recruited him, was a martyr to the politics of his institution, going so far as to suggest that Adams, in his struggles against the status quo, delayed treatment of his own fatal illness beyond the possibility of cure.

15. Letter C. R. Drew to J. Becker, July 11, 1944, https://profiles.nlm.nih.gov/spotlight/bg/catalog/nlm:nlmuid-101584649X105-doc. Beattie's original telegram appears to have been lost many years ago.

16. C. E. Wynes, *Charles Richard Drew: The Man and the Myth* (University of Illinois Press, 1988), 36.

17. *Report of the Blood Transfusion Betterment Association*, 4–5.

18. Stetten, "Blood Plasma for Great Britain," 33.

19. Stetten, "Blood Plasma for Great Britain," 36; Wynes, *Charles Richard Drew*, 60. Despite Stetten's characterization of the unanimous choice of Drew, some sources indicate that Scudder, who naturally had many of the same qualifications as his protégé and was, moreover, immediately at hand, was offered the position of medical supervisor first, but that his other responsibilities at the Rockefeller Institute and Columbia precluded his accepting the role.

20. Letter C. R. Drew to J. Becker, July 11, 1944, https://profiles.nlm.nih.gov/spotlight/bg/catalog/nlm:nlmuid-101584649X105-doc.

21. Stetten, "Blood Plasma for Great Britain," 34.

22. Wynes, *Charles Richard Drew*, 67.

23. Stetten, "Blood Plasma for Great Britain," 33.

24. *Report of the Blood Transfusion Betterment Association*, 50.

25. "Letter from a Distinguished Emeritus Member," 4.

26. Grace Drew gave birth to a son, Eric, on September 24, 1940.

27. Letter C. R. Drew to L. Drew, September 29, 1940. Personal collection of Charlene Drew Jarvis.

28. Stetten, "Blood Plasma for Great Britain," 29.

29. Stetten, "Blood Plasma for Great Britain," 33.

30. Letter C. R. Drew to N. Drew, October 25, 1940. Personal collection of Charlene Drew Jarvis.

31. *Report of the Blood Transfusion Betterment Association*, 23.

32. *Report of the Blood Transfusion Betterment Association*, 62–63. "This bottle was accepted as the standard container when the project first opened. In mass production, however, with many volunteer workers doing the phlebotomies certain disadvantages soon became obvious. These were: 1. A rather small but definite and constant percentage of bloods were lost through clotting as the result of the inability to mix thoroughly the citrate and the blood during the bleeding. 2. As a result of the very high percentage of women donors whose blood counts run far below those of the average male, the line of demarcation between the plasma and the cells in a large percentage of cases fell not in the narrow constricted neck but rather in the wide bulbous lower part of the bottle. This of course defeated the purpose for which the bottles were constructed. 3. Some cells in many cases settled on the slope of the upper bulb and at the time of removing or siphoning the plasma were often sucked into the pooling flask thereby causing a plasma less clear than desirable."

33. A. Yancey, "The Life of Charles R. Drew, M.D., M.D.Sc. and Perspectives of a Former Resident in General Surgery," in *A Century of Black Surgeons: The U.S.A. Experience*, ed. C. Organ and M. Kosiba (Transcript Press, 1987), 79.

34. Letter C. R. Drew to L. Drew, undated. Personal collection of Charlene Drew Jarvis.

35. Letter C. R. Drew to L. Drew, December 9, 1940. Personal collection of Charlene Drew Jarvis.

36. In addition to those individuals already mentioned, Drew had correspondence during the program with such leaders as Evarts Graham, a world-renowned thoracic surgeon at Washington University in St. Louis; Alton Ochsner, chief of surgery at Tulane University, Elliot C. Cutler, Moseley Professor of Surgery at Harvard University and the Peter Bent Brigham Hospital, Winford H. Smith, director of the Johns Hopkins Hospital, Mont Reid of the University of Cincinnati, and Roy McClure of the Henry Ford Hospital.

37. Letter C. R. Drew to L. Drew, February 10, 1941. Personal collection of Charlene Drew Jarvis.

38. At this time the association changed its name to omit the word "Betterment."

39. Letter C. R. Drew to L. Drew, February 10, 1941.

40. *Report of the Blood Transfusion Betterment Association*, 11.

41. Writing in his authoritative history composed long after the war, *Blood Program in World War Two*, then brigadier general Douglas Kendrick observed: "The blood for Britain project was a most valuable introduction to the later development of the American Red Cross blood donor service. The experience of the New York chapter served as a pattern for the organization and operation of the blood donor service which was to supply plasma for the armed forces and blood for overseas shipment. This chapter was ready to begin operations as soon as the Surgeons General of the Army and the Navy requested the American Red Cross to be responsible for the blood donor program. There were many mistakes made in the operation of the blood and plasma program during the United States participation in World War 2, but far more would have been made without the trial and error experience of the Blood for Britain project. The chief lesson learned was that blood and plasma, if they are to remain uncontaminated and safe for use, must be handled in a completely closed system. The vacuum system devised by Elliott in 1936 ended this particular problem. The gravity system of bleeding may be less damaging to red blood cells than a vacuum system, but only the completely closed system possible with the vacuum bottle ensures sterility." D. Kendrick, *Blood Program in World War 2*, Medical Department, United States Army (Washington, DC: Office of the Surgeon General, Dept. of the Army, 1964), 13.

42. In the weeks following Pearl Harbor, Drew was declared 3A by the Selective Service System, a classification of deferral because absence would cause hardship upon his family. Drew described himself at that time as six feet tall, weighing two hundred pounds, with hazel eyes, brown hair, and light freckled skin. Letter C. R. Drew to L. Drew, January 9, 1940. 1942 Selective Service Registration card, Charles R. Drew, Howard University, Moorland-Spingarn Research Center, Charles R. Drew Papers, 134: 1–10.

43. Letter C. R. Drew to L. Drew, January 9, 1940, personal collection of Charlene Drew Jarvis. Draft cards of Charles R. Drew, Charles R. Drew Papers, Moorland-Spingarn Research Center, Howard University, 134: 1–10.

44. *Report of the Blood Transfusion Betterment Association*, 107.

45. Minutes of Meeting of the Board of Medical Control, Blood Transfusion Betterment Association, January 8, 1941, https://profiles.nlm.nih.gov/spotlight/bg/catalog/nlm:nlmuid-101584649X28-doc.

46. Letter C. R. Drew to L. Drew, February 10, 1941. Personal collection of Charlene Drew Jarvis.

47. Letter C. R. Drew to L. Drew, February 24, 1941. Personal collection of Charlene Drew Jarvis.

48. "Transcript of Comments by Charles Drew at American Human Serum Symposium," June 2–3, 1941, https://profiles.nlm.nih.gov/spotlight/bg/catalog/nlm:nlmuid-101584649X64-doc.

49. "Comments by Charles Drew."

50. Letter C. R. Drew to L. Drew, March 10, 1941. Personal collection of Charlene Drew Jarvis.

51. Letter C. R. Drew to L. Drew, March 17, 1941. Personal collection of Charlene Drew Jarvis.

52. Yancey, "Life of Charles R. Drew," 79–80.

53. Letter C. R. Drew to L. Drew, March 17, 1941. Personal collection of Charlene Drew Jarvis.

54. Yancey, "Life of Charles R. Drew," 79.

55. Letter C. R. Drew to L. Drew, February 10, 1941. Personal collection of Charlene Drew Jarvis.

56. Letter C. R. Drew to L. Drew, March 24, 1941. Personal collection of Charlene Drew Jarvis, https://profiles.nlm.nih.gov/spotlight/bg/catalog/nlm:nlmuid-101584649X61-doc.

57. Howard University Press Release, February 1942. Personal collection of Charlene Drew Jarvis.

Chapter 9

1. B. Syphax, "The Howard Department of Surgery," *Journal of the National Medical Association* 59 (1967): 441–42.

2. L. LeFall and B. Syphax, "The Howard University Department of Surgery and Freedmen's Hospital," in *A Century of Black Surgeons: The U.S.A. Experience*, ed. C. Organ and M. Kosiba (Transcript Press, 1987), 13.

3. Syphax, "Howard Department of Surgery," 443.

4. Charles Drew quotes. Personal collection of Charlene Drew Jarvis.

5. LeFall and Syphax, "Howard University Department of Surgery," 15–16.

6. Syphax, "Howard Department of Surgery," 443.

7. J. E. White, "Dr. Charles Drew as I Saw Him," unpublished, 1965. Personal collection of Charlene Drew Jarvis.

8. "Letter C. R. Drew to L. Drew," personal collection of Charlene Drew Jarvis, March 24, 1941, https://profiles.nlm.nih.gov/spotlight/bg/catalog/nlm:nlmuid-101584649X61-doc.

9. Rosella was the middle name of Charles's mother, Nora.

10. Eva Drew Pennington, unpublished memoirs.

11. "The John A. Andrew Clinics," *Journal of the National Medical Association* 35 (1943): 106.

12. W. M. Cobb, "P. G. Numa, and M. D. Adams, 1885–1940," *Journal of the National Medical Association* 43 (1951): 45.

13. Cobb, "Numa and Adams," 46.

14. Department of Surgery, Freedmen's Hospital, Surgical Statistics, July 1, 1944–June 30, 1945, https://profiles.nlm.nih.gov/spotlight/bg/catalog/nlm:nlmuid-101584649X66-doc.

15. D. Kendrick, *Blood Program in World War 2*, Medical Department, United States Army, in World War 2 (Washington, DC: Office of the Surgeon General, Dept. of the Army, 1964), 101–6.

16. T. Guglielmo, "Red Cross, Double Cross: Race and America's World War II-era Blood Donor Service," *Journal of American History* 97, no. 1 (2010): 63–90.

17. Guglielmo, "Red Cross, Double Cross."

18. Howard University Press Release, February 1942. Personal collection of Charlene Drew Jarvis.

19. Since the release had no other apparent purpose, it seems to have been composed specifically as a response to the Red Cross policy.

20. J. Francis, "Negro Surgeon, World Plasma Expert, Derides Red Cross Blood Segregation," *Chicago Defender*, September 26, 1942, 1.

21. Charles Richard Drew, *Current Biography 1944* (Harold Wilson Company, 1945), 10–11.

22. Spencie Love, *One Blood: The Death and Resurrection of Charles R. Drew* (Chapel Hill: University of North Carolina Press, November 17, 1997), 156.

23. W. M. Cobb, "Charles Richard Drew, M.D., 1904–1950," *Journal of the National Medical Association* 42 (1950): 245.

24. C. R. Drew, "The Negro Physician in the Present War Effort," April 27, 1943. https://profiles.nlm.nih.gov/spotlight/bg/catalog/nlm:nlmuid-101584649X47-doc.

25. Douglass spoke these famous words as part of a speech given at National Hall in Philadelphia on July 6, 1863.

26. Drew, "Negro Physician."

27. Department of Surgery, Freedmen's Hospital, Surgical Statistics, July 1, 1944–June 30, 1945, https://profiles.nlm.nih.gov/spotlight/bg/catalog/nlm:nlmuid-101584649X66-doc.

28. H. Bims, "Charles Drew's Other Medical Revolution: Famed Pioneer in Blood Preservation Trained Vanguard of Black Surgeons," *Ebony* 30 (1974): 88.

29. "Drew's Achievements Are Almost Legendary," undated. Personal collection of Charlene Drew Jarvis.

30. J. E. White, "Dr. Charles Drew as I Saw Him," unpublished, 1965. Personal collection of Charlene Drew Jarvis.

31. Bims, "Charles Drew's Other Medical Revolution," 88.

32. Bims, "Charles Drew's Other Medical Revolution," 88.

33. Lenore Drew reminiscences. Personal collection of Charlene Drew Jarvis.

34. C. E. Wynes, *Charles Richard Drew: The Man and the Myth* (University of Illinois Press, 1988), 77.

35. Lenore Drew reminiscences. Personal collection of Charlene Drew Jarvis.

36. Love, *One Blood*, 165.

37. L. Drew, address to graduating medical students (undated), https://profiles.nlm.nih.gov/spotlight/bg/catalog/nlm:nlmuid-101584649X48-doc.

38. Cobb, "Charles Richard Drew," 244.

39. Cobb, "Charles Richard Drew," 244.

40. P. B. Cornely, "Charles R. Drew (1904–1950): An Appreciation," *Phylon* 11 (1950): 77.

41. Cobb, "Charles Richard Drew," 244.

42. "Dr. C. R. Drew Is Honored," *New York Times*, March 31, 1944, 23. In addition to his social activism, Joshua Elias Spingarn was a noted scholar in Renaissance comparative literature and an avid horticulturalist. He also cofounded the Harcourt, Brace and Co. publishing house and earned the rank of major in the US Army in World War I. His will included a bequest to fund the award that bears his name in perpetuity.

43. Lenore Drew reminiscences. Personal collection of Charlene Drew Jarvis.

44. Pennington, unpublished memoirs.

45. Program, Presentation of the 29th Spingarn Medal, July 16, 1944. Personal collection of Charlene Drew Jarvis.

46. Speech of Charles R. Drew at Spingarn Medal Award Ceremony, Chicago, Illinois, July 16, 1944. Personal collection of Charlene Drew Jarvis.

Chapter 10

1. A. Yancey, "The Life of Charles R. Drew, M.D., M.D.Sc. and Perspectives of a Former Resident in General Surgery," in *A Century of Black Surgeons: The U.S.A. Experience*, ed. C. Organ and M. Kosiba (Transcript Press, 1987), 92.

2. C. A. Miller, *A Time for All Things: The Life of Michael E. DeBakey* (London: Oxford University Press, 2019), 126.

3. Letter C. R. Drew to R. J. Coffey, January 18, 1950, https://profiles.nlm.nih.gov/spotlight/bg/catalog/nlm:nlmuid-101584649X119-doc.

4. Letter R. J. Coffey to C. R. Drew, January 25, 1950, https://profiles.nlm.nih.gov/spotlight/bg/catalog/nlm:nlmuid-101584649X120-doc.

5. J. A. Kenney, "Some Notes on the History of the National Medical Association," *Journal of the National Medical Association* 25, no. 3 (1933): 97–104.

6. P. J. Kernahan, "Medical Practice and Jim Crow," in *Black Surgeons and Surgery in America* (Chicago: American College of Surgeons, 2021), 72–73.

7. C. E. Wynes, *Charles Richard Drew: The Man and the Myth*, (University of Illinois Press, 1988), 85–86.

8. Letter C. R. Drew to M. Fishbein, January 13, 1947, https://profiles.nlm.nih.gov/spotlight/bg/catalog/nlm:nlmuid-101584649X126-doc

9. The International College of Surgeons was founded in Geneva in 1935. This organization began accepting Black American surgeons as members in 1945. Drew was inducted in 1946.

10. Charles Drew Curriculum Vitae, undated. Personal collection of Charlene Drew Jarvis.

11. Letter M. Fishbein to C. R. Drew, January 22, 1947, https://profiles.nlm.nih.gov/spotlight/bg/catalog/nlm:nlmuid-101584649X127-doc.

12. Letter C. R. Drew to M. Fishbein, January 30, 1947, https://profiles.nlm.nih.gov/spotlight/bg/catalog/nlm:nlmuid-101584649X128-doc.

13. Letter M. Fishbein to C. R. Drew, February 3, 1947, https://profiles.nlm.nih.gov/spotlight/bg/catalog/nlm:nlmuid-101584649X129-doc.

14. Letter C. R. Drew to G. Lull, January 31, 1947, https://profiles.nlm.nih.gov/spotlight/bg/catalog/nlm:nlmuid-101584649X134-doc.

15. Letter G. Lull to C. R. Drew, February 5, 1947, https://profiles.nlm.nih.gov/spotlight/bg/catalog/nlm:nlmuid-101584649X135-doc.

16. P. J. Kernahan, "Medical Practice and Jim Crow," in *Black Surgeons and Surgery in America* (Chicago: American College of Surgeons, 2021), 73. The AMA did not alter its bylaws to remove the control of membership from local societies, thus ending the policy that permitted race-based discrimination, until 1968.

17. Kernahan, "Medical Practice and Jim Crow," 74. Williams' reputation was so outstanding that white surgeons attended his clinics to watch him operate. He was also the first vice president of the National Association of Colored Physicians, Dentists, and Pharmacists, founded in 1895 in response to the AMA resistance. This organization became the National Medical Association in 1903. The John A. Andrew Clinical Society, which operated the annual Tuskegee Clinic, arose from the 1912 NMA conference.

18. Kernahan, "Medical Practice and Jim Crow," 90.

19. Letter C. R. Drew to J. Scudder, September 10, 1945, https://profiles.nlm.nih.gov/spotlight/bg/catalog/nlm:nlmuid-101584649X136-doc.

20. Letter C. R. Drew to R. J. Coffey, January 18, 1950, https://profiles.nlm.nih.gov/spotlight/bg/catalog/nlm:nlmuid-101584649X119-doc.

21. Letter R. J. Coffey to C. R. Drew, January 25, 1950, https://profiles.nlm.nih.gov/spotlight/bg/catalog/nlm:nlmuid-101584649X120-doc. In addition to Blades and Coffey, Drew's other referees were Whipple, Harry H. Kerr, and C. L. Hall.

22. "Stars of Stage, Radio, and Screen to Feature Newspaper Week Broadcasts," *Jackson Advocate*, February 23, 1946, 2.

23. Robert Gould Shaw, the son of Boston abolitionists, was colonel of the 54th Massachusetts Infantry Regiment, one of the first African American units in the Civil War. He was selected for this command by Massachusetts Governor John A. Andrew, for whom the Tuskegee Clinic was named. Shaw was killed in the regiment's assault on Battery Wagner near Charleston, South Carolina on July 18, 1863. The story of the regiment is dramatized in the 1989 motion picture *Glory*.

24. "Speech for the Temple Israel Brotherhood," Boston, Massachusetts, March 21, 1946, https://profiles.nlm.nih.gov/spotlight/bg/catalog/nlm:nlmuid-101584649X140-doc.

25. P. J. Kernahan, "Medical Practice and Jim Crow," in *Black Surgeons and Surgery in America* (Chicago: American College of Surgeons, 2021), 74.

26. C. R. Drew, "Annual Report of the Surgical Section of the National Medical Association," *Journal of the National Medical Association* 39, no. 6 (1947): 263–64.

27. Drew, "Annual Report of the Surgical Section," 265.

28. Drew, "Annual Report of the Surgical Section," 265.

29. Wynes, *Charles Richard Drew*, 117.

30. C. R. Drew, "World Health and the United Nations," *Journal of the National Medical Association* 40 (1947): 100.

31. *The Negro Problem* was an early twentieth-century collection of essays on race issues by prominent Black writers.

32. Letter C. R. Drew to J. F. Bates, January 27, 1947, https://profiles.nlm.nih.gov/spotlight/bg/catalog/nlm:nlmuid-101584649X113-doc.

33. Evans was an African American electrical engineer who was also on the Howard faculty. A graduate of MIT, he was instrumental in the efforts to integrate the armed forces.

34. C. R. Drew, "A Report to the Surgeon General, U.S. Army," September 15, 1949, https://profiles.nlm.nih.gov/spotlight/bg/catalog/nlm:nlmuid-101584649X46-doc. Subsequent details regarding the official aspects of Drew's 1949 European mission all derive from this report.

35. Drew, "Report to the Surgeon General," 17.

36. Letter C. R. Drew to L. Drew, July 3, 1949. Personal collection of Charlene Drew Jarvis.

37. Letter C. R. Drew to L. Drew, July 3, 1949. Personal collection of Charlene Drew Jarvis.

38. C. R. Drew, "Report to the Surgeon General."

39. Letter C. R. Drew to L. Drew, July 6, 1949. Personal collection of Charlene Drew Jarvis.

40. Letter C. R. Drew to L. Drew, July 10, 1949. Personal collection of Charlene Drew Jarvis.

41. Letter C. R. Drew to L. Drew, July 11, 1949. Personal collection of Charlene Drew Jarvis.

42. Letter C. R. Drew to L. Drew, July 17, 1949. Personal collection of Charlene Drew Jarvis.

43. Drew, "Report to the Surgeon General," 6.

44. Letter C. R. Drew to L. Drew, July 25, 1949. Personal collection of Charlene Drew Jarvis. Drew told his old friend W. Montague Cobb that this Europe trip was the "first real vacation he ever had." W. M. Cobb, "Charles Richard Drew, M. D., 1904–1950," *Journal of the National Medical Association* 42 (1950): 245.

45. Letter C. R. Drew to N. Drew, August 7, 1949. Personal collection of Charlene Drew Jarvis.

46. Letter C. R. Drew to L. Drew, July 29, 1949. Personal collection of Charlene Drew Jarvis.

47. Letter C. R. Drew to L. Drew, August 2, 1949. Personal collection of Charlene Drew Jarvis.

48. Letter C. R. Drew to L. Drew, August 9, 1949. Personal collection of Charlene Drew Jarvis. This hotel, an early modernist structure, was built in the 1930s and became popular with American officers during World War II. It still stands today as a "mixed-use development."

49. Letter C. R. Drew to L. Drew, August 9, 1949, personal collection of Charlene Drew Jarvis.

50. Letter C. R. Drew to L. Drew, August 9, 1949, personal collection of Charlene Drew Jarvis.

51. Letter C. R. Drew to O. Glaser, June 6, 1949, https://profiles.nlm.nih.gov/spotlight/bg/catalog/nlm:nlmuid-101584649X131-doc.

52. Letter O. Glaser to C. R. Drew, September 21, 1949, https://profiles.nlm.nih.gov/spotlight/bg/catalog/nlm:nlmuid-101584649X130-doc.

53. This organization was founded in 1915 by a group of scholars that included the eminent historian Carter Woodson. It continues today as the Association for the Study of African American Life and History.

54. C. R. Drew, "Negro Scholars in Scientific Research," *The Journal of Negro History* 35 (1950): 139.

55. C. D. Jarvis, "Remembering Special Times with Dad," *Washington Post*, December 25, 1981.

56. Charles Drew quotes, undated. Personal collection of Charlene Drew Jarvis.

57. Wynes, *Charles Richard Drew*, 78.

58. E. Cornwell, D. Chang, and L. Leffall, "The Southern Surgical Association History of Medicine Scholarship Presentation: Dr. Charles Drew, a Surgical Pioneer," *Annals of Surgery* 243 (2006): 616. Credit is due Dr. Edward Cornwell of the Howard University Department of Surgery for painstakingly reconstructing Drew's final day of March 31, 1950.

Chapter 11

1. Interview with LaSalle Leffall, Jr., November 19, 2010, https://profiles.nlm.nih.gov/spotlight/bg/catalog/nlm:nlmuid-101584649X143-doc.

2. W. Johnson, "April 1, 1950," *Journal of the National Medical Association* 76 (1984): 416–18.

3. C. E. Wynes, *Charles Richard Drew: The Man and the Myth* (University of Illinois Press, 1988), 2.

4. Johnson, "April 1, 1950."

5. Johnson, "April 1, 1950."

6. Wynes, *Charles Richard Drew*, 110.

7. Spencie Love, *One Blood: The Death and Resurrection of Charles R. Drew* (Chapel Hill: University of North Carolina Press, November 17, 1997), 21.

8. Love, *One Blood*, 23. Harold Kernodle later noted that the Alamance County physicians did telephone Duke, not to arrange transport but to ask for any recommendations as Drew's resuscitation proceeded.

9. Love, *One Blood*, 21.

10. Interviewed on September 19, 1985, Charles Kernodle recalled, "We started fluids on him, plasma probably. There was no time to give him whole blood. It took too long to crossmatch." Love, *One Blood*, 23. In February 1992, however, he stated, "No blood was given because it was not possible; the hospital had no blood bank." P. P. Craft, "Charles Drew: Dispelling the Myth," *Southern Medical Journal* 85 (1992): 1240. Both recollections, of course, came decades after the event.

11. Love, *One Blood*, 21. In a recollection from much later Ford reported that "his face was blown up like a balloon indicating a superior vena cava syndrome, as well as, I understand, many fractures." Craft, "Dispelling the Myth," 1240. In superior vena cava syndrome this large vein, which collects most of the venous blood

returning to the heart from the head, neck, and arms, is obstructed. This can lead, among other things, to the presentation described by Ford.

12. W. Johnson, "April 1, 1950," Drew's death certificate was signed by Harold Kernodle on April 1. He listed the Disease or Condition Directly Leading to Death as "automobile accident," with "1. Brain injury, 2. Internal hemorrhage lungs, and 3. Multiple extremity injuries."

Chapter 12

1. Spencie Love, *One Blood: The Death and Resurrection of Charles R. Drew* (Chapel Hill: University of North Carolina Press, November 17, 1997), 27–28.

2. Paul B. Cornely, "Charles R. Drew (1904–1950): An Appreciation," *Phylon* 11 (1950): 176–77.

3. Love, *One Blood*, 27.

4. Eva Drew Pennington, unpublished memoirs. Grayson McGuire operated the McGuire Funeral Home in Washington, DC. His father insisted on coming out of retirement to prepare Drew's body, feeling it to be an honor but also insisting that he was the best man for the job.

5. Yancey Arias, "The Life of Charles R. Drew, M.D., M.D.Sc. and Perspectives of a Former Resident in General Surgery," in *A Century of Black Surgeons: The U.S.A. Experience*, ed. Claude Organ and Margaret Kosiba (Transcript Press, 1987), 86.

6. Love, *One Blood*, 28.

7. Howard University, Moorland-Spingarn Research Center, Charles R. Drew Papers, 134–43.

8. William Montague Cobb, "Charles Richard Drew, M.D., 1904–1950," *Journal of the National Medical Association* 42 (1950): 245; "Thousands Pay Tribute to Drew," Baltimore Afro-American, April 11, 1950. Howard officials estimated that five thousand mourners passed through Rankin Chapel to see Drew.

9. Pennington, unpublished memoirs.

10. "Thousands Pay Tribute to Drew."

11. "Dentists, Medics Pay Drew Silent Tribute," *Baltimore Afro-American*, April 11, 1950.

12. L. D. Robbins, "Unforgettable Charlie Drew," *Reader's Digest* 112 (1978): 137.

13. Dr. Charles R. Drew, Congressional Record, Proceedings and Debates of the 81st Congress, Second Session, US Government Printing Office, 1950.

14. Dr. Charles R. Drew, Congressional Record.

15. Lenore estimated that the value of Drew's personal possessions and accounts was less than $3,000 at his death. Lenore Drew reminiscences, personal collection of Charlene Drew Jarvis.

16. Lenore Drew reminiscences; Lenore believed that Harold Ickes, the former secretary of the interior who was a staunch advocate for the rights of African Americans, was responsible for seeing the pension through. Ickes, however, left the cabinet several years before and was a private citizen at the time of Drew's death.

17. Letter G. W. Stephenson to L. D. Leffall, June 18, 1982, Archives of the American College of Surgeons, Chicago, Illinois.

18. P. P. Craft, "Charles Drew: Dispelling the Myth," *Southern Medical Journal* 85 (1992): 1240. "Please accept our many thanks for the efforts extended by you and your staff on April 1 in an attempt to save the life of Dr. Charles R. Drew. It is our understanding that at the time of treatment and care you were completely unaware of identification. Such kindness cannot go unmentioned. Though all efforts were futile, there is much comfort derived in knowing that everything was done in his fight for life. Again, we wish to express our deepest appreciation." For an in-depth discussion of the propagation of myths regarding Drew's death, see Love, *One Blood*.

19. H. Bims, "Charles Drew's Other Medical Revolution: Famed Pioneer in Blood Preservation Trained Vanguard of Black Surgeons," *Ebony* 30 (1974): 96.

Index

Adams, Numa P. G., 110, 114, 115, 120, 121, 138, 153, 154, 197, 202, 286n18, 289n47
Alamance, 253–58
Alamance County General Hospital, 256
Alpha Omega Alpha, 91, 100
American Board of Surgery, 150, 179, 181, 182, 193, 198, 207, 227
American College of Surgeons, 220, 227
American Federation of Labor, 7
American Human Serum Association, 192
American Journal of Physiology, 135
American Medical Association, 116, 220
American Occupied Zone of Europe, 238
American Red Cross, 171, 184, 185
American Review of Soviet Medicine, 210
Amherst Ambulance Corps, 26
Amherst College (1922–26), Drew's time at: African American classmate boundaries, 40; biology classes, 36; ceaseless course, 40; classes in theology and Bible literature, 24; classmates of 1926, 42; Cobb Pentathlon Trophy, 31; commencement, 43; enrollment day, 24; football team, 29, 32, 35, 37, 38; graduation portrait, Drew's, 43; interclass competitions, 25; language departments, 26; philosophy class, 35; underclass sporting, 27
Anderson, Marian, 91, 212
Annapolis Athletic Club, 58
Atlas of Surgical Operations, 125; 1939 ed., 207

Baker, Howie, 100
Baltimore (1926–28), Drew's time in, 45–66; *Baltimore Afro-American*, 58; basketball team, 59–60; Morgan College campus, 57
Banked Blood: A Study in Blood Preservation (thesis), 163
Banneker, Benjamin, 248
Bazin, Albert, 154, 283n74, 284n83, 289n49
Beattie, John, 77, 173
"Best Player I Ever Coached, The" 39
Blades, Brian, 219
Bliss, Raymond, 244
"bloodletting" team, 193
blood preservation studies, 154–67
Blood Transfusion Betterment Association, 159, 171, 174, 175, 177, 186
Board of Medical Control of the Association, 187

Board of Trustees of Morgan College, 46
Boles, May Ellis, 92
Bordentown Manual Training team, 49
Bordentown School, 58
Boston University, 101
Bronson, Kathryn Charlene Price, 267
Brooks, Walter H., 7
Brown University, 86
Bullock, Samuel, 3, 4, 208, 251, 255
Burdick Vocational School, 266
Burrell, Nora, 6, 19
Burwell, Hartford, 233
Bush, John F., 163, 171, 175, 177, 181, 182, 185

Cadet Review, 16
cardiogenic shock, 145
Cardoza, Warick, 173, 293n12
Carnegie, Andrew, 47
Carver, George Washington, 211, 248
Centenary Biblical Institute of the Methodist Episcopal Church, 47
Century Athletic Club of New York, 47
Challenger, 264
Charles R. Drew Memorial Foundation, 263
Charles R. Drew University of Medicine and Science, 268
Chicago Defender, 204, 213, 220
Chi Eta Phi Nursing Society, 252
Christian Association of Amherst College, 23
Civil Rights Movement, 216
Class of 1926 Freshman Bible, The, 23
Cleveland Call and Post, 204
Cobb, Samuel L., 31
Cobb, William Montague, 9, 24, 31, 34, 35, 38, 40, 41, 53, 78, 108–10, 202, 206, 211, 261
Cobb Pentathlon Trophy, 31
Coffey, Robert J., 219, 228–29, 298n4, 300n21
Collip, J. B., 78
Columbia University, 29, 118, 130, 131, 145, 153, 167, 197, 263, 266, 269; Medical Center, 131
Columbia University Presbyterian Hospital Blood Bank, 145, 172
Cook, W. Mercer, 24, 92, 136, 138, 206, 261, 278n14
Coolidge, Calvin, Jr., 34
Cornell University, 136
Cornely, Paul B., 231, 259
Corwin, E. H. L., 171
Crabtree, Lucille, 258, 264
Credentials Committee, American College of Surgeons, 264
Crump, Walter Gray, 135
Curtis, Austin M., 199
Cushing, Harvey, 174
Cutler, Elliot C., 125, 286n25

Davis, Edwin Porter, 62
Davis, Norman H., 175, 181
Davis, Robert C., 195
Denit, Guy, 244
District of Columbia Public Schools, 267
Douglass, Frederick, 206, 297n25
Drew, Eva Virginia, 19
Drew, Grace Ridgeley, 90, 271n1, 273n37, 281n33
Drew, Joseph, 13, 61
Drew, Lenore, 259
Drew, Minnie Lenore Robbins, 136, 137, 266, 287n13
Drew, Richard Thomas, Jr. 6, 9, 12, 79, 122
Drew, Sylvia, 267
Drury, A. N., 180
DuBois, W. E. B., 55, 92, 211
Duke University Divinity School, 267
Duke University Medical Center, 258

Dunbar High School, 15, 16, 30, 31, 48, 54, 80, 126, 157, 208, 261, 268; basketball team, 16; football team, 15; yearbook, 22
Durán-Jordà, Frederic, 158, 192

Edwards, Phil, 96
Effendi, Shoghi, 281n51
Ellington, Duke, 278n13
Elliot, John, 169
Ellison, Ralph, 91
E. S. Jones Prize for Meritorious Research, 202
Evans, John C., 237, 276n51
Evening Star, 11, 273n38

Fishbein, Morris, 222–27
Fitch, Albert Parker, 26
Flexner, Abraham, 116, 117, 285n6
Flexner Report, 116, 117, 221
Foggy Bottom (1904–22), 6–22; advantages of, 13; community of, 20; demographics of, 6
Fokine Ballet, 152
Ford, John R., 3, 4, 251
Foster, Stephen, 7
Francis Municipal Swimming Pool, 78
Francis Olympics, 87
Franklin, John Hope, 91
Frost, Robert, 43

Galento, Tony, 152
GEB Fellowship, 167
General Education Board (GEB), 117
George Washington University, 6, 228
Giddings School, 126
Glaser, Otto, 40, 44, 247, 301n50, 301n51
Great Depression, 79
Greene, Clarence S., 237
Gregory, Frederick Drew, 165, 264
Grey's Anatomy, 72

Halsted, William Stewart, 104, 124
Harrison, F. C., 86
Harvard Medical School, 61, 125
Hastie, William H., 24, 27, 41, 212, 261
Henderson, Edwin Bancroft, 14, 48, 53, 292n73, 292n74
Hill, Talmadge "Marse," 48, 49
Howard, Oliver Otis, 113
Howard Hill Mossman Trophy, 43
Howard University, 7, 17, 30, 53, 58, 60, 62, 63, 80, 84, 90, 92, 94, 108, 114, 118, 122, 130, 132, 167, 172, 178, 185, 195, 197, 198, 204, 212, 217, 222, 223, 229, 231, 249, 260–63, 267, 268; Board of Athletic Control, 63; Cancer Center, 251; College of Medicine, 3; Department of Surgery, 259; Medical School, 61, 78, 109, 110, 113, 115, 117, 136, 166, 173, 253, 267; School of Law, 267; student routines, general surgical wards, 128–30
Howes, Edward, 118, 197
Hughes, Langston, 92
Humphrey, Hubert, 262
hypovolemic shock, 147

Jarvis, Charlene Drew, 267
Jason, Robert S., 118
John A. Andrew Hospital, 4
John A. Andrew Society, 251
John H. Johnson School of Communications, 268
Johns Hopkins Hospital, 68
Johns Hopkins School of Medicine, 116–17, 124
Johnson, Joseph L., 198
Johnson, Mordecai, 114, 115
Johnson, Walter, 3, 4, 251
Johnson Chapel, 24
Jones, R. Frank, 199, 261, 263

Journal of the American Medical Association, 222
Jungle, The, 116

Kendrick, Douglas, 170, 295n41, 297n15
Kernodle, Charles, 258, 302n10

Landsteiner, Karl, 242
Laurey, Richard, 268
Law, Jim F., 48
Lee, Octo, 151
Lincoln Memorial, 10, 138
Lincoln University, 49
Lippard, Vernon W., 153, 164
Louis, Joe, 152
Love, Spencie, 64
Lucretia Mott Elementary School, 10
Lull, George F., 223, 225, 226, 299n14, 299n15

Mackenzie, John C., 65, 154
Marshall, Charles, 8
Maxwell, Mary, 92–94, 141, 281n51
Maxwell, William Sutherland, 92
McGill, James, 67
McGill Medical Society, 99
McGill Undergraduate Medical Journal, 99
McGill University, 3, 67, 105, 237, 267; Faculty of Medicine, 70, 128, 130
McLaughry, DeOrmand "Tuss," 28, 29, 32, 34, 37, 38, 48, 85, 86, 90, 260, 276n56
Medical Research Council of Great Britain, 178
Meiklejohn, Alexander, 21, 24, 43, 273n41
Mellanby, Edward, 178, 181
"Memory Song to Amherst," 43
Methodist Episcopal Church, 47
Miner Normal School for Colored Girls, 7, 126, 158
Montreal, Drew's time in: Alpha Omega Alpha, 100; Canadian medical career, 110; demoralizing response, 109; facility-based medical care, 109; training regimens, 104
Montreal Basketball League, 75
Montreal General Hospital, 105, 107
Moore, Jerry, 261
Moorland-Spingarn Research Center, 272n30
M Street High School, 7, 14

Naismith National Basketball Hall of Fame, 14
National Association for the Advancement of Colored People (NAACP), 55
National Board of Medical Examiners test, 108
National Medical Association (NMA), 221
The Negro in Sports, 164
Nelligan, Richard F., 27, 31, 41, 101
Newport, F. Dwight "Doc," 275n37
Niagara Movement, 55
Nineteenth Street Baptist Church, 10
Nviaser, Julius, 199

Ochsner, Alton, 294n36
Oertel, Horst, 89, 118
Olds, George D., 43
Old Testament, *Song of Solomon*, 93
Olio yearbook, 42
One Blood: The Death and Resurrection of Charles Drew, 63–64
Osler, William, 68, 104, 285n15

Parks, Gordon, 91
Pasteur, Louis, 169
Paul Laurence Dunbar High School, 13
Pearl Harbor, 203
Penfield, Wilder, 237

Pennington, Eva Drew, 266
Pennsylvania's Cheyney Training School, 58
Pinckney, Leslie, 233
Pittsburgh Courier, 53
Pratt, George, 43
Preparatory High School for Colored Youth, 13
Price, Bebe Drew, 267
Price, Kline A., Jr., 267

Queen's University, 90
Quick, C. Mason, 259, 264

Rappleye, William C., 166
Rawlins Park, 272n13
Red Cross Blood Donor Service, 203
Red Cross / Blood Transfusion Association, 187
Reich, Rudolph, 238
Rhoads, Cornelius P., 187, 251
Richardson, Louisa C., 62
Ridgeley, Albert, 90
Robbins, Minnie Lenore, 136–37, 266
Rockefeller Foundation, 121
"Role of Soviet Investigators in the Development of the Blood Bank, The" 210
Roosevelt, Franklin D., 262
Rosenwald, Julius, 91, 92
Rosenwald Fellowships, 91
Rosenwald Fund, 96
Rowland, William Tingle, 26

Samuel L. Cobb Pentathlon Trophy, 27
Saturday Evening Post, 37
Scudder, John, 132, 134, 142, 145, 154, 156, 157, 175, 176, 182, 188, 227, 262, 290n63
Shaw, Robert Gould, 300n23
Siglo del Oro, 26
Simpson, J. C., 64, 72, 91, 279n28
Sloan, Lawrence W., 135, 287n9
Smith, DeWitt, 186
Smith, Grafton Elliot, 77
Smith, Lee Waller, 278n16
Smith, Margaret E., 135
Song of Solomon, 93
"Soul of Old Amherst, The" 43
Spencer, John Oakley, 46–47
Spingarn Medal, 213
Squier, J. Bentley, 156, 186
Stehle, R. L., 86
Stetten, DeWitt, 171, 175, 177
Stimson, Henry, 204
Stoddard, Helen, 288n27
Stubbs, Frederick Douglass, 233, 235
Student Christian Association, 71
Study of Anatomy, 72
Syphax, Burke, 123, 233, 260–61, 268

Taft, William Howard, 12
Tait, John, 77, 78
Tait-Mackenzie Trophy, 73, 101
Taylor, Earl, 195
Textbook of Biochemistry, A, 79
Thaddeus Stevens Elementary, 8
Thomas, Dick, 48, 49, 59
Thomas W. Ashley Memorial Trophy, 32
Tovell, Ralph M., 238
"Transfusion Trailer" team, 194

USNS Charles Drew, 269
US Public Health Service, 250

Virchow, Rudolph, 285n15
Virginia Avenue, 11
Voorhees, Tracy, 171, 186

Walker, James E., 16
Waller, Garnett Russell, 55
Waller, Lelia, 55, 56, 95, 141
Ward Athletic Club of Annapolis, 49
Washington, Booker T., 91
Washington Herald, 11
Washington Times, 11
Watts, Charles D., 268
Wayne State University, 118
Webster, Noah, 24
Weissmuller, Johnny, 158
Wesleyan University, 29
Whipple, Allen Oldfather, 132, 142, 147, 149, 150, 152, 262, 286n1
White, Jack E., 200
Whitnall, Samuel Ernest, 72
Williams, Esther, 158
Williams, J. Francis, 100
Wilson, Woodrow, 292n6
Wormley, Lowell Cheatham, 136, 138, 152

Yancey, Asa, 194, 216, 251

Zollinger, Robert M., 125

About the Author

Craig A. Miller, MD, FSVS, FACS, was educated at Northwestern University, The Ohio State University, and the University of California, San Francisco. He is the author of three previous books, *The Making of a Surgeon in the 21st Century*, *The Big Z: The Life of Robert M. Zollinger, MD*, and *A Time for All Things: The Life of Michael E. DeBakey*. He has been a scholar-in-residence at the Medical Heritage Center of The Ohio State University College of Medicine and held the Michael E. DeBakey Fellowship in the History of Medicine at the National Library of Medicine. Dr. Miller has received many awards and accolades for his work in research and clinical medicine, as well as in scientific history and biography. He is an attending vascular surgeon with the United States Veterans Administration and lives in Dublin, Ohio, with his wife, Mandy, and sons, Kellen and Jack.